THE DOCTORS BOOK OF
HOME
REMEDIES

II

Over 1,200 New
Doctor-Tested Tips and Techniques
Anyone Can Use to Heal Hundreds of
Everyday Health Problems

By Sid Kirchheimer

and the Editors of *PREVENTION* Magazine Health Books

RODALE PRESS, EMMAUS, PENNSYLVANIA

Library of Congress Cataloging-in-Publication Data

    The Doctors book of home remedies II : over 1,200 new doctor-tested tips and techniques anyone can use to heal hundreds of everyday health problems / by Sid Kirchheimer and the editors of Prevention magazine health books.
        p.   cm.
  Includes index.
  ISBN 0-87596-158-4 hardcover
    1. Medicine, Popular.   I. Kirchheimer, Sid.   II. Prevention (Emmaus, Pa.)   III. Title: Doctors book of home remedies 2.
  RC81.D65   1993
  610—dc20   93-7754
                                                    CIP

Distributed in the book trade by St. Martin's Press

2 4 6 8 10 9 7 5 3 1   hardcover

OUR MISSION

We publish books that empower people's lives.

RODALE ✣ BOOKS

Notice

This book is intended as a reference volume only, not as a medical guide or manual for self-treatment. If you suspect that you have a medical problem, please seek competent medical care. The information here is designed to help you make informed choices about your health. It is not intended as a substitute for any treatment prescribed by your doctor.

THE DOCTORS BOOK OF HOME REMEDIES II

Editor: Edward Claflin
Writers: Sid Kirchheimer, with:

Douglas Dollemore   Laura Wallace-Smith
Marcia Holman   Joe Wargo
Brian Kaufman   Mark Wisniewski
Gale Maleskey   Pat Wittig
Sheila Skaff

Senior Editors: John Feltman, Russell Wild
Editorial Researcher: Bernadette Sukley
Researchers and Fact Checkers: Susan Burdick, Carlotta B. Cuerdon, Christine Dreisbach, Melissa Dunford, Melissa Gotthardt, Dawn Horvath, Anne Remondi Imhoff, Paris Mihely-Muchanic, Deborah J. Pedron, Sally Reith, Sandi Salera-Lloyd, Anita Small
Book and Cover Designer: Vic Mazurkiewicz
Production Editor: Jane Sherman
Copy Editor: Susan G. Berg
Office Manager: Roberta Mulliner
Office Staff: Julie Kehs, Sylvia Membrino, Mary Lou Stephen

PREVENTION MAGAZINE HEALTH BOOKS
William Gottlieb, **Editor in Chief**
Debora Tkac, **Executive Editor**
Jane Knutila, **Art Director**
Ann Gossy Yermish, **Research Chief**
Ann Snyder, **Copy Manager**

Contents

Ten Million Reasons to Read This Book

Sometimes I feel a little like Newton when the apple dropped on his head.

Only my apple was the kind that keeps doctors away.

What was my momentous discovery?

I discovered that millions of people wanted a way to treat their everyday health problems *without* going to the doctor—they wanted to treat those problems at *home*.

I discovered that those same people didn't want to choose from one or two remedies for each of their problems—they wanted *dozens* of remedies, a cornucopia of options.

And—perhaps most importantly—I discovered that even though people would rather skip a high-priced office visit, they still wanted their home remedies *from* doctors. Because those remedies (unlike folk remedies and other dubious cures) would *work,* and they'd be virtually risk-free.

Newton made his discovery sitting under a tree. I made mine sitting at a desk. That's where, in 1988, I "discovered" the idea for what has become one of the best-selling health books of all time: *The Doctors Book of Home Remedies.* Ten million people bought that book. Ten million families have an everyday, practical reference volume in their homes that can save them hundreds of dollars (and maybe even their lives).

But good apple trees bear a lot of fruit.

What you have in your hands—*The Doctors Book of Home Remedies II*—is our second discovery. To create this book, we called 500 *new* doctors, the top experts in every field. We expanded the list of diseases and conditions, including over 100 new areas of health concern. And we added over 1,200 new remedies—1,200 new ways to heal yourself and your family. If you are one of the ten million people who bought the original *Doctors Book of Home Remedies,* you'll find a whole new world of feel-better possibilities. If you didn't buy the first book, you have a lot to look forward to: The top health authorities in America have given you thousands of effective self-treatment tips for hundreds of common complaints.

Go ahead, take your first bite. You'll make a discovery, too—the exciting discovery of better health.

William Gottlieb
Editor in Chief
Prevention Magazine Health Books

Age Spots

T alk about a spotty reputation! Heck, most people can't agree on what to *call* these unappealing but otherwise harmless dark spots that usually occur on the forehead and the back of the hands and arms.

Some folks think age spots are caused by old age—an understandable mistake, since the spots are extremely common *after* age 55 and rarely appear before middle age. Others know them as liver spots.

The appearance of these dark, blotchy spots can be scary—resembling the early forms of skin cancer to the untrained eye. But genuine age spots are really nothing more than "adult freckles" that result from overexposure to the sun. (However, if you notice an increase in size or "bizarre" color changes, see your doctor immediately.)

"Age spots should really be called sun spots, because they are caused by being out in the sun," says D'Anne Kleinsmith, M.D., a cosmetic dermatologist at William Beaumont Hospital near Detroit. "They have absolutely nothing to do with your liver and little to do with your age, other than the fact that they usually occur on older people."

Still, they *are* unbecoming. Sometimes they may be raised and look like tiny moles. Usually, though, they're just like dark, smooth freckles. If you've had them, you've probably noticed that they seem to appear suddenly on sun-exposed skin areas (usually areas *not* protected with sunscreen). So here's what to do about liver spots . . . er, age sp . . . uh, *lentigines* (their medical name).

Get help from hydroquinone. This safe "lightening agent" is found in products such as Porcelana and Esoterica that you can obtain without a prescription. Hydroquinone helps lighten age spots until they become unnoticeable. "Dab it on the individual spots with a cotton ball," says Dr. Kleinsmith.

1

Sunscreen Each Day Keeps Age Spots Away

The best way to avoid *ever* having age spots is to use a good-quality sunscreen each time you go outdoors, including when it's overcast. And if you already have age spots, sunscreen will keep them from darkening and will help prevent new ones.

Either way, remember the "15" rules.

Look for a sun protection factor (SPF) of at least 15. Unprotected, the average person's skin turns red—a signal of overexposure—after just 30 minutes. But with SPF 15 sunscreen, you can stay out 15 times as long, or seven hours, with the same effect (although it's not recommended).

Apply sunscreen at least 15 minutes before going outdoors. That way, the skin has a chance to absorb it.

But don't expect overnight success: This therapy usually takes a month or two before you see any results. Follow the directions on the package and try to dab the medication right on the spots, so you don't "bleach" the pigment in nonaffected skin.

Shed away "spotted" skin. Lac-Hydrin Five lotion, another nonprescription remedy, contains lactic acid. "The acid can help bleaching agents work faster by enhancing the normal shedding of upper, 'dead' skin layers," says Michael Ramsey, M.D., clinical instructor of dermatology at Baylor College of Medicine in Houston. This leaves a lighter layer of skin underneath.

Reach for lemon aid. "The juice of a fresh lemon is acidic enough to safely peel off the upper layer of skin, which will remove or lighten some age spots," says Jerome Z. Litt, M.D., assistant clinical professor of dermatology at Case Western Reserve University School of Medicine in Cleveland. "Rub it on with a cotton ball twice daily where the age spots are, and in six to eight weeks, they should begin to fade away."

How about an onion rub? Rubbing a piece of sliced *red* onion on age spots can have the same fading effect, "since it has the same peeling acid as fresh lemon juice," adds Dr. Litt.

Use castor oil for smooth relief. "If the surface of individual lesions appears rougher than surrounding skin—which often occurs with age spots—applying castor oil twice daily with a cotton swab will sometimes bring about improvement," says Dr. Ramsey. On larger lesions, a bandage applied with the castor oil at nighttime may speed improvement.

Be a shady character. "Since age spots are caused by excessive sun exposure, avoid the sun and you'll avoid age spots," suggests Albert M. Kligman, M.D., Ph.D., professor of dermatology at the University of Pennsylvania School of Medicine in Philadelphia. "You will never see an age spot on someone who stays in the shade." If you already have age spots, limiting sun exposure will help prevent them from darkening and will minimize a recurrence or the appearance of new ones.

Cover 'em up. If all else fails in trying to remedy them, hide them. "Many types of makeup can cover the spots," says Edward Bondi, M.D., a dermatologist who is affiliated with the University of Pennsylvania Hospital in Philadelphia. "If they are really dark spots, a heavier-based makeup will work, but if they're not so bad, then many water-based types will do the trick. A product called Covermark has routinely been used to hide age spots." *Note:* If you suffer from acne, avoid heavier oil-based makeups, because they can worsen blemishes.

Aging Eyes

It happens to a lot of people around age 40. You begin to realize it takes a Herculean effort to read the newspaper or the tiny type on a food package or an aspirin bottle. As for threading a needle or removing a splinter—forget it! These simple tasks have become impossible feats.

That's because anything closer than an arm's length from your eyes is now one big blur.

You're not alone. If your far-away vision is fine (with or without corrective eyewear) but your close-up vision is fuzzier than a teddy bear's coat, blame it

When to See the Doctor

Gradual changes in vision as you age are normal, but a sudden change in your vision—no matter what your age—isn't, says Bruce Rosenthal, O.D., professor and chief of low vision services at the State University of New York College of Optometry in New York City. "Blurred vision can be a first sign of eye diseases such as glaucoma, macular degeneration or cataracts, which can seriously impair your vision."

Other conditions that can cause cloudy vision include diabetes, pregnancy, side effects of medications, anemia, kidney disease and optic nerve disease. So it's important to see a doctor as soon as possible if there's any sudden blurriness in your near or distant vision.

on an inflexible lens. And it's a problem as common as crow's feet and silver hair.

Around age 40, you may find it's more difficult to focus on near objects, particularly printed words when you're reading. Doctors call this presbyopia.

But before you shell out the green stuff for special prescription glasses, these tips may help you fine-tune your focusing.

Do the fine print sprint. "Part of the problem of the aging eye is that the lens becomes less flexible," says Bruce Rosenthal, O.D., professor and chief of low vision services at the State University of New York College of Optometry in New York City. "If you exercise the muscles that control the shape of the lens, it may be possible to delay near-point fuzziness to some degree."

One exercise involves cutting headlines of decreasing size out of the newspaper and affixing each one to a pencil. Then hold the largest headline about a foot away from your face. Gradually bring it in toward your nose, trying to keep the print in focus. Move the headline back out again. Repeat with the next smaller headline, then the rest, until you have looked at all the headlines.

"With practice, you may be able to read even the tiniest labels on medicine bottles with no difficulty," says Dr. Rosenthal.

Follow the bouncing thumb. To keep your eye muscles fully flexed, hold out your thumb at arm's length. Move it in circles, then in figure eights, closer and farther away. Follow it with your eyes. This helps keep the fine motor system of your eyes in working order, says Dr. Rosenthal.

Switch frequently from near to far. If you keep your eyes fixed for long periods on a computer screen, for example, your eye muscles can temporarily become stuck. This slows focusing when you try to zoom from near to far and back again, says Dr. Rosenthal. To keep your eye muscles loose, look up every ten minutes and focus on a poster located about eight feet away. Then look back at the words on the computer screen. Shift your focus back and forth repeatedly for 30 seconds.

Invest in brighter bulbs. As your eyes age, you may begin to need more light for everyday activities. In fact, by age 60, you could need six times as much light as you did at age 20 to perform the same tasks, according to Dr. Rosenthal. "If you have better lighting, the pupils become smaller, and the

How to Adjust to Bifocals

If you have trouble with both near and distant vision, you may eventually end up with bifocals. But getting used to bifocals can be a lot like stumbling through a fun house filled with wavy mirrors.

Be patient, says Joseph P. Shovlin, O.D., an optometrist at the Northeastern Eye Institute, with headquarters in Scranton, Pennsylvania, and chairman of the Contact Lens Section of the American Optometric Association. "It can take from a few days to several weeks to get used to multifocal lenses." Be prepared for possible return visits to the optometrist for adjustments, since a dual-prescription lens often requires more precise measurements than a single-vision lens.

Here are tips to focus on.

- Wear the glasses all day for the first week or two until you're accustomed to them, even though you may not need them for all tasks.
- Avoid looking at your feet when walking.
- Hold reading material closer to your body and lower your eyes, not your head, so that you are reading out of the lowest part of the lens.
- Fold the newspaper in half or quarters and move it, rather than your head, to read comfortably.

amount of blur you experience may be less," says James Sheedy, O.D., Ph.D., associate clinical professor at the University of California, Berkeley, School of Optometry. You may find that high-wattage incandescent bulbs will help you see better than harsh fluorescent lights.

Check out off-the-rack reading glasses. All you may need to read and see close up are simple magnifiers, says Richard P. Mills, M.D., professor of oph-thalmology at the University of Washington School of Medicine in Seattle. "The drugstore demi-glasses that come in about ten different powers are medically acceptable," says Dr. Mills. "Just make sure they have no optical distortion."

To find out, hold the glasses at arm's length, then look through them as you move them in a circular motion. If there's some "swim," or distortion, get another pair. If you find that these reading glasses give you a headache or tired eyes, however, you're better off with prescription glasses.

Anal Fissures

When it comes to pain, embarrassment and inconvenience, these painful tears in the sensitive skin around your anus are truly a thorn in your (back)side. Fissures are usually caused by trying to pass hard, large stools. Since more fiber in your diet means looser stools, anal fissures are

When to See the Doctor

If you've tried self-help measures and still have anal fissures, or if you notice blood in your stool or experience any bleeding while trying to pass your stool, see your doctor as soon as possible. While some bleeding occurs because of hemorrhoids or trying to pass hard stools, rectal bleeding may be a warning sign of colon cancer or another serious problem. But you'll need a doctor's examination to find out the cause.

Maybe a Spray Will Do

As anyone with anal fissures can tell you, wiping with dry tissues is no picnic. To make personal hygiene a little easier on your tender bottom, there's ClenZone. This small cleansing device hooks up to your bathroom faucet; just spray yourself clean with a narrow stream of water aimed at the anal area. There's no need for toilet paper, except to pat yourself dry.

"This is a neat little appliance that offers a real nice way to get clean after a bowel movement," says colon-rectal surgeon John A. Flatley, M.D., clinical instructor of surgery at the University of Missouri/Kansas City School of Medicine. It can be used for both fissures and hemorrhoids. It's available through Hepp Industries, 687 Kildare Crescent, Seaford, NY 11783.

a sharp reminder to eat shredded wheat with newfound gusto. But here's how to fizzle your anal fissures.

Go high on fiber. Maybe oat bran doesn't go down as easy as a thick, juicy steak, but consuming a high-fiber diet is the best way to soften stools. Besides eating more grains, you should also eat plenty of fresh fruits and vegetables, all of which are naturally high in fiber. "Fruits, vegetables and whole grains are the best remedy and preventive measure" for fissures, says J. Byron Gathright, Jr., M.D., chairman of the Department of Colon and Rectal Surgery at the Ochsner Clinic in New Orleans and president of the American Society of Colon and Rectal Surgeons.

Drink a lot of water. Drinking six to eight glasses a day adds bulk to your system and softens stools, says Dr. Gathright. In addition, drinking a lot of water may help reduce some of the stomach discomfort you may experience when starting a high-fiber diet.

Try over-the-counter vitamin creams. To soothe the pain and help heal fissures, try over-the-counter ointments that contain vitamins A and D, suggests Marvin M. Schuster, M.D., chief of the Department of Digestive Diseases at Francis Scott Key Medical Center in Baltimore. Hydrocortisone creams, available at drugstores, are also helpful, adds Dr. Gathright.

Soothe your sit-upon. You can also protect your anal canal by lubricating it before each bowel movement. A gob of petroleum jelly inserted about ½ inch into the rectum may help the stool pass without causing any further damage, advises Edmund Leff, M.D., a proctologist in Phoenix and Scottsdale, Arizona.

Wipe yourself with facial tissue. The best toilet paper isn't toilet paper at all. Facial tissues coated with moisturizing lotion offer the least amount of friction to your fissure-plagued anal area, says Dr. Leff.

Talc yourself up down there. Following each shower or bowel movement, dust yourself with baby powder. This will help keep the area dry, which can help reduce friction throughout the day, says Dr. Schuster.

Angina

N early three million Americans have experienced an angina attack, which usually lasts about ten minutes. It's not the same as a heart attack, but because of its chest-crushing severity, it often seems like one. And failing to control angina makes you an ideal candidate for a heart attack. Angina is one of the first signs of serious heart disease.

If you've already been diagnosed with angina, your doctor probably has you on medication. But here are some home treatments that can help you manage or even *reverse* angina.

Eat vegetarian. A steak-and-potatoes diet (with extra butter and sour cream) may have caused your angina by boosting the levels of cholesterol in your blood, but a strict vegetarian diet may help cure it—often sooner than you may think. Dean Ornish, M.D., director of the Preventive Medicine Research Institute in Sausalito, California, and author of *Dr. Dean Ornish's Program for Reversing Heart Disease,* recommends that people make comprehensive changes in their diet and lifestyle. He suggests a low-fat vegetarian diet that includes *no* animal products except for skim milk, egg whites and nonfat yogurt.

"When they follow this diet, most people find that the severity and frequency of angina pain diminish markedly within a few weeks, or even a few days," says Dr. Ornish. A vegetarian diet can also prevent angina pain and help keep arteries clean, because dietary cholesterol is present only in meat, milk, egg yolks and other animal products. And those foods also are high in saturated fat, which your body converts to cholesterol.

If you eat meat, go lean and light. If you still want to eat meat, fish or poultry, you should limit it to no more than six ounces daily. Also, choose cuts that are lean and trimmed of all visible fat. If you eat ground beef, it should be labeled extra lean. Be sure to avoid cholesterol-rich organ meats such as liver, kidney and heart. And remove all skin from poultry before cooking.

Boost your vitamins—A, C and E. Here's another benefit of a low-fat vegetarian diet: It's rich in the antioxidant vitamins A, C and E—three nutrients that have been found to help prevent or control angina.

"If your diet consists mainly of vegetables, fruits and whole grains, then you're getting all the key nutrients you need," says Frank E. Rasler, M.D., an emergency room physician and a researcher at Emory University School of Public Health in Atlanta.

Take aspirin. Taking aspirin regularly, according to a dosage regimen recommended by your physician, can reduce heart attack risk. A dose as small as

When to See the Doctor

Although you should remain under a doctor's regular care once you've been diagnosed with angina, here are some warning signs that should prompt you to see your doctor at once.

- You experience chest pain that lasts more than 15 minutes (and is not relieved by three nitroglycerin tablets taken in succession 5 minutes apart). This could suggest a heart attack rather than angina, and you should go to the hospital immediately.
- You had gotten attacks only with exertion before but are now experiencing attacks during rest.
- You'd been able to exercise at a certain level *without* any angina pain, but now you feel pain when you exercise at that same level.
- You're experiencing pain when you exercise at a level that's *less* than before.

one baby aspirin daily has helped patients with unstable angina—the kind that can hit you when you're resting or even sleeping.

"It appears that aspirin helps prevent blood clots," says George Beller, M.D., professor of medicine and head of the Division of Cardiology at the University of Virginia School of Medicine in Charlottesville. If clots form too easily, your blood can't get through the narrowed artery, and that blockage could trigger a heart attack.

A caution: Be sure to get your doctor's approval before starting on aspirin. Even though it is an over-the-counter drug, aspirin can have side effects, and it could interact with other medications you may be taking.

Get a regular workout. Even though angina pain is *sometimes* triggered by exercise, you should still work out regularly. Exercise helps improve blood flow to the heart, and it also relieves the stress that helps trigger angina attacks.

"When patients start an exercise program, they may experience angina with increased exercise levels," says Dr. Beller.

The answer: Exercise until you begin to feel the onset of discomfort or pain, then stop until the pain subsides—which may require taking a nitroglycerin pill. Often you can then continue, and the pain will not return. Ultimately, an exercise regimen will *improve* exercise tolerance, with angina occurring only with greater exercise stress than when you first started.

Exercise good judgment. People with angina need to exercise certain precautions. For instance, inhaling carbon monoxide can trigger an angina attack, so if you run, do it *away* from traffic.

If you live in an urban environment, try to exercise indoors. In fact, just being exposed to everyday levels of carbon monoxide can cause angina prematurely in some people, says Sidney Gottlieb, M.D., a cardiologist and associate professor of medicine at Johns Hopkins Medical Institutions in Baltimore.

Also, exercising in the bitter cold can trigger angina attacks in some people. So for winter workouts, be sure to cover your face with a scarf.

Raise your headboard. If you experience angina attacks at night, raising the head of your bed three or four inches can reduce the number of attacks, says cardiologist R. Gregory Sachs, M.D., assistant professor of medicine at Columbia University College of Physicians and Surgeons in New York City. Sleeping in this position makes more blood pool in your legs, so not so much returns to the heart's narrowed arteries. And it may help reduce the need for nitroglycerin, the drug of choice for stopping angina pain. You should check with your doctor, however, before reducing any regular medication.

What You Should Know about Nitro

Placing a nitroglycerin tablet under your tongue is frequently pre-scribed to halt an angina attack. Unfortunately, some studies have shown that *two in three* people who use nitro don't know how to use it properly. Here are some recommendations given to angina patients by Frank E. Rasler, M.D., an emergency room physician and a researcher at Emory University School of Public Health in Atlanta.

Have a seat. You should be sitting or lying down when you take nitro. "Some patients have a drop in blood pressure that can cause them to faint if they're standing," says Dr. Rasler.

Keep pills sealed. Exposing pills to light or air decreases their effec-tiveness. So *always* keep them in a sealed brown bottle and close the bottle tightly after taking the pills you need. They should be replaced after three or four months.

Take pills that cause a burning or tingling sensation on the tongue. This indicates they're still working. "If you don't notice some sensation, it indicates the pills have lost their effectiveness and should be replaced or the pill is not dissolving due to lack of moisture under the tongue," says Dr. Rasler.

Drink water or juice. For a variety of reasons, some people have a very dry mouth during an angina attack. In this case, it is essential to moisten the mouth with a small cup of liquid before you will have any pain relief.

Put your foot down. If you do get angina attacks at night, Dr. Sachs suggests an alternative to reaching for a nitroglycerin tablet. Simply sit on the edge of the bed with your feet on the floor. "It is equivalent to the effect of nitroglycerin," he says. If you don't feel your symptoms begin to subside quickly, then reach for your medication.

Take time to relax. Practicing some sort of *daily* relaxation technique—be it yoga, meditation, stretching or positive imagery—is a proven way to manage stress and relieve angina pain, says Dr. Ornish. "Which method you choose is less important than doing it regularly."

11

Dr. Ornish doesn't think classes in relaxation techniques are necessary for everyone. "A good book or tape can teach you what you need to know," he says, "but a class can be very helpful."

Animal Bites

S ometimes man's best friend doesn't act like one. Actually, when you consider that dogs cause more than one million bites each year—half of them to children—you have to figure that "sometimes" is more frequent than you may think. Now add those times when kitty acts catty, when the family bird gets his feathers ruffled, when your pet hamster tries to bite off more than he can chew . . .

When to See the Doctor

A lthough small bites from household pets can be treated at home, you should see the doctor immediately if you have a deep bite or if the wound bleeds continuously, says the Advisory Committee on Immunization of the Centers for Disease Control and Prevention in Atlanta. Also see the doctor for any kind of animal bite—even if it's from a household dog or cat—if you have any swelling, pain or redness around the area of the puncture.

Sometimes a doctor will recommend a tetanus shot as insurance against infection, particularly if you have not had a booster within the past five to eight years.

In rare cases, there is a danger of rabies from animal bites. As a precaution, you should see the doctor immediately if you are bitten by any wild animal, including a squirrel or raccoon. If the animal cannot be tested for rabies, the doctor may recommend that you have a rabies vaccine immediately as a precaution.

Animal bites should not be taken lightly. Many pets—dogs and cats in particular—have bacteria in their saliva that can cause infection, and deep bites can mangle tissues. For these reasons alone, a bite that punctures the skin, even if it's a bite from your household pet, should be seen by the doctor. But for those injuries where the bite is only slightly worse than the bark, here's what to do.

Thoroughly wash the wound. Once you control bleeding—by pressing firmly against the wound with your hand—cleanse the wound thoroughly with soap and water to remove saliva and any other contamination as soon as possible, advises George Shambaugh, Jr., M.D., professor emeritus of otolaryngology/head and neck surgery at Northwestern University Medical School in Chicago. Continue washing for five full minutes.

Cover it. A loosely applied bandage protects the wound from infection, so cover it with a sterile gauze pad or bandage, adds Dr. Shambaugh.

Take a pain reliever. Even bites that don't break the skin can be painful, so take aspirin or acetaminophen (Tylenol) to reduce pain, says Peg Parry, a certified emergency room nurse at the Lehigh Valley Hospital Poison Control Center in Allentown, Pennsylvania. Don't wait for swelling. Elevate the area, if possible, and apply ice or a cold pack wrapped in a towel. Remember: Don't give aspirin to children because of the risk of Reye's syndrome.

Arthritis

Here's a disease that's so common that nearly one in seven Americans already has it—and a new case is diagnosed every 33 seconds. In fact, arthritis is *the* most widespread chronic disease in people over age 45, even when you consider the untold millions who never see a doctor about that blasted pain in their joints.

When you *do* see a doctor about that blasted pain, he will usually tell you what kind of arthritis you have. Although there are more than 100 different types, most fall into two broad categories.

Inflammatory arthritis (or rheumatoid arthritis) is best treated with anti-inflammatory drugs, though diet and lifestyle changes may help. Noninflammatory arthritis (or osteoarthritis) results when cartilage in joints deteriorates from injury or excessive use. Weight control, proper exercise and pain relievers are the key treatments here.

Although arthritis is potentially crippling, there are things you can do that may help control it. Here's what doctors recommend.

Eat your vegetables. Researchers at the University of Oslo in Norway discovered that people with rheumatoid arthritis who began a vegetarian diet saw dramatic improvements in their conditions within *one month* after cutting out meat, eggs, dairy products, sugar and foods with gluten, such as wheat bread. "A vegetarian diet is good, because the goal for arthritis sufferers is to cut as much saturated fat from their diets as possible and replace it with more polyunsaturated fat," says Paul Caldron, D.O., a clinical rheumatologist and researcher at the Arthritis Center in Phoenix.

Try something fishy. One of the best sources of polyunsaturated fat is cold-water fish such as salmon, sardines and herring. "They are rich in omega-3 fatty acids, which have been shown to have some minor beneficial effect on reducing the inflammatory aspects of arthritis," says Dr. Caldron.

Get hot on hot pepper cream. Research shows you can ease the pain by rubbing the joint with an over-the-counter ointment called Zostrix, made from capsaicin—the stuff that puts the hot in hot peppers. "You need to apply it three or four times a day on the affected area for at least two weeks before you'll see any improvement. An initial burning sensation at the site is not unusual for the first few days, but this goes away with continued application," says Esther Lipstein-Kresch, M.D., an assistant professor of medicine at the Albert Einstein College of Medicine of Yeshiva University in New York City who has done research at Queens Hospital Center in Jamaica, New York, and who has studied the effectiveness of capsaicin cream. "I also advise washing your hands immediately after you apply it—or even wearing gloves when you apply it—because it can sting and you don't want to get it in your eyes." (Sorry, but *eating* hot peppers won't help relieve arthritis.)

Use a dehumidifer. If the humidity is kept constant in your house, it can help calm arthritis pain caused by weather changes, says Joseph Hollander, M.D., professor emeritus of medicine at the University of Pennsylvania Hospital in Philadelphia. When rain is on the way, the sudden increase in humidity and decrease in air pressure can affect blood flow to arthritic joints, which become increasingly stiff until the storm actually starts. If you close the windows and turn on a dehumidifer—or run the air-conditioning in summer—you may be able to eliminate this short-term but significant pain.

Remedies for Your Specific Aches

From head to toe, there are specific arthritis treatments for specific body parts, according to Paul Caldron, D.O., a clinical rheumatologist and researcher at the Arthritis Center in Phoenix.

Give your neck a break. Don't extend your neck by looking up for long periods. If you're painting, hanging curtains or doing other work that requires you to look up for long a time, get a ladder and bring yourself to the same level as the work.

Support your shoulders. Don't sleep with your arms *over* your head, because that strains your shoulders. Dr. Caldron advises women to lighten their handbags so that they carry *only* what they need. And big-busted women are advised to get bras with more support to ease shoulder strain.

Glove your hands. Wear gloves with a thick palm padding—like work gloves—whenever you're holding something tightly. With thick gloves you don't have to exert as much force on the hand joints to hold a heavy skillet, a broom or a wrench. Also, you can build up handles of tools and garden supplies with foam rubber padding or terry cloth, so you're exerting less force on the joints.

Never squat or kneel. That's about the worst thing you can do to arthritic knee and hip joints.

Wear running or walking shoes whenever possible. To ease the pressure on aching feet, you want footwear that provides comfort and support. When shopping for dressier footwear, look for shoes that have a wide toe box and good, built-in arch support. The best shoes have heels approximately 1 to 1½ inches high, and they come up high on the instep. For men, a lace-up oxford, as opposed to a slip-on, is the preferable dress shoe.

Stay active. "Probably the most important thing you can do for osteoarthritis is exercise as much as you're able to," says Halsted R. Holman, M.D., director and professor of medicine at the Stanford University Arthritis Center in Stanford, California. "You'll find that the better your physical condition, the less arthritis pain you'll have."

Dr. Caldron recommends low-impact aerobic exercises and, if tolerated, very light weight lifting with one- to two-pound dumbbells. "Build up the muscle and tissue surrounding the joint," he suggests. "You can exercise on a floor mat, in a chair, on a stationary bicycle or in the water. The key is regularity, doing it no less than three times a week but preferably daily."

Learn your food "triggers." "Some people with rheumatoid arthritis seem to flare up after eating certain foods—especially alcohol, milk, tomatoes and certain nuts," says Dr. Caldron. "Although there's really no telling what your trigger might be, if you notice your condition worsens after eating a certain food, then listen to your body and avoid that food." The same goes for foods that improve arthritis, such as fish and fiber; try to eat them more regularly.

Take time to smell the roses. When you're tensed up, you hurt more. "Many people use relaxation as an effective way of diminishing arthritis pain," says Dr. Holman. "It really doesn't matter what you do—biofeedback, meditation, even listening to music—whatever helps *you* relax. The point is to practice a regular relaxation period and then also to use relaxation when pain is particularly severe."

Slim down. "Being overweight can enhance damage to joints by putting excess pressure on them, resulting in worsening osteoarthritis, so I advise losing any excess weight you're carrying," says Richard M. Pope, M.D., an arthritis researcher and chief of arthritis/connective tissue diseases at Northwestern University Medical School in Chicago. In fact, being overweight increases your risk of developing osteoarthritis, even if you don't have it now.

Try slow dancing. Dancing is a good way to combine weight loss, exercise and stress reduction. "Many of my patients participate in easy dance routines created as part of an overall education and activity program that shows them how to exercise while protecting their affected joints," adds Dr. Pope. "Easy, slow dancing is perfect for those with inflammatory arthritis, or osteoarthritis, because it's low impact."

Reach for the "right" pain reliever. Not all pain relievers are the same—at least for those with arthritis. "People with inflammatory arthritis should get more relief from aspirin or ibuprofen (Advil) but may get more stomach irritation with these," says Dr. Caldron. For over-the-counter pain relief without stomach irritation, he recommends acetaminophen (Tylenol). Recommended doses of these drugs should not be exceeded, nor regular dosing continued, for more than three weeks without consulting your physician.

Immobilize the pain. "Splints, slings, cervical collars and other protective devices are extremely useful when an area is particularly painful or inflamed," says Dr. Caldron. But he cautions that you can't leave on these devices for more than two days at a time. Even though these devices help reduce pain, your muscles can "rely" on them and weaken very quickly.

Use ice and heat judiciously. Although both ice packs and heat packs can provide some relief, don't use either for more than ten minutes at a time, advises Dr. Caldron. Usually ice is used to prevent swelling but may also douse pain; heat in small doses may promote muscle relaxation and soothe pain.

Asthma

Unless you happen to be lovestruck, that sudden bout of breathlessness is more likely to be caused by asthma than by Cupid's trusty arrow. A snort of dust or smoke or a whiff of the "wrong" flower, pet dander or perfume can instantaneously start you—along with one in ten other Americans—wheezing, coughing and gasping for air. Besides these allergens and irritants, other common asthma triggers include exercise, pollution or smog, a drastic change in weather or a cold or another infection in the airways.

Sure, an asthma attack is scary. But it doesn't mean you have to move to the desert or forever live in fear of your "twitchy" airways. Besides taking your doctor-prescribed medication, there are plenty of ways to avoid or treat asthma attacks. As a first step, it's a good idea to guard against dust mite

When to See the Doctor

Although asthma can usually be kept under control by following a doctor's advice, each year several thousand people in the United States die from asthma attacks.

To manage asthma, you need to control your environment as much as possible and use preventive medications, according to Peter S. Creticos, M.D., medical director of asthma and allergic diseases at the Johns Hopkins Asthma and Allergy Center in Baltimore. In conjunction with this regimen, other tools such as your bronchodilator inhaler (or tablets) are often needed to optimize control or to treat wheezing episodes.

But pay special attention if you find you have to use your bronchodilator much more frequently or if you are having attacks more "easily" than in the past. For instance, if you normally took a couple of puffs of your inhaler in a week but are now taking that much in a day, see your doctor as soon as possible, suggests Dr. Creticos.

Of course, any time that you have more severe difficulty breathing or an asthma attack that you can't control, go to the nearest hospital immediately.

allergies and hay fever (see pages 181 and 257). Then add the following actions to your anti-asthma repertoire.

Take up yoga. Practicing a simple yoga breathing technique in which you exhale for twice as long as you inhale can protect you from future attacks by building resistance. This technique has been found effective when practiced daily.

"The improvement in asthma control from this type of breathing is similar to what you would find using a corticosteroid inhaler," says Mary Schatz, M.D., a pathologist at Centennial Medical Center in Nashville, Tennessee, and a certified yoga instructor.

If you want to try this technique, the steps are "elegantly simple," as explained by Dr. Schatz in her book *Back Care Basics: A Doctor's Gentle Yoga Program for Back and Neck Pain Relief.*

1. Close your eyes.
2. Inhale naturally.
3. Exhale naturally.

Enjoy Exercise *without* Asthma Attacks

Just because you have asthma doesn't mean you can't enjoy a regular workout. But you do need to exercise some good judgment.

Swimming is probably the ideal exercise, because the high humidity of pools won't dry out your throat, says California allergist William Ziering, M.D., instructor of health sciences at Fresno State University and a past president for the Section on Allergy of the California Medical Association. Sports that require continuous, vigorous activity in dry air, such as running, are no longer discouraged if, under a doctor's supervision, special precautions are taken. According to Dr. Ziering, these involve using a "rescue inhaler" containing albuterol (prescribed by your doctor) 5 to 15 minutes before starting, taking a 5- to 10-minute warm-up and starting the activity at a slow pace for the first 5 to 15 minutes. Also good are sports that require shorter bursts of exercise, such as baseball, doubles tennis and golf.

If you must exercise in the cold, wear a mask or scarf over your face. And always have a warm-up period: By doing warm-ups, you may avoid asthma symptoms that typically occur during the first 15 minutes of exercise.

4. Pause without holding your breath for one or two seconds before your next inhalation. This will allow the exhalation to come to a natural completion.

Don't try to breathe slowly or deeply. But if you feel the need to inhale deeply, do so until you can return to the breathing exercise.

Avoid night noshing. Going to sleep on a full stomach might also feed your asthma.

"Asthma can be caused by stomach reflux," explains Peter S. Creticos, M.D., medical director of asthma and allergic diseases at the Johns Hopkins Asthma and Allergy Center in Baltimore. Reflux occurs when stomach acid backs up into the esophagus.

"Stomach contents may leak out and actually regurgitate into your mouth and then drip down into your airways while you're lying down or sleeping," he says. "Besides avoiding snacks, you could also take an antacid before bedtime to cut down on your stomach's acidity." Theophylline medications, which are sometimes prescribed to help control asthma, may actually aggravate your condition by increasing stomach reflux, says Dr. Creticos. If you are taking this medication and are having reflux problems, be sure to check with your doctor, so the dosage level can be adjusted.

Prop up your bed (or yourself). Besides cutting out midnight snacks, other ways to prevent reflux-induced asthma include elevating the head of your bed by placing it on bricks or wood blocks. Or prop yourself up with pillows to prevent acid's moving from your stomach to your esophagus, suggests H. James Wedner, M.D., chief of clinical allergy and immunology at Washington University School of Medicine in St. Louis.

Be sensitive to food sensitivity. Eating or even *smelling* foods that cause a reaction can trigger an asthma attack. "Some of the most common types of foods that trigger asthma are milk, eggs, nuts and seafood," says allergist John Carlston, M.D., associate professor of medicine at Eastern Virginia Medical School in Norfolk.

Go the fish route. Since Eskimos get asthma about as often as they get heat-stroke, some theorize that a fish-rich diet may help *prevent* asthma. Although tests aren't conclusive, Walter Pickett, Ph.D., senior research biochemist/group leader of the Medical Research Division at Lederle Laboratories in Pearl River, New York, says it is conceivable that eating sardines, herring, mackerel

---

Beware of Aspirin!

If you have asthma and suffer from sinusitis and nasal polyps, you should get your pain relief from acetaminophen, *not* from aspirin or other nonsteroidal anti-inflammatory drugs (NSAIDs) such as ibuprofen (Advil).

"Taking aspirin or NSAIDs could make your asthma worse or may even be life-threatening," warns Peter S. Creticos, M.D., medical director of asthma and allergic diseases at the Johns Hopkins Asthma and Allergy Center in Baltimore. Acetaminophen products such as Tylenol, Aspirin-Free Anacin and Panadol are considered safe, he says.

Also, if you have arthritis as well as asthma, Dr. Creticos recommends seeing your doctor before taking any of the usual medications to ease pain and inflammation. Ask the doctor to prescribe an anti-inflammatory medication that will help the symptoms without causing asthma problems.

and other fish rich in omega-3 fatty acids at least once a week may help lessen asthma's impact.

Multiply your vitamins. Taking a good multivitamin/mineral supplement and eating plenty of fruits and vegetables may also help, since some nutrients have been found to lessen symptoms associated with asthma attacks. Reviewing data from more than 9,000 people, researchers found that those with reduced levels of vitamin C and zinc suffered more from wheezing and other bronchial problems. Good food sources of vitamin C include citrus fruits, broccoli and peppers. Oysters, beef and crab are among the foods highest in zinc.

Get relief from caffeine. Although coffee has been shown to contribute to some health problems, it may be more helpful than harmful for many people with asthma. Caffeine, it turns out, has nearly the same effect as theophylline.

"A couple of cups of strong, regular black coffee will have a beneficial effect on asthma," says allergist Allan Becker, M.D., an associate professor of medicine in the Section of Pediatric Allergy and Clinical Immunology at the University of Manitoba in Winnipeg who tested the effects of caffeine on asthma. But *don't* use caffeine as a substitute for—or in combination with—your medication, he advises, because it is good only for emergency use. "In an emergency, when you don't have your medication around, two cups of strong, regular black coffee (sugar and milk slow absorption) can provide effective temporary relief until your regular medication is available," says Dr. Becker. Relief can also be provided—but the effect will be slower—with two cups of hot cocoa or eight ounces of milk chocolate candy.

Athlete's Foot

Considering that this ailment is most often associated with stalwart Schwarzeneggerites, it's no wonder that most people *don't* refer to athlete's foot by its wimpy clinical name: "ringworm of the feet."

But truth be told, this nasty little bugger could care less whether you pump up or punk out, whether your running is done in marathons or just into the kitchen for a halftime snack. If you want to see what encourages ringworm of the feet, just look down. Whether Nikes or ortho-walkers are your preferred footwear, your shoes are ringworm's idea of a happy home.

"Athlete's foot is caused by a fungus that thrives in warm, moist conditions— and the closed shoes present a good 'incubator' for these organisms," says Michael Ramsey, M.D., clinical instructor of dermatology at Baylor College of Medicine in Houston. "That's why athlete's foot is quite *un*common in primitive cultures where shoes are not worn." But if you wear shoes more often than a bushman does, here's how to get a toehold on this irritating but relatively harmless infection.

Sock it to 'em. "Whenever you take off or put on your socks, it's a good practice to rub a sock up and down your toe webs," says Rodney Basler, M.D., a

---

Is It *Really* Athlete's Foot?

Y ou may be able to run like the wind, pump iron until it rusts and make your heart beat faster than Dan Cupid's target practice, but even the most versatile jock-of-all-trades is a lousy Marcus Welby when it comes to diagnosing athlete's foot.

"A lot of people who think they have athlete's foot actually have another condition—usually eczema, dermatitis or some kind of allergic reaction to their shoes," says Rodney Basler, M.D., a dermatologist and assistant professor of internal medicine at the University of Nebraska Medical Center in Omaha. "One way to tell if it's *really* athlete's foot is if there's an infection in the toe web between your fourth and fifth toe— your 'ring' toe and pinkie. If it's *not* there, the problem is usually *not* athlete's foot."

It's also *not* athlete's foot if:
- The infection is identical on both feet. "Then it's probably eczema or an allergic reaction to your shoes," says Dr. Basler.
- It's only on the top of your toes. "Contact dermatitis may be caused by shoe material," he adds.
- It occurs on a child below the age of puberty. Athlete's foot rarely strikes before adolescence.
- The foot is red, swollen, blistered and sore. Again, severe dermatitis is the likely culprit.

dermatologist and assistant professor of internal medicine at the University of Nebraska Medical Center in Omaha. "That keeps the areas between your toes dry, which is essential in preventing and treating athlete's foot."

Get cooking with baking soda. Baking soda is a cheaper alternative to expensive foot powders, yet it does essentially the same thing. Either sprinkle it on dry or make a paste by moistening one tablespoon of baking soda with lukewarm water, suggests Suzanne M. Levine, D.P.M., a clinical assistant podiatrist at the Wycoff Heights Medical Center and adjunct clinical instructor at New York College of Podiatric Medicine, both in New York City. Rub the mixture on your feet and between your toes. After about 15 minutes, rinse it off and dry thoroughly.

The answer is blowin' from your dryer. "Use your hair dryer on your feet to dry them more effectively than you can with a towel," adds Dr. Basler. "And blowing air from your hair dryer into your shoes is a good way to dry them out after you wear them."

Find relief in sheep's clothing. "Placing lamb's wool between the tips of your toes (after removing your shoes) allows air to reach the affected skin, which helps make conditions less favorable for fungal growth," says Dr. Ramsey. So if the day's almost over and you can kick back for a while, prop up your bare feet with some lamb's wool between your toes.

Put on some antiperspirant. "Rubbing or spraying antiperspirant on your feet can keep them from sweating," says Dr. Basler. "You can use the same brand you use on your underarms. As long as it contains aluminum chlorohydrate, the active drying ingredient, it will work."

Disinfect your shoes. Neal Kramer, D.P.M., a Bethlehem, Pennsylvania, podiatrist, says that Lysol and other household disinfectants can kill off any living fungus spores. After you take off your shoes, rub the insides with a cloth or paper towel that has a dab of disinfectant. (Then use that hair dryer to dry out the insides of the shoes!)

The right solution: Don't use creams. Antifungal creams have the right ingredients but the wrong way of presenting them. "The problem with creams is that they *help* trap moisture, especially between toes," says Dr. Basler. "Solutions are much better than creams." *Note:* While solutions are more effective for remedying, creams can be used to help *prevent* athlete's foot.

23

Use the power in powder. If you're going with an over-the-counter powder—the most common remedy—Dr. Ramsey says some of the best are Zeasorb-AF, Desenex, Tinactin and Micatin. "I recommend *against* using cornstarch, because it sometimes sets you up for a yeast infection," adds Dr. Basler, who also recommends Mycelex as a nonprescription remedy.

Foot brine is fine. A mixture of two teaspoons of salt per pint of warm water provides a foot soak that zaps excess perspiration and hampers fungus growth, says Glenn Copeland, D.P.M., who is podiatrist for the Toronto Blue Jays professional baseball team and a staff member at the Toronto Women's College Hospital. Simply soak your feet for five to ten minutes at a time, repeating often until the condition clears. *Added bonus:* This saline solution helps soften the affected area, so antifungal medications can penetrate deeper for better results.

Remove dead skin. When your condition starts to improve, remove any dead skin. According to Frederick Hass, M.D., a general practitioner in San Rafael, California, and author of *The Foot Book*, dead skin houses fungus that can reinfect you. To remove it, use a bristled scrub brush on the entire foot and a baby bottle "nipple brush" on toe webs. And brush in the shower, so the dead skin goes down the drain without touching other parts of your body.

Be a shoe swapper. "In theory, you're supposed to wear a pair of shoes only once every five days in order to allow shoes to *really* dry out between wearings," adds Dr. Basler. "If people don't have enough shoes to do that, I suggest that they wear different pairs as often as possible."

Backache

C onsidering all the grief and bother it causes people, back pain ranks right up there with the common cold. And like the common cold, which responds just as well to chicken soup as to antibiotics, "treating chronic low back pain effectively requires the consistent use of seemingly simple remedies, not rocket science methods," says Brent V. Lovejoy, D.O., an occupational medicine specialist in Denver and a medical consultant to the construction industry.

Only about 20 percent of acute back pain can be traced to some obvious cause, such as a herniated disk. So most back pain is considered a "mechanical" problem. And it's not all that easy to diagnose.

"Talk with ten different doctors and you will get ten different opinions as to exactly where in the back this pain originates," says Scott Haldeman, M.D., D.C., Ph.D., associate clinical professor in the Department of Neurology at the University of California, Irvine, and adjunct professor at the Los Angeles Chiropractic College. Muscle spasms, jammed back joints and stretched ligaments have all been implicated.

What *is* known for sure is that in addition to having a medical evaluation, there are lots of things you can do for yourself, both to ease flare-ups and to ward off future backaches. In fact, a few of these things are so important that doctors who treat back pain successfully consider them *essential,* not optional!

Raise your fitness level. "If you have a back injury that does not require surgery, studies indicate your aerobic capacity level is the single most important predictor of getting better," Dr. Lovejoy says. In other words, if you're physically fit, you're much more likely to recover.

That's why daily aerobic exercise is the "treatment of choice" in the view of Dr. Lovejoy and many other doctors. "For the construction workers I treat, I recommend brisk walking with hand weights and strength training with free weights," Dr. Lovejoy says. Adds Dr. Haldeman: "Do anything and everything that you can do comfortably and continuously."

Cushion your dogs. The pounding stress that running, and even just walking, normally produces is transmitted right up your back. And for a weak back, that can mean pain.

"Shoes designed specifically to absorb shock, such as running shoes, or special shock-absorbing inserts available at sporting goods stores may reduce back pain," says researcher Arkady Voloshin, Ph.D., professor of engineering in the Department of Mechanical Engineering and Mechanics at Lehigh University in Bethlehem, Pennsylvania. In one study, Dr. Voloshin found that 80 percent of back pain sufferers reported rapid and significant relief when they switched from basic street shoes to lightweight, flexible-soled shoes with simple shock-absorbing cushions.

Get horizontal—then get going. Rest, not exercise, is what most doctors recommend *initially* for acute back pain. "But we tell people that in order to get their circulation going, they need to be up and walking around for 45 minutes of every three hours," Dr. Lovejoy says. "Otherwise, they stiffen up like a board, and everything they do hurts."

Don't overdo a rest stop. More than two days' bed rest may not be helpful, according to Richard A. Deyo, M.D., D.P.H., professor in the Departments of Medicine and Health Services at the University of Washington in Seattle.

He found that back pain sufferers who were advised to stay in bed just two days missed 45 percent fewer days of work during the following three months than patients advised to rest for a full week. Muscles may weaken quickly with bed rest, and weak muscles can perpetuate an aching back.

Turn to aspirin, Advil or Tylenol. Any over-the-counter painkiller that contains aspirin, ibuprofen (Advil) or acetaminophen (Tylenol) could ease your back pain, according to Dr. Haldeman. But don't use painkillers before the fact. "If you know you are going to have back pain if you do something such as running, it's better not to do the activity than to mask your pain with drugs," says Dr. Haldeman. And do not give aspirin to children because of the risk of Reye's syndrome.

Get a posture check. Neither a fence post nor a spaghetti noodle be. An erect but *relaxed* stance, both standing and sitting, puts the least stress on back muscles, experts say.

Find your most restful position. Is your lower back acting up? Try this relaxation tactic: Lie on the floor with your knees bent at a 90-degree angle and your calves resting on the seat of a chair. "This position reduces pressure in your back more than anything else," Dr. Haldeman says. "Most people find it very comfortable."

Warm up your muscles before you hit high gear. Like old rubber bands, stiff muscles can fray when they're stretched by sudden movement. So warm up first with a few minutes of relaxed walking. Swing your hips and arms as you walk, then try a few slow side-to-side twists. If you're planning a specific activity, such as a golf swing, go through the motion several times, slowly, before you add speed and force.

Try some aqua- and yoga-laxation. Water exercises, especially an arthritis range-of-motion program, are a safe and effective way to knock the rust off back muscles that haven't been stretched for a while, says Dr. Haldeman.

When to See the Doctor

Seventy to 90 percent of back pain goes away by itself or with some minor home treatment," says Scott Haldeman, M.D., D.C., Ph.D., associate clinical professor in the Department of Neurology at the University of California, Irvine, and adjunct professor at the Los Angeles Chiropractic College.

See a doctor if your back pain doesn't improve after three days—or if the pain is so bad you can't budge from the bed. You'll also need a doctor's advice if your legs are weak or numb or if back pain is accompanied by fever. Other call-the-doctor symptoms include stomach cramps, chest pain and difficulty breathing.

In some cases, back pain may be associated with loss of bowel or bladder control. This demands immediate attention: It may indicate a severely herniated disk or spinal cord or nerve damage.

Check with your doctor, hospital or health center to find out where these programs are offered. Many people with back problems benefit from yoga, too, according to Dr. Haldeman—provided they begin slowly and advance according to their tolerance and ability.

Roll on a tennis ball. It's possible to relieve pain with "acupressure" or "trigger point" treatment using a tennis ball, says Robert King, co-director of the Chicago School of Massage Therapy and a nationally certified massage therapist. (He also recommends some of the wooden "pain relievers" designed for people who have aches and pains—such as a Backnobber.)

For the tennis ball treatment: Lie on a hard surface and position the tennis ball under you so that it is pressing against a tender spot. Roll onto the ball gradually, utilizing your body weight until the pain and tenderness subside.

To decrease back pain, don't smoke. Experimental work has shown that smoking reduces the amount of oxygen that travels, via osmosis, to spinal disks at night while you sleep. "If you smoke a pack of cigarettes a day, you'll probably double the amount of back pain you would have if you didn't smoke," Dr. Lovejoy says.

Ice it up. To get ready for a gentle icing, first freeze some water in a small paper cup. When you're ready to use it, Dr. Haldeman says, peel back the side of the cup to expose about ½ inch or so of ice. Lie on your stomach with a towel on your back, and have a friend or spouse massage your aching spots with the ice. (The ice should not be applied directly to the skin.) You can also lie down on your back with your knees bent and slide a bag of crushed ice (wrapped in a wet towel) under the sore spot, Dr. Lovejoy says.

Warm up the ache. A heating pad or hot water bottle can help. Or simply curl up in front of a hot wood stove to ease your aches. How do you decide whether your aching back needs heat or cold? "You pick one or the other, try it for a while and see if it helps," Dr. Haldeman says.

Bad Breath

Even with regular brushing and flossing, even with mints, mouthwashes and other breath fresheners, are there times when that h-h-h-horrendous h-h-h-halitosis h-h-h-has (*ugh!*) made some of those around you consider career opportunities in Arctic Circle weather stations?

If your mate or colleagues start inquiring about getting your mouth declared "endangered swamplands," don't take it *too* personally. After all, bad breath hits just about *everyone* sometime—and, unfortunately, everyone around us as well. "There are so many causes of bad breath, literally dozens of them, that it is occasionally difficult to pinpoint," says Joseph Tonzetich, Ph.D., professor of oral biology at the University of British Columbia in Vancouver.

Fact is, just about anything we put in our mouths, from antihistamines and other drugs to food and drink, can make your breath smell a tad uglier. Stress, sinus problems, mouth sores, talking, even our hormones can intensify bad breath. But breathe easy, folks, because here's how to kiss that nasty halitosis goodbye.

Eat an orange. "Some cases of bad breath—particularly those caused by stress and taking drugs—are the result of your mouth being too dry," says Dr. Tonzetich. "Citrus fruits and other foods high in citric acid are very good at stimulating saliva. The acid also helps suppress the activity of some odor-

When to See the Doctor

When bad breath continues despite your best efforts to remedy it, your problem may be more than just going a little too heavy on the onions. It can be a warning sign of a serious medical condition.

Bad breath is to be expected if you have a mouth sore, tooth or gum disease, sinus or tonsil infections or other problems in the oral/nasal cavity. It is also normal after dental surgery.

But it can also indicate gastrointestinal disorders, "problem" stress, tuberculosis, syphilis, dehydration, zinc deficiency, even cancer.

So it makes sense to do a self-check every now and then. Cup your hands over your nose and mouth, give a puff as if you were blowing into a balloon, and sniff your own breath. If it's bad, you can tell immediately by the smell.

Advice: If you've tried everything to remove bad breath and it still won't go away, then see your dentist or doctor, advises dentist Roger P. Levin, D.D.S., president of the Maryland Academy of General Dentistry.

causing enzymes, while the 'tangy' taste of lemons, oranges and grapefruit helps freshen your mouth."

Be a picker. "Probably one of the best ways to control bad breath is to use an oral irrigation device such as a Water Pik to 'irrigate' your teeth," says Fred G. Fedok, M.D., assistant professor of otolaryngology/head and neck surgery at University Hospital of Pennsylvania State University in Hershey. "Using a Water Pik helps remove food and other debris that cause a lot of bad breath."

Try the baking soda solution. You can add extra punch to your Water Pik by using a baking soda solution to clean your teeth. "You can brush on baking soda with a toothbrush and then rinse with water or use your Water Pik," says Dr. Fedok. "Or what I *really* recommend is mixing baking soda with warm water, pouring that solution into the Water Pik and using it to irrigate your teeth and mouth."

According to Dr. Fedok, "Baking soda is a great remedy for bad breath, because it changes the pH in your mouth and makes it a less friendly environment for many bacteria." He adds that baking soda is especially helpful to those with bad breath caused by gingivitis.

Brush your tongue. "Perhaps the most *overlooked* way of eliminating bad breath is to brush the top surface of the tongue when you brush your teeth," says Dr. Tonzetich. "Although there are many causes of bad breath, usually the odor arises from the surface of the tongue." That's because the tongue is covered with microscopic, hairlike projections that trap and harbor plaque and food, says Eric Shapira, D.D.S., assistant clinical professor and lecturer at the University of the Pacific School of Dentistry in San Francisco. A daily, gentle brushing (including the top of your tongue) unlodges these odorous particles.

Or give it a wipe. Don't have a toothbrush handy? Not to worry. "Simply take a hanky or a piece of gauze and give your tongue a good wiping," advises David S. Halpern, D.M.D., a dentist in Columbia, Maryland, and a spokesdentist for the Academy of General Dentistry. "Even a quick wipe is good for removing the coating on your tongue that can cause bad breath."

Clean your sinuses. Since bad breath can be caused by any number of sinus problems, some people get relief by "washing" out the area inside your nose where the sinuses drain, says Dr. Fedok. If you want to try it, use a saline solution in a blue-ball syringe—the kind used to clean out ears. (Both the solution and the syringe are available at most pharmacies.) "You'll have to refill the syringe several times. Spray the saline up each nostril, letting the solution drain out the other nostril and your mouth. It may take up to a pint of saline to wash out your sinuses," says Dr. Fedok.

Use the *right* mouthwash. Just about any type of mouthwash will temporarily mask the odors of bad breath—usually for about 20 minutes. But to eliminate the foul smell with the efficiency of Rambo in a bad mood, choose a mouthwash that contains zinc. "Zinc has a tendency to do a lot of things to inhibit the production of sulfur compounds that cause bad breath," says Dr. Tonzetich. "And zinc mouthwashes don't taste as metallic as copper-containing oral products."

Eat breakfast. Miss breakfast and it's a good bet you may have tainted breath *all* morning long, adds Dr. Tonzetich. "You usually have tainted breath until you take in some food," he says. "A lot of people who go without breakfast have bad breath at least until lunchtime."

Complete your dining with water. Whether you're having a quick snack or a multicourse meal, a water chaser is the ideal after-dining drink. "Swishing a mouthful of water is a great way to get rid of odors caused by food and drink," says Dr. Halpern.

This is especially recommended after having coffee, tea, soft drinks or alcohol, which can leave a residue that can attach to plaque in your mouth, causing bad breath.

Settle your stomach. Indigestion or stomach problems can cause you to burp, expelling foul gaseous odors, says Dr. Halpern. To relieve this problem, take antacids to settle your stomach.

Don't even *handle* garlic. Sure, everybody knows that *eating* garlic causes breath that can stop a clock. But *handling* it during food preparation can also cook up some foul odors, says Ronald S. Bogdasarian, M.D., an otorhino-laryngologist and clinical assistant professor at the University of Michigan School of Medicine in Ann Arbor who has done research into the causes and cures of bad breath. That's because aromatic substances in garlic seem to enter the body through the pores, arrive in the bloodstream and get released in the lungs before being exhaled.

Chew your "greens." Besides being instant breath fresheners, parsley and wintergreen also release pleasant aromatic substances into the lungs. The result: They'll be freshening your breath some 24 hours later, adds Dr. Bogdasarian.

Watch your diet. Some research indicates that a high-fat diet may contribute to bad breath. The theory is that certain fats—particularly those in cheeses, butter, whole milk and fatty meats—may contain certain aromatic substances that we metabolize and exhale, says Dr. Bogdasarian. If other causes of bad breath have been eliminated, try cutting back on deli meats and dairy products and replacing them with more carbohydrates, fruits, vegetables and whole grains.

Know your medications. Many prescription and over-the-counter drugs contribute to bad breath by having a "drying" effect on the mouth. That's because saliva, being slightly acidic, normally suppresses bacteria. But some drugs cause saliva to dry up. When it does, the bacteria in your mouth start reproducing like rabbits in springtime. Antihistamines, decongestants, anti-anxiety drugs, diuretics and certain heart medications lead the list of drugs that have a mouth-drying effect. If you're taking any of these drugs, be sure to *increase* your intake of water. Chewing gum or sucking on hard candies will also keep saliva flowing.

Bedsores

Bedsores, which usually afflict the bedridden and handicapped, are purplish skin ulcers that result when skin is squeezed against bony parts of the body such as heels or hips. In some cases, the damage extends deep into muscle and bone, causing extremely serious infection.

People who have bedsores—also called pressure ulcers—need to be under a doctor's care. And anyone who has diabetes must be especially alert for this condition. Bedsores are often treated with antibiotics, and some doctors also recommend a special diet that's high in vitamin C, protein and zinc. But here are some other treatments you might want to know about if you're caring for someone who may be developing bedsores or who already has them.

Make "shifts" last no more than one hour. "Patients with bedsores need to be rotated, or shifted to a new position, constantly," says Nelson Lee Novick, M.D.,

---

A Sweet Cure?

For extreme cases of bedsores, don't be surprised if your doctor reaches for the sugar jar instead of the medicine cabinet. Sugar has been found to help hard-to-heal areas such as bedsores by acting as a scavenger of sorts—picking up dead bacteria and white blood cells. This debris is later flushed away when the wound is cleansed with water.

Sugar also absorbs moisture from the wounds and creates an unfavorable environment for bacterial growth, says Alvin B. Segelman, Ph.D., former professor of pharmacognosy at Rutgers University College of Pharmacy in New Brunswick, New Jersey, and now vice president for research and development for Nature's Sunshine Products, based in Utah. But *never* try using sugar on any wound yourself, unless you're under the care of a health professional.

associate clinical professor of dermatology at Mount Sinai School of Medicine in New York City. He suggests shifting the patient every 30 minutes to relieve pressure that can cause bedsores.

Try a new mattress. Air mattresses, like those used by campers, help reduce pressure under bony areas of the body that are often afflicted with pressure ulcers, according to a study by gerontology researchers at the University of Alabama in Birmingham. Lying on a "cushion of air" offers less pressure than lying on a spring mattress.

Keep skin moist. Running a humidifier or regularly applying moisturizers to bedridden people can prevent skin dryness and irritation and make skin more resistant to bedsores and other infections.

Bed-Wetting

L ike failing the Big Test or dropping that high fly ball in the bottom of the ninth inning, bed-wetting is among the more humiliating experiences of childhood.

And it's something that many kids have to endure—about one in every seven, in fact.

But unlike math class or Little League, bed-wetting—or enuresis, as it's medically known—is likely to be part of a family tradition. If both parents were bed-wetters, chances are three in four that their offspring will be, too. If one parent was, the odds are about one in two.

Usually, bed-wetting is due to a small bladder, and most children will "outgrow" the problem. In fact, parents don't need to give bed-wetting a second thought until the child is about five years old—the age when most children have adequate control of urination.

Even though, in most cases, bed-wetting isn't caused by psychological problems, it could affect the child's self-esteem. It's important to avoid humiliating or punishing children who wet their beds. In fact, doctors say that punishment can *worsen* the problem because of additional stress. Instead, give your child a little understanding. And here's what else you can do to help your kid have a drier dream time.

Hit the sack. After heredity, the biggest culprit is sleep loss. "Not getting enough sleep will make bed-wetting worse," says Thomas Roth, Ph.D., president of the National Sleep Foundation and director of the Henry Ford Hospital Sleep Disorders and Research Center in Detroit. "I don't think napping is a good idea, because it spreads out the sleep you should be getting at night, but I do advise that bed-wetters increase their sleep by going to bed earlier."

Address those allergies. "Another reason why kids wet their beds at night is allergies," says Marc Weissbluth, M.D., director of Children's Memorial Hospital Sleep Disorders Center in Chicago and author of *Healthy Sleep Habits, Happy Child.* "A child with allergies has more difficulty sleeping and fewer deep-sleep periods." During the time when they are going from a deep sleep to a light sleep, the sphincter around the urinary passage relaxes, and they wet their beds.

"If you're not sure whether allergies are the cause, check for signs of snoring, mouth breathing or night sweating," says Dr. Weissbluth. Then treat the allergies.

Let them slurp a lot during the day. Rather than depriving your child of fluids at night, some experts recommend giving extra drinks during the day to "stretch" the bladder and improve its capacity. One way that may be helpful is to encourage the child to "hold off" urinating as long as possible, according to the *Journal of Pediatrics.*

Reward them for results. An easier method (at least as far as kids are concerned) is to have the child keep a diary and to award gold stars on the calendar for each dry night. In one study, 70 percent of bed-wetters who were treated this way wet their beds less. One in four stopped bed-wetting entirely.

Get "alarmed." There are various safe and effective bed-wetting alarms that are worn on the body and help wake up the child at the first sign of bed-wetting, says Barton D. Schmitt, M.D., professor of pediatrics at the University of Colorado School of Medicine in Denver. A moisture sensor is attached to the child's underwear, with a buzzer or an alarm near the child's ear. When a few drops of urine are released, the alarm sounds, and the child awakens and uses the toilet to finish emptying the bladder. Eventually the child will awaken to the sensation of a full bladder. One drawback: The alarm may have to be used for four to five months before it has the desired result (a doctor's guidance may be helpful).

Bee Stings

Bees usually don't go looking for trouble. If you don't bother them by poking around their nests, chances are you'll never get stung. And even if you do, most bee stings cause little pain, usually lasting from a few hours to a few days.

Unless, of course, you're allergic—in which case you need emergency care. But for the vast majority of the population, a little tender loving care is all you'll need.

Scrape out the stinger. One of the best ways to remove a stinger—and avoid any *additional* pain—is to "scrape" it out of the skin with a credit card, a knife or a long fingernail, advises John Yunginger, M.D., professor and pediatrics consultant at the Mayo Clinic in Rochester, Minnesota. "The biggest mistake people make is trying to pull the stinger out. In doing that, you squeeze the tiny venom sac attached to the stinger and accidentally release more venom into your skin." If you scrape the stinger out, this sac goes undisturbed.

Rub an aspirin on the sting. "Rubbing a wet aspirin on the area where you were stung can help neutralize some of the inflammatory agents in the venom," says Herbert Luscombe, M.D., professor emeritus of dermatology at Jefferson Medical College of Thomas Jefferson University and senior attending dermatologist at Thomas Jefferson University Hospital, both in Philadelphia. If you are allergic or sensitive to aspirin taken by mouth, though, you shouldn't try rubbing it on your skin.

Get tender relief with meat tenderizer. "Make a paste with meat tenderizer and water and apply it to the sting," says Philip Koehler, Ph.D., an entomologist at the U.S. Department of Agriculture Laboratory at the University of

When to See the Doctor

Allergic reactions to bee stings can be life-threatening. In fact, as many as 100 people a year die from bee stings. That's more than the number who die from the bites or stings of all other animals combined, says wilderness medicine specialist Kenneth W. Kizer, M.D., M.P.H., professor of emergency medicine at the University of California, Davis. How do you recognize an allergic reaction? If you or your child experiences *any* of these symptoms, seek emergency care immediately.

- You have trouble breathing, tightness in the throat or chest, dizziness, nausea or other symptoms of serious allergic reaction.
- Swelling spreads to a large area—for example, your entire arm swells, or a *large* section of the trunk puffs up.
- Pain and swelling continue for more than 72 hours without any relief.

Whenever they're outdoors, people who know they're allergic should always carry a bee sting kit recommended by their physician. These kits contain antihistamine pills and/or adrenaline injections that should be administered immediately after the sting. "Usually you take the pills first, and if there is no improvement in a few minutes and you cannot get to professional medical help, then you can administer the injection," says Dr. Kizer.

Florida in Gainesville. "The reason meat tenderizer works is because insect bites and stings are made up of protein—and meat tenderizer breaks down this protein." Use Adolph's, McCormick or another product that contains papain—the active venom-busting ingredient.

Try baking soda. Some doctors say baking soda can help ease bee sting pain. Claude Frazier, M.D., an allergist in Asheville, North Carolina, recommends applying a paste of baking soda and water directly on the sting for 15 or 20 minutes.

Kill the sting with Sting-Kill. Another towelette product that works well is called Sting-Kill. "This product is sold at some pharmacies and at beekeeper supply stores, and I'm told it's *very* effective," says Dr. Yuninger. Wonder where to find such a store? Call a local beekeeper and ask where you can purchase Sting-Kill; there are beekeeper supply stores in most metropolitan areas.

Wipe out the pain with ammonia. Sometimes dabbing some household ammonia on the sting also does the trick, says Dr. Luscombe. In fact, ammonia is a key ingredient in a product called After Bite, which is sold over the counter and comes in convenient towelettes that you rub on the sting.

Swallow a pain reliever. "One of the best ways to relieve the pain of a bee sting is to simply take a mild pain reliever such as aspirin, ibuprofen (Advil) or acetaminophen (Tylenol)," says wilderness medicine specialist Kenneth W. Kizer, M.D., M.P.H., professor of emergency medicine at the University of California, Davis. Do not give aspirin to children because of the risk of Reye's syndrome.

Take an antihistamine. Benadryl or another nonprescription antihistamine will ease swelling and pain in adults. An antihistamine-containing cough syrup such as Benylin works better for children, advises Dr. Koehler.

Dress plain, not flashy. Bees are attracted to brightly colored clothing— particularly floral prints and dark colors. Wearing white, khaki and other light colors is a good way to keep bees away.

Don't smell so sweet. The sweet smell of flowers isn't the only fragrance that attracts bees. Wearing perfume or after-shave may entice bees to come your

ID Your Bees

No matter the species of bee, the spot it stings will feel red and swollen. But all bees are not the same, and neither is their method of stinging, according to Edgar Raffensperger, Ph.D., professor of entomology at Cornell University in Ithaca, New York.

Honeybees, which have a fuzzy, golden brown body, sting only once and then die. That's because their stingers remain embedded in your skin.

Wasps and *hornets* can sting repeatedly because they have smooth stingers that can exit pierced skin easily. Wasps and hornets are shiny, and their thorax (middle section) is characteristically slim.

Yellow jackets resemble wasps and can also sting repeatedly. Don't smash them, because when destroyed, their venom sac releases a chemical that incites other yellow jackets to attack.

way. Most experts agree that you should skip the refined scents if you know you're venturing into bee-filled territory.

Up your zinc intake. Certain nutrients appear to offer protection against some insects, possibly by altering body odor. "My sister had a terrible problem with yellow jacket bees until she started taking zinc," says George Shambaugh, Jr., M.D., professor emeritus of otolaryngology/head and neck surgery at Northwestern University Medical School in Chicago. "Now she never gets stung."

He advises taking 60 milligrams a day—about four times the Recommended Dietary Allowance. Good dietary sources of zinc include oysters, red meats and fortified cereals. Besides zinc, thiamine (vitamin B₁) may also help. But if you do go the supplement route, check with your doctor, because high levels of any nutrient can cause problems.

Belching

In some parts of the world, the ultimate compliment you can pay the host after a hearty, sumptuous feast is one prolonged, expressive belch.

Unfortunately, that kind of complimentary noise won't earn you the Best Manners Award at Aunt Martha's Sunday buffet. But polite or not, belching *does* come naturally: A study has shown that healthy young people belch an average of 11 times in 20 hours—*excluding* mealtimes.

The gas you release while belching comes from your upper gastrointestinal tract. It got there because you swallowed it while talking, eating or drinking. The air that goes down with every swallow just adds to the air already in your stomach—and all this trapped air speaks loud and clear when it comes back up.

What to do when belching becomes a bother? Try these tips from our experts.

Eat modest meals at a measured pace. "Eat small meals, and eat slowly," advises Nicholas Talley, M.D., Ph.D., a gastroenterologist and associate professor of medicine at the Mayo Clinic in Rochester, Minnesota. Dr. Talley also recommends not eating and drinking at the same time to reduce repetitive swallowing.

Banish balloon food. Certain foods and beverages are particularly gassy or puffed up with air. Watch out for "carbonated or foaming beverages, or dishes made with beaten eggs or whipped cream," says Ronald L. Hoffman, M.D., director of the Hoffman Center for Holistic Medicine in New York City.

Break those air-grabbing habits. How else do you swallow air when you're not eating? According to Dr. Hoffman, smoking, sipping through a straw, chewing gum and sucking hard candies can add to the trapped air in your stomach and contribute to belching problems. Drinking from water fountains, cans and bottles can also be blamed. Try to avoid munching or chewing when you're on the go. And when you want a sip of something, try to drink calmly rather than grabbing a gulp on the go.

Relax for relief. "Work to reduce your anxiety level," recommends Dr. Talley. "Sometimes you're swallowing air because you're anxious." Among the best

Try These Belch-Busting Exercises

Plenty of fourth-graders learn how to gulp air and produce a command performance of belching. And it stands to reason that any talent that can be learned can also be unlearned—so why not train your innards *not* to belch?

Here's a way to take the belch potential out of your sips and swallows, recommended by Marvin L. Hanson, Ph.D., chairman of the Department of Communication Disorders at the University of Utah in Salt Lake City. To get more control of your swallowing, Dr. Hanson recommends practicing these steps as you swallow any liquid.

1. Lift your tongue up.
2. Keep your teeth together *or* slightly parted.
3. Sip, but don't slurp, the liquid. (Don't swallow yet.)
4. Close your lips and pull them in a bit.
5. Squeeze your tongue up.
6. Swallow.

Though these steps may feel forced at first, just keep practicing until you're swallowing smoothly. With repetition, belch-free sipping can become a habit.

stress relievers are regular exercise, meditation and soothing activities such as taking a hot bath.

Don't try to belch. Many people don't realize that a forced belch will backfire, says Dr. Talley. When you try to force up the trapped air, he says, you often swallow more air at the time or just afterward, so you end up getting more air down than you actually remove. The bottom line: "Don't force yourself to belch," says Dr. Talley.

Do a trial run of anatacids. Some people who feel they have excess stomach gas may benefit from over-the-counter antacids in standard doses, says Dr. Talley. That's because stomach acid sometimes reacts with food to create excess carbon dioxide in your stomach. If you do take antacids, begin with a short "trial run" to see whether they're effective, he suggests.

Forget the plop-plop-fizz-fizz. Effervescent over-the-counter remedies like Alka-Seltzer are no help to belchers, says Dr. Hoffman. Like carbonated beverages, these remedies make you belch even more, because you're swallowing more air along with the remedy.

Defoam those bubbles with simethicone. An ingredient in over-the-counter products like Maalox Plus and Mylanta, simethicone is a "defoaming" agent. "Simethicone works well for gas in the small intestine and reduces belching," Dr. Hoffman says. This belch blaster smashes up the biggest gas bubbles and breaks them into smaller ones that burst more easily.

Let your coffee cool a bit. "When you slurp a hot beverage, you swallow air," says Marvin L. Hanson, Ph.D., chairman of the Department of Communication Disorders at the University of Utah in Salt Lake City. To get around that problem, simply let your coffee cool a bit before you take a steamy sip.

Binge Eating

There are generally two triggers to an eating binge: Either you're on a diet and your body needs the extra food or you overeat because you're trying to suppress some emotion—stress, loneliness, depression or anger," says Adam Drewnowski, Ph.D., director of the Human Nutrition Program at the University of Michigan in Ann Arbor. "Either way, the end result is usually feelings of guilt."

While doctors say understanding and resolving your feelings is the best way to get off these feeding frenzies, here's some immediate help.

Write about your feelings. "I tell my patients who binge-eat when they're angry or depressed to write down their feelings in a letter they *don't* intend to send," says Karyn Scher, Ph.D., director of training for the Graduate Hospital Eating Disorders Service in Philadelphia.

"One reason why women are much more likely than men to go on eating binges is because our society has trained them to suppress their anger or other 'negative' emotions. Simply write how you feel, or pen a sample dialogue as you would like it to unfold for two people—yourself and the person causing those feelings," suggests Dr. Scher.

Besides keeping you from bingeing (both your mind and hands are occupied), this technique has another benefit: You'll learn healthier ways to deal with negative emotions.

Antibinge hotline: Call a friend. If you binge-eat out of boredom, it may be a sign of loneliness or social isolation, so Dr. Scher suggests you call a friend or relative. "I tell my patients to create a phone chain with at least six people they can call when they feel lonely or bored."

Count to 20. The next time you get a food craving, make yourself wait 20 minutes before you succumb. Most food cravings that *aren't* due to hunger will subside in that time. If not—if you're still hungry after 20 minutes—then you probably do need food.

41

"Ideally, you should do something that's incompatible with eating, such as taking a walk," suggests Linda Crawford, a certified eating disorders counselor at Green Mountain at Fox Run, a weight and health management center in Ludlow, Vermont.

Take to the sidewalk. Walking and other forms of aerobic exercise are among the best ways to kill food cravings, adds Dr. Scher. Vigorous exercise

When to See the Doctor

Almost everyone sneaks an extra goody now and then. But if you find you often eat until you're so overstuffed that you can't go on, you might be a victim of binge-eating disorder or bulimia. Both of these are serious conditions that require psychiatric counseling, according to Robert L. Spitzer, M.D., professor of psychiatry at Columbia University and director of biometric research at the New York State Psychiatric Institute, both in New York City.

Those with bulimia eat to excess and then induce vomiting to avoid gaining weight. For those with binge-eating disorder, the eating pattern is the same, but they don't try to vomit afterward.

Both disorders, doctors say, are usually caused by emotional stress or self-esteem problems. Left untreated, bulimia can cause serious metabolic problems, and binge-eating disorder can lead to physical ailments associated with obesity.

You should seek a doctor for counseling, according to Dr. Spitzer, if you have at least two "binges" a week, for a period of six months or longer, in which you consume about 2,000 calories when you're just snacking. That amount of calories is roughly the equivalent of a full day's worth of meals at one sitting. You should also talk to a doctor if you're:

• Eating much faster than normal.
• Eating to a point where you feel uncomfortably full.
• Eating large amounts of food when you're not physically hungry or when it's not a regular mealtime.
• Eating alone because of embarrassment or because you feel disgust or guilt about the way you eat.

Also, be sure to get medical attention as soon as possible if you induce vomiting after meals, says Dr. Spitzer.

may break a cycle of stress-induced bingeing. Lots of people report a sense of physical well-being after 20 minutes of aerobic exercise that offsets the urge to binge.

Drown your sorrows. Even if emotion rather than hunger is driving you to eat, drinking lots of water can help—by freshening your taste buds and filling your belly, which reduces your food cravings, according to George Blackburn, M.D., Ph.D., chief of the Nutrition/Metabolism Laboratory at New England Deaconess Hospital in Boston.

Choose low-fat alternatives. "If you totally deny yourself, you'll go crazy and just binge out even more later on," says Dr. Drewnowski. "Instead of forbidding yourself to eat, indulge in a smaller portion of a lower-fat substitute. For instance, if you're craving a bowl of ice cream, give in to a scoop of frozen yogurt."

Although many people suggest carrying around a bag of carrots or celery sticks for when the munchies hit, Dr. Drewnowski has found that these crunchy substitutes don't work. "You need to eat something along the same lines as what you're craving, only in smaller portions," he advises.

Sizzle your taste buds with spicy foods. Ever try to wolf down mass quantities of chili or peppers, horseradish or curry? It can't be done. So when the urge to eat is overwhelming, reach for a hot Mexican, Thai or Indian snack.

"The flavor is so intense that you'll find yourself eating much smaller portions than you would of bland or sweet foods," says Maria Simonson, Ph.D., Sc.D., professor emeritus and director of the Health, Weight and Stress Program at the Johns Hopkins Medical Institutions in Baltimore. Another bonus: Since they heat your entire body (not just your mouth), spicy foods speed up metabolism—so you won't gain as much.

Eat three squares *every day.* "A lot of people set themselves up for binges by restricting their food while dieting," says Dr. Scher. "When you skip breakfast and have nothing but a salad for lunch, by the time dinner rolls around, you're literally starving for food and will eat anything and everything. But if you consume three sensible meals each day—even while dieting—your body won't experience this intense starvation, and you'll be better able to control nighttime binges."

Black Eye

For some, a black eye is a badge of honor, a symbol of having principles and being willing to fight for them. But for others, it's an emblem of embarrassment—the result of foolishly walking into a door, challenging a guy named Turk to a fight or going for a pony ride on a fire-snortin' bronco known as The Widow Maker.

Well, never mind *how* you got that shiner. Here's how to heal it and hide it quicker than you can say "Knockout!"

Give it a Hawaiian punch. "Eating pineapple or papaya—or better yet, a fruit cocktail made of both—can help remedy a black eye," says Las Vegas orthopedic surgeon Michael Rask, M.D., chairman of the American Academy of Neurological and Orthopedic Surgeons and the American Board of Ringside Medicine and Surgery. According to Dr. Rask, "An enzyme found in those fruits 'changes' the molecular structure of the blood, so it's more easily absorbed by the body." If you have a black eye, eat three papayas a day for faster healing. Or you can take up to 600 milligrams of papaya in capsule form (sold in health food stores) four times a day. Loading up on pineapple will also do the trick, according to Dr. Rask, and both fruits give you a healthy dose of vitamin C.

Let vitamin C show its muscle. It's well documented that vitamin C promotes healing—and for anyone who bruises easily, getting plenty of vitamin C in your diet is a must. If you're sporting a black eye, take a daily vitamin C supplement and increase your intake of vitamin C–rich foods such as broccoli, mangoes, peppers and sweet potatoes, as well as pineapple and papaya, to speed the healing process.

Chill your shiner with frozen corn. Remember when tough guys used to slap a slab of raw steak over a black eye? Well, it isn't the *steak* that brings relief; it's the *coldness* of the piece of meat that helps decrease blood flow and relieve swelling. But you can save yourself some money (as well as a nice piece of

When to See the Doctor

Whenever you get a black eye, it's best to see your doctor to make sure your eyesight doesn't take a worse beating than your ego. "A black eye can be very serious and a threat to your permanent vision. Don't just assume 'it's no big thing,' " says Las Vegas orthopedic surgeon Michael Rask, M.D., chairman of the American Academy of Neurological and Orthopedic Surgeons and the American Board of Ringside Medicine and Surgery.

You need immediate medical care if:

- You have blurred or double vision or your eyesight is impaired in any way.
- You have pain *in* your eye as well as *around* it.
- You become light-sensitive.
- You have "floaters" or other specks in your field of vision.

meat) by using *anything* icy. "I recommend you use a bag of frozen vegetables wrapped in a washcloth," advises Rodney Basler, M.D., a dermatologist and assistant professor of internal medicine at the University of Nebraska Medical Center in Omaha. "It contours to your face better than a steak, and when you're done using it, you can just throw the bag back into the freezer and save it for the next day's treatment." Keep the cold compress on your blackened eye for about 20 minutes, or until the skin begins to feel numb; then remove it for about 10 minutes. You may continue this procedure on and off for three days, or until swelling subsides.

Avoid aspirin. It's an anticoagulant, which means it prevents the blood from clotting. "If you take aspirin, you may have a harder time stopping the bleeding that causes discoloration," says ophthalmologist Jack Jeffers, M.D., director of emergency services and director of the Center for Sports Vision at Wills Eye Hospital in Philadelphia. "So you may wind up with a bigger bruise." If you need a pain reliever, it's better to stick with Tylenol and other acetaminophen products.

Hide the damage. A makeup product called Dermablend, available over the counter, is effective at hiding birthmarks and skin discoloration caused by broken blood vessels. "Dermablend certainly helps cover a black eye," says Dr. Basler.

Blemishes

You may have thought it was over, another chapter of adolescence that could be forgotten as easily as algebra or your high school gym teacher. But now, as you stare in the mirror at that huge red dot on your chin, you have more than memories to remind you of the bother of blemishes.

And you're not alone. Although considered to be primarily a torment of teenagers, blemishes continue to provide plenty of angst in adulthood, and they can occur in varying degrees of severity. Anyone with hormones can get blemishes—and of course, we've *all* got hormones.

"The severity of most blemishes is related to heredity, amount of oil secretion, hormones and, to some extent, stress," says Michael Ramsey, M.D., clinical instructor of dermatology at Baylor College of Medicine in Houston. But here's how you can put a quick end to your own private Zit Parade.

Don't scrub. The biggest mistake by the acne-prone is thinking that washing with might is washing right. "In fact, the friction you create by overscrubbing can stir up new blemishes and aggravate existing ones," says dermatologist Edward Bondi, M.D., who treats the acne-ridden at the University of Pennsylvania Hospital in Philadelphia. "You shouldn't even wash with a washcloth. Instead, gently clean your face with your hands."

Use an over-the-counter medication with benzoyl peroxide. This active ingredient is "the first line of treatment and the *best* over-the-counter medication you can use," says Dr. Bondi. Oxy-5, Oxy-10, Fostex and Clearasil products are among those containing this active ingredient. But note that benzoyl peroxide is better at preventing new lesions than at getting rid of what you already have. "One common mistake is to dab it on the blemishes themselves," adds Dr. Bondi. "What's *more* effective is to spread it all over the face, especially in areas where acne is prone to be present."

In a pinch, try calamine. If you feel a blemish flourishing and you're all out of benzoyl peroxide, there's no need to run to the all-night minimart. Calamine lotion absorbs excess skin oil and can help nip that blotch in the bud, advises Thomas Goodman, Jr., M.D., assistant professor of dermatology at the University of Tennesee Center for Health Sciences in Memphis.

Chill out to avoid blemishes. Controlling the stress in your life is one of the best ways to control acne and other blemishes. "There's no question that stress plays a key role in the development of new blemishes and continuance of existing ones," says Dr. Bondi. If you're prone to acne, find a relaxation technique that works for you—such as exercise, meditation or listening to music—and practice it daily, particularly when you're stressed out.

Put on a cube—cosmetically. Placing an ice cube on blemishes for about 60 seconds after washing can help make them less noticeable, because cold reduces inflammation, adds Dr. Goodman.

Avoid the big squeeze. Sure, you may be lucky enough to remove that nasty pimple by squeezing it—but in the process, you'll probably cause several more to develop. "Although you may get one lesion to open and clear up quicker, there may be two or three smaller lesions beside it that you *don't* see that you can rupture from squeezing," says Dr. Bondi. "And if you squeeze the wrong way, you can get permanent scarring."

Get in the shade. Although sunshine tends to "camouflage" blemishes by tanning your hide, there's no scientific evidence that sunshine helps remedy pimples. And the sunlight may cause adverse skin reactions to some acne medications. If you notice your skin turning red and blotchy, "minimize exposure to sunlight, infrared heat lamps and even sunscreens," cautions Thomas Gossel, Ph.D., R.Ph., professor of pharmacology and toxicology and associate dean at Ohio Northern University College of Pharmacy in Ada and an expert on over-the-counter products.

Watch your diet. "Iodine *has* been associated with acne, so iodine-rich foods such as beef liver, clams, crabs and other shellfish should not be ingested in large quantities," says Dr. Ramsey. "And although scientific studies *haven't* shown that chocolate, sodas, greasy foods or milk aggravates acne, if you find that you break out after eating certain foods, then forget the studies and avoid those foods." Among the other likely suspects are cheeses, nuts and other high-fat foods, as well as caffeine.

Don't put too much hope in special soap. "Acne soaps tend to be very good at drying your skin, but many do *nothing* to treat acne," adds Dr. Bondi. "Rather than buying a special 'acne' soap, you're better off getting the *right* soap for your skin." That means a gentle soap like Dove if you have dry skin—*especially* in the winter—and maybe a stronger soap if your skin is excessively oily.

Read the labels on your cosmetics. Oil-based makeups have long been known to trigger blemishes, because the oil is usually a derivative of fatty acids more potent than your body's acids.

"If you're prone to blemishes, you're better off with a makeup that lists water as one of its main ingredients," says Michael Stein, a Hollywood makeup artist whose company has touched up famous movie faces. Specific ingredients too rich for blemish-prone skin include lanolins, isopropyl myristate, laureth-4 and sodium lauryl sulfate.

Blisters

You've heard of body language? Well, consider blisters more like body *profanity*—the skin's response to getting too much friction. Don't believe it? Just try to break in a new pair of shoes and you'll end up with an *(expletive deleted)* friction blister on your heel. Or spend too much time raking leaves and you'll curse the fat blisters that show up on the palms of your hands.

But since there will always be new shoes to break in and lawns in need of care, there will always be blisters—*unless* you take some precautions. So here's how to banish that blister before it articulates new meanings for the nastiest four-letter word of all—*pain*. Let's start with the most prevalent kind—foot blisters.

Give your feet a lube job. "Blisters are the result of too much friction. To avoid some of that friction and prevent a blister, liberally rub Vaseline over your feet," says Robert Diamond, D.P.M., a Pennsylvania podiatrist affiliated with Muhlenberg Hospital Center in Bethlehem and Allentown Osteopathic Hospital. "If the shoe doesn't fit correctly and your foot is slipping, you'll have better glide, so there's less friction—and therefore less chance of developing a friction blister."

Quit the cotton. Sorry, but much-ballyhooed cotton sweat socks *don't* offer the best protection against blisters. In fact, sports podiatrists say that man-made acrylic socks are best for preventing blisters. "Cotton fiber becomes abrasive with repeated use, and it also compresses and loses its shape and 'cushion' when wet," says Douglas Richie, Jr., D.P.M., clinical instructor of podiatry at Los Angeles County–University of Southern California Medical Center in Los Angeles. According to Dr. Richie, "The shape of the sock is critical when it's inside a shoe." So a sock that loses its shape is just what your blister-vulnerable foot *doesn't* need.

Silken your skin. "Wearing a silk undersock can help prevent foot blisters and relieve the pain once you get them, since silk is less damaging to the skin than other fabrics," says Nicholas J. Lowe, M.D., clinical professor of dermatology at the University of California, Los Angeles, School of Medicine and director of the Skin Research Foundation of California in Santa Monica.

Use powder power. Rubbing baby powder on your feet *before* any blister-promoting activity is another good preventer. "Make powdering part of your daily routine," says Richard Cowin, D.P.M., director of Cowin Foot Clinic of Orlando, Florida. Reason: Like petroleum jelly, it helps reduce friction and eases glide.

Put new footwear in your handbag. "Probably the biggest cause of foot blisters in women comes from trying to break in a new pair of shoes," says dermatologist Joseph Bark, M.D., past chairman of the Department of Dermatology at St. Joseph's Hospital in Lexington, Kentucky. "My advice to women who get a new pair of shoes? Wear them for only 30 minutes at a time. It's all right to wear the shoes several times a day, but only for 30 minutes—at least for the first few days." (So carry an extra pair of broken-in shoes in your handbag and trade off a few times during the day.)

Pad it with moleskin. A moleskin pad (available at most drugstores) is the best *preventive* measure for the blister-prone, and it's also great for *relieving* pain once the blister forms. Cut the moleskin into a doughnut shape and place it over the blister (or the area where you're prone to get it). "Leave the central area open over the blister," advises Suzanne Tanner, M.D., assistant professor of orthopedics at the University of Colorado Sportsmedicine Center in

The Right Way to "Pop" Blisters

Some doctors say that leaving a blister alone will reduce the risk of secondary infection. Others say that if a blister hurts, you should prick it with a pin to drain the water or blood that builds up under the "roof" of the skin. Draining it, they say, will ease the pain.

Since blisters usually hurt, most folks vote to pop—but often do it wrong and risk infection. Here's the proper procedure.

"One of the biggest mistakes people make is to pull off the skin from the top of the blister," says Rodney Basler, M.D., a dermatologist and assistant professor of internal medicine at the University of Nebraska Medical Center in Omaha. Instead, he suggests a specific procedure that has been proven to be most effective: After pushing the fluid to one end of the "bubble," prick the blister on the side containing the fluid, using a pin that's been sterilized with alcohol, a lighted match or boiling water. The pin should prick the blister horizontally, just above the skin. Dr. Basler suggests doing it three times—when you first see the blister, again 12 hours later and then 12 hours after that.

The buildup of fluid *does* cause pain, and by removing *all* the fluid, you reduce the pain. But remember: To avoid infection, always sterilize the needle with a flame, alcohol or boiling water before lancing your blister, says Dr. Basler.

Denver. The surrounding moleskin will absorb the shock and friction that cause or aggravate blisters.

Try a heel lift. Blisters on the back of the foot? They could be blamed on the heel counter—the tough shoe leather that covers your heel. If the counter rubs the wrong area of your foot, you'll have blister trouble fast. The fix? "All you usually have to do is put in a heel lift," says Dr. Cowin. Make sure to use the same size heel lift in *both* shoes unless advised differently by your doctor, even if only one heel is blistering.

Use an insole. To avoid blisters on the heel and other parts of the foot, many doctors recommend a Spenco insole. These store-bought inserts cut down on friction to prevent new blisters and help ease the pain of existing ones, says Dr. Diamond.

Soak 'em in Epsom. "If you perspire too much, you're more prone to getting blisters," adds Dr. Diamond. "If that's your problem, soaking feet in Epsom salts can help dry excessive sweating." Dissolve Epsom salts in warm water and soak your feet for about five minutes at the end of the day. Then dry thoroughly.

Give a double dose of healing gel. Research shows that triple antibiotic ointments can eliminate bacterial contamination after *two* applications. Neosporin and other nonprescription antibiotic ointments are sold in all drugstores. Avoid old standbys such as iodine and camphor-phenol, because they delay healing. After applying the antibiotic, you should cover the area with a gauze pad—but change that covering each time it gets wet to avoid contamination.

For hands—try a combination play. If your problem is hand blisters rather than foot blisters, the Epsom salts relief can be a big help. Also, wear heavy-duty work gloves whenever you have yard work to do. Another way to prevent blisters on your hands: Follow the advice of Dr. Cowin and rub some baby powder on your hands.

Bloodshot Eyes

P arty into the wee hours of the morning and the town isn't the only thing that will be painted red: Don't be surprised if your morning-after eyes resemble a ruby-colored road map.

Of course, heavy partying is not the only way to make your eyes burn red the next morning. Colds, allergies, even swimming in a chlorinated pool turns eyes bloodshot. But rest assured, the damage is usually minor and temporary. Here's how to whiten up those eyes again.

Apply a cold compress. If your eyes itch, the bloodshot look is probably caused by allergies. "A cold washcloth placed over your eyes will soothe the pain and shrink the blood vessels if your eyes are bloodshot because of allergies," says Eric Donnenfeld, M.D., associate professor of ophthalmology at North Shore University Hospital/Cornell Medical College in Manhasset, New

York. Hold the cold compress over your eyes until the itchiness subsides. You can repeat as often as convenient during the day.

For tired eyes—use a warm compress. If your eyes are red but don't itch, then a warm compress is the answer, adds Dr. Donnenfeld: "Warmth is best for bloodshot eyes caused by fatigue, staying up too late or a cold." Just place a warm washcloth over your closed eyes for 10 to 20 minutes.

Try artificial tears. If your bloodshot eyes are stinging, try soothing them with nonpreservative artificial tears, suggests Paul Vinger, M.D., assistant clinical professor of ophthalmology at Harvard University in Cambridge, Massachusetts. He recommends the single-dose packages.

Contacts wearers: Read the label. If you're a contact lens wearer and you notice more eye redness than in the past, read the label on your contact lens cleaner. If you're not using one labeled "preservative-free," switch to one that is. Preservatives in the cleaner can cause reddened eyes.

Put a lid on "red-out" products. "Eyedrops that promise to remove redness should be used only occasionally, because they can become habit forming," warns Dr. Donnenfeld. "After using them for a while, you may develop a 'rebound' effect, so if you *don't* use the drops, your eyes become red." His advice: Avoid using these over-the-counter products for more than four consecutive days, and try not to use them more than once daily.

Avoid known allergens. Steer clear of anything that has caused you to have allergies in the past: It could be causing your red-eye to flare up. Also, wash your hands after petting pets or applying makeup and shampoo, advises Thomas Platts-Mills, M.D., Ph.D., head of the Division of Allergy and Clinical Immunology at the University of Virginia Health Sciences Center in Charlottesville.

Body Odor

B ack when our ancestors were walking on their knuckles, when there were no Johnny Mathis records or candlelight dinners to help set the mood, most folks had a nice, natural ripeness that may have turned on their dinner companions more than it turned them off.

How times change. These days, that same natural body odor can leave you lonelier than ol' Uncle Ugh before his end-of-month bath night. Of course, the smell-good departments of pharmacies and supermarkets are well stocked with a scented array of deodorants, which kill the bacteria that cause the odor or mask the smell that the bacteria create.

But many people get irritations from deodorants and antiperspirants. The aluminum salts and other drying agents may be too strong for the sensitive glands in the armpits, says William Epstein, M.D., professor of dermatology at the University of California, San Francisco, School of Medicine. Luckily for you (and for everyone around you), there are other ways to banish body odor—sans deodorant. Among the most effective ways:

Don't stink with zinc. Some people find that body odor problems can be remedied simply by consuming more zinc, says Morton Scribner, M.D., a dermatologist in Arcadia, California. He suggests that you boost intake with a daily supplement of 25 to 50 milligrams of zinc. Or steer toward zinc-rich foods such as oysters, lean beef, king crab and wheat germ.

"Roll on" some baking soda. "Sodium bicarbonate, better known as baking soda, kills the odor-causing bacteria and absorbs moisture," says Arthur Jacknowitz, Pharm.D., professor and chairman of clinical pharmacy at West Virginia University School of Pharmacy in Morgantown. "Many people find that baking soda is just as effective as a deodorant." Simply sprinkle a generous amount into your bath and soak yourself, or mix it with a little talcum powder and apply it directly to underarms.

When to See the Doctor

When deodorants can't do the job and washing seems like a waste, you may have a body odor problem that requires some heavy artillery—namely, your doctor's expertise.

"If you've done everything you can and nothing seems to help, then you really need to see a dermatologist who specializes in body odor problems," advises George Preti, Ph.D., a researcher at the Monell Chemical Senses Center in Philadelphia. "You may have an underlying condition that requires certain antibiotics to kill the bacteria, or your doctor may prescribe a special soap."

Clean yourself the way doctors do. Surgeons scrub with antibacterial soap before an operation in order to kill bacteria. These soaps are "great for people with problem body odor or a tendency to get irritated from deodorants," says John F. Romano, M.D., a dermatologist and clinical assistant professor of medicine at The New York Hospital–Cornell Medical Center in New York City. And they're available over the counter at most drugstores. "Just ask the pharmacist for a surgical 'scrub' soap, then wash with it to kill the bacteria that cause body odors," says Dr. Romano. Scrub soap is very effective, yet gentle enough to use in the groin and underarm areas, he adds.

Do don some Domeboro. Another over-the-counter product that's an effective alternative to deodorant is Domeboro, says D'Anne Kleinsmith, M.D., a cosmetic dermatologist at William Beaumont Hospital near Detroit. Domeboro is a powder that you mix in cool or lukewarm water and apply to your problem areas. "It will relieve odor and wetness in those areas—whether it's your underarms, groin or feet or under your breasts," says Dr. Kleinsmith.

Shave excess hair under your arms. "The presence of hair increases body odor, because it serves as a collection site for secretions, debris and bacteria," says Dr. Jacknowitz. "Shaving your armpits is one way to reduce body odor problems. However, antiperspirants should not be used on newly shaved skin."

Hold the spices. Extracts of proteins and oils from certain foods and spices remain in your body's excretions and secretions for hours after you eat them.

These extracts can impart an odor. Fish, cumin, curry and garlic lead the list. "So if you have body odor problems, you'll have *more* problems if you eat a lot of these foods," says Dr. Kleinsmith.

Boils

You may recall that Pharaoh didn't think much of the idea of giving Moses and company their freedom. Even when a bundle of plagues were cast upon Egypt, Pharaoh didn't let those folks go. (If you don't remember, you can rent *The Ten Commandments* on video and relive it all with Yul Brynner and Charlton Heston.) But when Pharaoh saw *boils* among the plagues, the next thing you know, he was crying *"Enough!"*—and Moses was crossing the border.

Boils are the result of bacteria that invade through a microscopic break in the skin and infect a blocked oil gland or hair follicle. An abscess results when white blood cells, sent to kill the invaders, produce pus. Sounds nasty, but even though boils are sometimes painful and ugly, they're rarely dangerous.

Keep it wet and warm. "A warm compress is the best way to treat a boil, but you have to keep it very wet and very warm," says John F. Romano, M.D., a dermatologist and clinical assistant professor of medicine at The New York Hospital–Cornell Medical Center in New York City. "It's not enough to wring out a washcloth and place it on the boil. You should leave the compress on for 10 to 15 minutes, but keep wetting it every few minutes to make sure the boil stays wet and warm." He suggests this 15-minute compress four or five times daily to bring the boil to a head, which leads to its draining and then healing.

Lead staph to slaughter. If you're prone to boils, you may be able to lessen their frequency by cleaning your skin with an antiseptic soap such as Betadine, says dermatologist Adrian Connolly, M.D., clinical assistant professor of medicine at the University of Medicine and Dentistry of New Jersey in Newark.

Don't monkey with cysts. When cysts become infected, they often have a nasty way of turning into boils. So leave cysts alone, or have them excised by a doctor.

When to See the Doctor

You can treat most small boils (less than ½ inch) at home, but boils that are larger than that or that don't respond to simple remedies require a doctor's attention. You should never squeeze a large boil or a boil of any size around certain "danger zones": face, armpits, groin and the breasts of a nursing woman.

Be sure to consult a doctor if you see red lines radiating from the boil or if you get fever, chills or swelling in other parts of your body. You may also need a doctor's care if the boil is extremely tender or is under a thick layer of skin, as with some boils on the back. And if you have diabetes, you should always consult with your doctor any time boils appear: You might need antibiotics that are available only by prescription.

Hit the showers. When a boil is draining, keep the skin around it clean by taking showers instead of baths. This reduces the chance of spreading the infection to other parts of the body. After treating a boil, wash your hands well before preparing food, because staph bacteria can cause food poisoning.

Head for the kitchen. Applying pieces of warm, milk-soaked bread directly on the boil is an old folk remedy—and some people find it works quite well, according to Varro E. Tyler, Ph.D., professor of pharmacognosy at Purdue University in West Lafayette, Indiana, and author of *The Honest Herbal*.

Try vegetables . . . or tea. Other home remedies for boils include "compresses" of heated slices of tomato—or raw onion, mashed garlic or the outer leaves of cabbage. You can press these cut vegetables directly on the boil and see for yourself how well they work. Another kitchen compress: Place a warm tea bag of black tea directly on the boil for 15 minutes several times a day.

Breastfeeding

To your baby, your breasts are much more than a meal ticket. Study after study has shown that breastfed babies consistently seem to fare better than their formula-fed counterparts. In later years, they may score higher on IQ tests, and they're more immune to a host of problems ranging from diaper rash to cancer.

While mother's milk seems to offer Junior a smorgasbord of benefits, it isn't always a picnic to you: When you're nursing, your breast may get hard and heavy, achy and swollen. Your nipples may feel more than a little bit chewed up. But if you want your baby to have the benefits, you probably want to go on breastfeeding. So here are some remedies to make the whole process smoother.

Eat garlic. Breast pain aside, perhaps the hardest part of breastfeeding is trying to convince the little tyke to eat well; some babies gnaw, bite and "play" with nipples, and they may not ingest enough milk for a good meal.

Researchers at the Monell Chemical Senses Center in Philadelphia found that mothers who ate 1.5 grams of garlic extract two hours before nursing got an odor in their milk that prompted infants to suck longer and possibly ingest more milk. Besides that, the babies experienced *no* abdominal cramps or other problems associated with spicy foods. If straight garlic isn't your idea of a tasty snack, try eating garlicky dishes before nursing.

Reposition your baby. The key to problem-free feeding is positioning. "The baby should face you entirely: head, chest, genitals, knees," suggests Marsha Walker, R.N., an international board-certified lactation consultant who is president of Lactation Associates in Weston, Massachusetts. According to Walker, you should grip the baby so that his buttocks are in one hand and his head is in the bend of your elbow. Let your other hand slip under your breast, with all four fingers supporting it. But don't put your fingers on the areola (the darker area around the nipple). Then tickle the baby's lower lip with your nipple to get his mouth open wide. When his mouth opens, pull his body in quickly so that his mouth fixes on the areola.

Go for depth. The nipple should be deep in the baby's throat, adds Carolyn Rawlins, M.D., an obstetrician in Munster, Indiana, and a member of the board of directors of La Leche League International, a support group for breastfeeding mothers, in Franklin Park, Illinois. "This way, there is no movement of the nipple when the baby sucks."

Use *both* breasts. Nurse on one side until it appears that the baby is losing interest, advises Walker. Then offer your baby the other side. Next time you feed, start with the side you ended with the time before. Some babies—especially newborns—won't take both breasts at one feeding, so Walker advises you offer the other side after about an hour, when the baby rouses a little.

Say *ahhhh* with vitamin E. To soothe cracked nipples associated with breastfeeding, break open a vitamin E capsule and rub a small amount of the liquid on your nipples, advises Dr. Rawlins. The secret, however, is to use only a drop or two—and apply it only after you've finished nursing.

Or soothe with your own milk. Another effective treatment for hurting nipples is to express a little bit of milk and rub it in. Milk left at the end of the feeding is very high in lubricants and contains an antibiotic substance, says Dr. Rawlins.

Choose the *right* nursing bras. The best advice for buying a nursing bra is to go one cup size larger than your size during pregnancy, says Walker. Cotton fabrics are easier on your breasts than nylon, and the nursing opening should be wide enough that it doesn't compress the breast. And avoid using breast pads with plastic, because they retain moisture, which can be irritating.

Keep nipples from drying out. That means *no* soap on your nipples when you're showering, cautions Dr. Rawlins. "Do you see the little bumps around the areola? Those are glands that produce oil with natural antiseptic in it. So you don't need to use soap."

And after your shower, to prevent irritation, *don't* towel nipples dry; let them air-dry.

Breast Lumpiness

A s if being swollen and tender weren't bad enough, your breasts can also become lumpy. With many women, lumps often show up before menstruation. That's because hormones stimulate fluid buildup in the breast's milk glands and ducts. This buildup, in turn, creates lumps that can feel like masses of grain, peas, grapes or even golf balls.

Women who regularly experience this know that in a few days, when their period begins, the lumps will melt away. But women who feel pain along with the swelling may find this premenstrual problem intolerable. Here are some ways to reduce the lumps and raise your comfort level with ready remedies at home.

Steer clear of caffeine. The caffeine in black tea, coffee, cola and chocolate is often blamed for breast lumpiness. If you want to avoid caffeine completely, also avoid soft drinks like Mountain Dew and over-the-counter medications such as Dexatrim, Extra-Strength Excedrin, Midol, Anacin and Sinarest.

"Some women swear this works, and there's some research to indicate it may help," says David Rose, M.D., Ph.D., D.Sc., chief of the Division of Nutrition and Endocrinology and associate director of the Naylor Dana Institute for Disease Prevention at the American Health Foundation in Valhalla, New York. Dr. Rose suggests that you try to avoid caffeine for two or three months as a trial run: "If it works for you, then stay away from these things. If there is no improvement, obviously it is not going to help you—so you may as well go back to your coffee."

Take it easy on salt. A high-salt diet makes it harder for your body to counteract the hormone-induced fluid retention that occurs during the two weeks leading up to your period. "Try to keep your sodium intake to under 1,500 milligrams a day," advises gynecologist Robert L. Shirley, M.D., clinical

When to See the Doctor

There's always concern that lumps may signal, or hide, a more serious condition such as breast cancer. Although that's seldom the case, a woman who sees a doctor for lumpy breasts should make sure her breasts are checked for dominant, solitary or asymmetric masses.

While premenstrual breast lumpiness usually appears symmetrically and in both breasts, you should see your doctor if you detect any change from this pattern. Doctors recommend that all women have a yearly breast exam and perform self-exams monthly. Yearly or biyearly mammograms are recommended for all women once they reach age 40.

professor of medicine at Harvard Medical School in Boston. Also, read the labels of processed foods and avoid the ones that have more than 300 milligrams of sodium per serving. If you miss the flavor of salt, use spices to make up for lost taste.

Don't bring home the bacon. Some women placed on a relatively lean diet, with no more than 20 percent of calories from fat, have reported that it seems to help relieve the pain in lumpy breasts. You can significantly reduce fat in your diet by avoiding fatty meats, oils and dairy products. Substitute fruits, vegetables and whole grains whenever possible. And if you eat wheat bran, there's an added plus: This type of fiber reduces estrogen, the hormone that stimulates breast tissue.

Get support. No, not the touchy-feely kind—the Maidenform kind. Find a good, sturdy sports bra, suggests California nurse Kerry McGinn, R.N., author of *The Informed Woman's Guide to Breast Health.* When you try on a bra for fit, do some running in place in the changing room—and get the bra that minimizes bounce. "You want a bra that holds you firmly and comfortably, without biting and binding," McGinn says.

Try heat, ice or both. A warm bath or shower or a heating pad relieves pain for some women, McGinn says. Others find respite with anything cool—an ice pack wrapped in a towel, or fingertips chilled in cold water. And some women find alternating between a heating pad and an ice pack works best for them, McGinn says.

Do a soap massage. "Soap your breasts well in the bath or shower, and then move your fingers gently in small circles all over each breast," McGinn suggests. (The circles should be about the size of a coin.)

Then, holding your hands vertically on each side of one breast, gently press in and up to raise the breast. This helps move fluid out of the breast and into the lymph ducts under the arms and around the collarbone, where it can be transported out of the body.

Take a multivitamin/mineral supplement. Among the vitamins and minerals that may have some benefits are vitamin A, the B-complex vitamins, vitamin E, iodine and selenium, according to Susan Lark, M.D., medical director of the PMS and Menopause Self-Help Center in Los Altos, California. Adds Dr. Rose: "It's a shotgun approach that has not been studied in clinical trials, but it can't do any harm at safe dosages, and it might help."

Exercise every day. An hour of aerobic exercise daily can make a difference. Studies have shown that exercise helps reduce premenstrual water retention and thus ease the pain of swollen breasts. If running or even walking causes pain (even when you're wearing a well-fitting sports bra), try biking or swimming.

Shed excess pounds. The more body fat a woman carries around, the higher her blood levels of estrogen. And since estrogen is the hormone that stimulates breast tissue, "losing some weight does seem like a reasonable thing to do," says Dr. Rose.

Breast Tenderness

Diet, nutrition, water, weight, time of life, time of the month and hormones—some combination of these factors is likely to lead to breast tenderness some time in a woman's life. In fact, nearly three in four women suffer from breast pain and discomfort at least once in their adult lives. And some have this problem quite frequently.

Want relief?

Make your burgers rare. "The more animal proteins you eat, the slower your body will excrete estrogen," says Susan Doughty, R.N., a nurse practitioner at Women to Women, a clinic in Yarmouth, Maine. This excess estrogen often winds up in breast tissue, which is particularly sensitive to hormones.

Dehydrogenate your menu. Besides reducing meat and poultry, eliminate or drastically cut back on your intake of margarine and other hydrogenated fats, advises Christiane Northrup, M.D., assistant clinical professor of obstetrics and gynecology at the University of Vermont College of Medicine in Burlington. Hydrogenated fats interfere with your body's ability to convert essential fatty acids from the diet into gamma linoleic acid (GLA). Since your body needs GLA to help prevent breast pain, you may be asking for discomfort if you overdo hydrogenated fats and suppress the production of GLA.

Eliminate caffeine. The role of caffeine in contributing to breast discomfort has not been proven, but many doctors recommend no caffeine anyway. "I've seen women with pain and other symptoms of benign breast changes get markedly better after abstaining from caffeine," says Thomas J. Smith, M.D., director of the Breast Health Center at New England Medical Center in Boston. But you have to cut it *out*, not just *down*. Besides coffee and tea, other caffeinated items include soft drinks, chocolate, ice cream products and many over-the-counter pain relievers.

When to See the Doctor

Breast tenderness is generally not threatening, but if you have persistent tenderness accompanied by redness and you feel a mass, you should see your doctor, says Christiane Northrup, M.D., assistant clinical professor of obstetrics and gynecology at the University of Vermont College of Medicine in Burlington.

Ellen Yankauskas, M.D., director of the Women's Center for Family Health in Atascadero, California, adds that there are three symptoms—the three Hs—that should send you to your doctor if they all occur at the same time: The breast is hot, it's hard, and it's hurting. She also advises that bloody discharge from the nipple is cause to see your physician right away.

Get your vitamins. A good multivitamin/mineral supplement and a diet with plenty of foods rich in calcium, magnesium, vitamin C and B-complex vitamins are effective weapons against breast tenderness. Most of these vitamins indirectly affect the production of a hormone that can cause breast pain, says Dr. Northrup. Another helpful nutrient is vitamin E. "Many women find relief when they take a vitamin E supplement of 200 to 400 international units a day, particularly when they're experiencing pain," according to Ellen Yankauskas, M.D., director of the Women's Center for Family Health in Atascadero, California.

Slim down if you need to. If you're overweight, simply dropping some of that excess weight may be enough to cure breast tenderness, says California nurse Kerry McGinn, R.N., author of *The Informed Woman's Guide to Breast Health.* In women, extra body fat makes the body produce more estrogen than it needs.

Try these herbal teas. "Corn silk, buchu and uva ursi teas—available at most health food stores—are three very mild diuretics that seem to relieve breast tenderness in some women," says Dr. Yankauskas. By flushing fluid from your system, diuretics can help reduce breast swelling.

Or go the over-the-counter route. If you prefer to go with an over-the-counter pain reliever, look for one containing the active ingredient pamabron, Dr. Yankauskas advises. Pamabron acts as a mild diuretic.

Brittle Nails

Trying to put a finger on the cause of frail nails? You could blame dry, overheated houses: When we stoke up the dry heat in winter, dry nails are one of the results. Or you could blame Father Time: After age 35, the natural aging process makes nails more brittle.

Mostly, though, you *should* blame water. "People don't realize that when your hands are soaking, your nails can absorb between 20 and 25 percent of their weight in water," says Herbert Luscombe, M.D., professor emeritus of dermatology at Jefferson Medical College of Thomas Jefferson University and senior attending dermatologist at Thomas Jefferson University Hospital, both in Philadelphia. "So if you do a lot of dishes, or swimming, or even bathing, you're more prone to brittle nails."

Nails expand as they absorb water, then contract when hands are dry. The more water you expose nails to, the more they expand and contract—and that weakens them. But here's how to keep them firm, so they're tough enough to withstand the rigors of clean living and water sports.

Chow down on cauliflower. A little-known nutrient called biotin can thicken nails to help prevent splitting and cracking. "Biotin is absorbed into the core of the nail, where it may encourage a better, thicker nail to grow," says Richard K. Scher, M.D., professor of dermatology and head of the Nail Section at Columbia University–Presbyterian Medical Center in New York City. Cauliflower is a rich source of biotin, as are legumes such as peanuts and lentils. One study showed that people consuming 2,500 micrograms (2.5 milligrams) of biotin daily had marked increases in nail thickness after six months. To get this much biotin, you'll need to take it in supplement form.

Get cookin' with cooking oil. "A regular soaking with vegetable oil is very effective. It replenishes the moisture lost from having your hands in and out of water frequently," says Dr. Luscombe. In fact, vegetable oils are *better* than many

Thumbnails Down on Strengtheners

Nail strengtheners may be touted as the way to turn weak and brittle nails into unbreakables. In reality, most claims for these products are excessive, according to Richard K. Scher, M.D., professor of dermatology and head of the Nail Section at Columbia University–Presbyterian Medical Center in New York City.

Nail strengtheners supposedly contain an ingredient that binds to damaged nails and makes them thicker. But you can't change the nail structure simply by applying something to the surface, says Paul Kechijian, M.D., clinical associate professor of dermatology and chief of the Nail Section at New York University Medical Center in New York City. "At best, nail strengtheners protect the nail plate, so they won't peel," he says. "They merely camouflage the brittleness."

commercially sold nail care products because they don't have the alcohol-containing fragrances that can dry out nails.

Messy soaking in oil isn't necessary: Just brush on the oil and massage it into the nail. "I put some safflower or vegetable oil in a clean, empty nail polish bottle and brush it on my nails several times a day," says hand model Trisha Webster, who works for the Wilhelmina Modeling Agency in New York City. "And don't forget to put a drop of oil on the underside of the nail at your fingertip."

Use an over-the-counter moisturizer. You should moisturize nails right after you wash your hands. "And do it every time," says Paul Kechijian, M.D., clinical associate professor of dermatology and chief of the Nail Section at New York University Medical Center in New York City. If you use a commercial moisturizer, look for the kind that contains urea or lactic acid, two ingredients that attract and bind moisture to your nails.

Trim nails short. If you're plagued by brittle nails, trim them shorter, advises Dr. Kechijian. Longer nails are just more likely to crack or tear. Trim your nails right after washing or bathing, when they're softer and less likely to crack or break.

Massage your fingertips. "Regularly massage your fingertips to improve blood circulation around your nails," says Webster. She suggests three or four times a day—or at least in the morning and evening. If you use some petroleum jelly while you're at it, you'll moisturize as you massage.

Don't play taps. Forget that old folk remedy that calls for tapping your nails on a hard surface in order to toughen them. "If you traumatize them in some way, they *will* grow faster," says Dr. Scher. "And because they are newer, younger nails, they may seem like they are stronger, but they're really not." For the same reason, avoid nail biting: Your nervous nibbling is just another trauma for your nails.

Glove 'em if you love 'em. Washing dishes? "*Always* wear rubber gloves with separate cotton gloves inside," says Dr. Kechijian. "The rubber keeps water off your nails, and the cotton absorbs sweat, so nails won't get soggy *inside* the gloves."

He suggests keeping a half-dozen pairs of cotton gloves on hand and washing and drying them after each use. That way, you'll always have a clean, dry pair each time you do the dishes.

Broken Bones

Ever since Sir Isaac Newton figured out why apples fall *down* and not *up,* we've known the hard truths about gravity—and one of the hardest is that when you hit the ground, you can break a bone. With 206 bones in the human body, there's a lot of potential for breakage.

If you're on the mend from a fracture, there are some ways you can speed healing and make yourself more comfortable.

Butt out. Smoking can delay the healing of bones—up to five months longer for serious fractures and less for minor breaks, says orthopedic surgeon George Cierny III, M.D., of Atlanta. He has shown experimentally that nicotine and other substances in cigarette smoke reduce the amount of oxygen reaching bone tissue, causing the delay in healing. So if you're a smoker, expect a longer-than-average healing time.

Watch what you drink. It's still unknown what effect alcohol and caffeine have on *healing,* but researchers know that people who consume beverages containing these two substances are more likely to endure fractures. That's because caffeine and alcohol affect bone mass and interfere with calcium absorption, which builds stronger bones.

When to See the Doctor

The most important thing you should know about broken bones is that they require *immediate* medical attention. If you even *suspect* a fracture, have a doctor check it out. Otherwise, you may further damage the broken bone. There's also risk of infection and delayed healing.

Use Gravity to Stop Itchy Casts

Bothered by that annoying itch from inside a cast? Don't try to scratch it with a ruler, clothes hanger or other device—you'll just get more itching from the tiny cuts caused by your scratching.

"Instead, simply elevate the fractured area so that it's above the level of your heart," suggests Philip Sanfilippo, D.P.M., a San Francisco podiatrist who specializes in sports injuries and treatment. "By doing that, you'll diminish blood flow to the area and reduce swelling. Often that's enough to relieve the itching."

"In our study, there was an increased risk of getting fractures in those who drank more than four cups of coffee daily or about two glasses of alcohol—wine, beer or a highball," says Graham A. Colditz, M.D., a researcher at Harvard Medical School in Boston.

RICE is nice. On the first-aid front, most experts suggest some big chill—even after your doctor has treated you. The acronym RICE—rest, ice, compression and elevation—describes the best way to hasten healing and prevent further damage. If you have a minor fracture that's protected by an air cast or soft cast, your doctor might let you remove the cast now and then to apply ice directly.

"Put a bag of frozen vegetables on the fracture for about 20 minutes, then remove it for 10," suggests Steven Subotnick, D.P.M., a sports podiatrist in Hayward, California, and author of *Sports and Exercise Injuries.* "But make sure you put a washcloth between your skin and the ice bag to prevent an ice burn." Since you want to avoid pressure on the area, the cold compress should be applied lightly.

Even if you can't take off a soft cast, you can apply ice to the outside of the cast, and it will help chill the area underneath.

Bronchitis

It may produce some of the nastiest-looking phlegm you've ever seen, but bronchitis's bark is usually worse than its bite. Granted, it's quite a bark, as mucous membranes lining the air passages in your chest become irritated. To soothe the irritation, your body makes secretions to coat the airways. This produces a buildup of gunk in your lungs, which must be cleared by your coughing and sputtering more than a '67 Rambler in dire need of a tune-up.

Like the common cold, bronchitis affects most everyone sometime in his life. Acute cases are usually caused by a virus and will clear up on their own in a week or two. Chronic cases, however, are almost always caused by smoking—either your own habit or long-term exposure to secondhand smoke—and these cases may last for months. Bronchitis may also cause soreness, tightness or wheezing in the chest, chills, fatigue or a slight fever. But here's how to quiet all your symptoms.

Liquefy the problem. "Drinking fluids may help the mucus become more watery and easier to cough up," says Barbara Phillips, M.D., associate professor of pulmonary medicine at the University of Kentucky Medical Center in Lexington. Four to six glasses is probably plenty.

And while warm liquids like Mom's chicken soup may make you feel better, a cool glass of water, juice or any other nonalcoholic beverage works just as well. "All beverages are the same temperature inside your body," says Douglas Holsclaw, M.D., professor of pediatrics and director of the Pediatric Pulmonary and Cystic Fibrosis Center at Hahnemann University Hospital in Philadelphia. To avoid losing fluids from your body, doctors advise staying away from booze, because it can actually cause dehydration. Also avoid caffeinated products such as coffee, tea and cola, because they make you urinate more and you may actually lose more fluids than you gain.

When to See the Doctor

Bronchitis is usually not a serious problem, but you should see your doctor if:
- Your cough doesn't improve or it worsens after one week. (Sometimes the only way to distinguish bronchitis from pneumonia is with an x-ray.)
- You are coughing up blood.
- You are elderly and get a hacking cough on top of another illness.
- You are short of breath and have a very profuse cough.
- You have a very high fever (over 101°F) *or* one that lasts more than three days.

Reach for the red pepper. Hot peppers, curry and other spicy foods that make your eyes water or nose run can help bring an early end to bronchitis. "Hot, spicy foods help mucous membranes all over, not just in your nose, to secrete more liquids, which can help thin mucus," says Varro E. Tyler, Ph.D., professor of pharmacognosy at Purdue University in West Lafayette, Indiana. The advantage of thinner mucus is that it's easier to cough up.

Get away from cigarettes. Even being *near* someone who smokes can make bronchitis worse or cause return episodes. "You need to avoid all tobacco smoke," says Dr. Phillips. "Even if you don't smoke but you're exposed to exhaled smoke, you are doing what's called passive smoking, and that can give you bronchitis."

If you do smoke, quitting is the *most* important thing you can do, since this habit has been linked to as many as 95 percent of all cases of chronic bronchitis. "Your bronchitis will improve when you stop smoking," says Gordon Snider, M.D., chief of medical service at Boston Veterans Administration Medical Center. Some new ex-smokers experience increased coughing and sputum production for a week or two after quitting, adds Dr. Phillips. This is actually a good sign—the airways are sweeping out a lot of accumulated secretions. Symptoms usually subside after two to four weeks.

Plug in the vaporizer. "If you have mucus that is thick or difficult to cough up, a vaporizer will help loosen the secretions," adds Dr. Phillips. If you don't have a vaporizer, either run a hot shower with the bathroom door closed or fill the sink with hot water, put a towel over your head and the sink to create a tent, and inhale the steam for five to ten minutes every couple of hours, suggests Dr. Snider.

Don't rely on expectorants. Over-the-counter cough medicines may suppress your cough—the opposite of what you want. Besides, there's no evidence that they help dry up mucus. You'll get better—and cheaper—results by drinking lots of liquids.

Bruises

It seems only fitting that we're welcomed to this world with a rousing smack on the butt. After all, what better way to prepare us for the next 75 years or so of stumbling, tumbling and fumbling our way through life—running smack into table ends, bedposts and doorknobs?

But as often as we encounter "objects in the way," our battered bodies never quite get used to it. So we all have to deal with the discoloration and pain of bruises.

What can we do about it? Naturally, it's helpful to stop bumping into things. But when we just can't help it:

Reach for the frozen goods. Icing an injury is the best way to stop a bruise in its tracks—as long as the ice is applied within 24 hours of an injury, and the sooner, the better, says Hugh Macaulay, M.D., emergency room physician at Aspen Valley Hospital in Aspen, Colorado. The cold constricts blood vessels, so less blood spills into the tissues around the injury. That reduces inflammation and pain and makes it less likely that you will develop a blackish blotch.

Apply an ice pack wrapped in a towel for about 15 minutes, then allow the skin to "warm" naturally for about 10 minutes before you put on the ice pack again. You can repeat the ice-pack application four or five times the first day. (If you don't have a conventional ice bag, ice cubes in a washcloth or a bag of frozen vegetables will do fine.)

Wrap and elevate. "Use an elastic bandage, and elevate the bruised limb to help drain blood from that area," says Las Vegas orthopedic surgeon Michael Rask, M.D., chairman of the American Academy of Neurological and Orthopedic Surgeons and the American Board of Ringside Medicine and Surgery. Since blood is affected by gravity, propping up your foot or arm will help your bruise heal faster.

Heat what's hurt. The day *after* applying ice packs, switch to heat to dilate blood vessels and improve circulation, says Sheldon V. Pollack, M.D., a dermatologist and associate professor on the Faculty of Medicine at the University of Toronto. A heating pad or a warm, wet washcloth will help.

Eat more broccoli. "If you're prone to bruising, it's a good idea to eat more foods rich in vitamin C," says Dr. Rask. Foods high in vitamin C may help prevent bruises and heal them faster. Studies show that vitamin C helps build collagen tissues (that is, skin tissue) around blood vessels in the skin. Besides broccoli, foods high in vitamin C include sweet potatoes, cauliflower and citrus fruits. "You can also take vitamin C in supplement form, but don't exceed 2,000 milligrams a day," says Dr. Rask, and only for the duration of the injury. High doses of vitamin C are not recommended for long-term use without medical supervision.

Comfort with comfrey. Some people say that bruises heal faster if you place heated pieces of crushed comfrey directly on the bruise. Make a poultice by placing the comfrey leaves in hot water, then spreading them on a warm, moist washcloth. Press the poultice to the bruise. But don't ingest this easy-to-grow herb (also available at many health food stores), because it can be dangerous when taken internally. Don't place it on open wounds, either, says Varro E. Tyler, Ph.D., professor of pharmacognosy at Purdue University in West Lafayette, Indiana.

Bunions

A bunion is an overgrowth of bone that causes your big toe to thrust out beyond the normal profile of your foot. And while a lot of people blame the shoes they wear, bunions are actually a hereditary problem: People in the same family are likely to have similar bone structure. Along with the overgrowth comes pain, as that bunion encounters the everyday assault and battery of shoe leather.

Bunions are ten times more common in women than in men. And because of the kinds of shoes that women wear, the pain is worse. The first sign is growth at the base of the big toe—the result of years of wearing too-tight shoes that cause pressure. Eventually, in some people, the enlargement of that growth forces your big toe to deviate toward the second toe. Since high heels make the front of your foot slide forward, every time you slide a pair on, you're putting your bunion-prone or bunion-afflicted big toe under pressure. Eventually the pressure may become so painful that just walking can be difficult.

The only way to remove bone overgrowth like bunions is with surgery. But if you don't like the thought of the scalpel, here are some homegrown healers to help keep you one step ahead of the pain.

Wear running shoes. "I recommend that my patients with bunions wear running shoes as often as possible," says Pennsylvania podiatrist Robert Diamond, D.P.M., who is affiliated with Muhlenberg Hospital Center in Bethlehem and Allentown Osteopathic Hospital. "Running shoes have a roomier toe box, which is essential for people with bunions. And since they're made from softer materials than regular shoes, there's not as much pressure." (Walking shoes work just as well, adds Terry Spilken, D.P.M., a podiatrist and adjunct faculty member at the New York College of Podiatric Medicine in New York City, and you might prefer them for appearance' sake.)

Heat it up. "Applying a heating pad to bunions on a regular basis helps increase blood flow, which breaks up the inflammation," says Dr. Spilken.

Are You Bunion-Prone?

Those with flat feet or low arches are most likely to develop bunions, says Terry Spilken, D.P.M., a podiatrist and adjunct faculty member at the New York College of Podiatric Medicine in New York City. "That's because flat-footed people are the most likely to pronate, which is an inward rolling of the foot. And that inward rolling puts more pressure on the area where bunions tend to develop."

The answer: If you're severely flat-footed or a pronator, wearing specially made orthotic devices can help keep you from pronating and thus developing bunions. The devices must be prescribed by a podiatrist and cost between $200 and $400.

Try hands-on healing. Regular massage in a perpendicular motion also helps ease bunion pain, says Dr. Spilken. He recommends that you massage *across* the bunion (and across the foot): "That offers more relief than massaging *along* the foot."

Ease the pressure with sling pads and spacers. There are various over-the-counter products that take the pressure off the bunion and ease the pain. A sling-type pad "pulls" the big toe away from the second toe. "It takes the pressure off the bump. And there are spacers that you place between the big and second toes," says Dr. Diamond. "They won't straighten the big toe, per se, but they do help relieve some of the pressure." Though moleskin pads are often used by bunion sufferers, Dr. Diamond says that they're less effective than the sling-type pads and spacers.

Go barefoot or wear sandals. The real culprits are shoes that rub your toes. So if you want to prevent pain from bunions, go without shoes as much as possible to ease pain and prevent a worsened condition. Whenever you're home (or in any situation where footwear is optional), go shoeless. If you can't, wear sandals or other open-toed shoes as much as possible.

Make sure your shoes fit correctly. When you must wear shoes, make sure they fit as well as possible. When you have the proper fit, the end of your longest toe should be a finger-width short of the end of your shoe, according to Dr. Spilken. "Width-wise, the shoe should be just wide enough to allow you

When Is Surgery Necessary?

Bunion surgery can be a simple outpatient procedure that can eliminate a bothersome bunion for good. Recovery usually takes about four weeks, but you'll probably need only a few days of complete rest and elevation.

"There are no hard-and-fast rules for determining who needs surgery, but if the bunion is painful or deforming your toes, then surgery is generally recommended," according to Pennsylvania podiatrist Robert Diamond, D.P.M., who is affiliated with Muhlenberg Hospital Center in Bethlehem and Allentown Osteopathic Hospital.

Most experts agree that if your bunions interfere with your lifestyle, causing you pain and keeping you from doing what you'd like, you *should* have surgery.

to fit a finger between the inside of the shoe and the side of your foot. In front, the shoe should not rub against your big toe or littlest toe," he says.

If you already own shoes that don't pass this measurement test, you can stretch them. Shoe repair stores provide this service for a reasonable price.

Soak your feet, saltlessly. A good hot soak in Epsom salts is the most popular home remedy for bunions. But perhaps you don't need *any* salt. "Just soaking your feet in hot water is enough to reduce inflammation and ease pain," says Dr. Spilken.

Burns

While close encounters of the third-degree kind require immediate medical attention, most everyday household burns are *not* too hot for you to handle.

There are no burned-in-stone rules about what to do when you've encountered searing ovens, sizzling fireplaces or super-hot steam. But here's the rule of thumb: First- and second-degree burns can usually be self-treated if they're smaller than a quarter on a child or a silver dollar on an adult. You should see a doctor, however, for larger burns or for burns on infants under 1 year of age or on adults over age 60.

No matter the cause, the key to quick relief is *quick* relief. Since your cells continue to toast even after you separate yourself from the heat source, what you do in the first few minutes after being burned can make all the difference in how well your skin heals. Here's how to make the most of that time—and shorten the healing process.

Milk it. "Milk is an excellent compress for minor burns," says Stephen M. Purcell, D.O., chairman of the Department of Dermatology at Philadelphia College of Osteopathic Medicine and assistant clinical professor at Hahnemann University School of Medicine in Philadelphia. "Simply soak the burned area in milk for 15 minutes or so, or apply a milk-soaked washcloth to the area." Whole milk is effective: Its fat content soothes burns and promotes healing. But make sure to rinse your skin and the washcloth in cool water afterward, because the milk will smell.

Keep it clean. A clean burn is a faster-healing burn. After 24 hours, wash the area gently with soap and water or a mild Betadine solution daily, suggests John Gillies, an emergency medical technician and program director for health services at the Colorado Outward Bound School in Denver. Keep the burn dry and clean and covered with a bandage such as a thick gauze pad between washings.

Prep it with Preparation H. No ifs, ands or buts, this hemorrhoid treatment can slice up to 3 days off the usual 7 to 15 days it takes for most burns to heal, says Jerold Z. Kaplan, M.D., medical director of Alta Bates Burn Center in Berkeley, California. Preparation H works because it contains a yeast derivative that helps speed healing. Simply dab a little on the burn and cover with a fresh sterile bandage every day.

Chill out, but not too much. You probably will instinctively reach for cold water to soothe a new burn. But *don't* make it *too* cold. Using ice water can risk making the burn even worse, because extreme cold can kill just as many skin cells as extreme heat. (That's why frostbite damage is very similar to the skin damage caused by a bad burn.) Cool, not cold, water will stop the burning from spreading through your tissues and will act as a temporary painkiller. So instead of running to the freezer, head to the kitchen faucet.

When to See the Doctor

How bad is your burn? Do you need medical assistance? To avoid getting burned because of a lack of knowledge about burns, here's how you can gauge.

First-degree burns are painful and red. They occur from sunburn, scalding and other minor accidents. You can usually treat them at home.

Second-degree burns ooze, blister and are painful. They result from severe sunburn or from brief contact with hot oven coils or other household accidents. These may be treated at home if the burn is confined to a small area of surface skin.

Third-degree burns are extremely dangerous—even if they don't hurt (the result of destroyed nerve endings). They leave skin charred and turn it white or cream-colored. Third-degree burns can be caused by fire, chemicals, electricity or any prolonged contact with hot surfaces. For these, you'll need immediate medical help.

Elevate it. One way to help take the sting out of that singe is to position yourself so that the burned area is above the level of your heart, advises Linda Phillips, M.D., assistant professor in the Plastic Surgery Division at the University of Texas Medical Branch at Galveston. This helps prevent swelling.

Say aloe. Who *doesn't* have an aloe plant in his house just for these types of emergencies? This cactuslike member of the lily family is thought to shorten the healing process up to 40 percent—and the coolness of its "juice" brings welcome relief when you have burn pain. Two or three days after the burn, simply open a leaf and smear its liquid directly on the burn, advises D'Anne Kleinsmith, M.D., a cosmetic dermatologist at William Beaumont Hospital near Detroit. Reapply four to six times daily, with or without a bandage covering.

Chow on vitamin C. Consuming more vitamin C aids in the healing process for burns and other wounds, so eating plenty of citrus fruits, potatoes and broccoli is helpful, says Las Vegas orthopedic surgeon Michael Rask, M.D., chairman of the American Academy of Neurological and Orthopedic Surgeons and the American Board of Ringside Medicine and Surgery.

Get vitamins A and E for healing. Vitamins A and E, which are antioxidants, can also speed healing, according to Dr. Rask. Good sources of vitamin A include green fruits and vegetables. Cereals and nuts are high in vitamin E—and you can also apply vitamin E directly to the burn. In fact, many people experience faster healing by rubbing the liquid from a vitamin E capsule on the burn once it begins to heal. It will feel good and may prevent scarring.

And discover the zinc link. For healthier skin *after* the burn (as well as quicker recovery time), consume plenty of foods rich in zinc, suggests Dr. Rask. Oysters are a great source of zinc. Crabmeat, wheat germ and low-fat dairy products also have a good supply.

Go antibiotic. There are many good over-the-counter antibiotic ointments that help heal burns and prevent infection, adds Dr. Kleinsmith. In choosing one, look for the active ingredients polymyxin B sulfate or bacitracin. Before applying the ointment, though, Dr. Kleinsmith recommends cleaning the wound with hydrogen peroxide if you find soap too abrasive.

Leave the butter for your bread. Forget the old spouses' tale of putting butter on burns. Although milk is soothing, butter and margarine retain heat in tissues and can make the burn worse; plus, that greasy stuff is perfect for breeding infectious bacteria.

Bursitis

It's one of those *-itis* problems with the power to make you cringe and reach for the aspirin. A common condition, bursitis rarely causes serious damage if it is recognized early and treated properly.

Bursitis occurs when the bursae—small sliding pouches that allow parts of the body to move smoothly—become inflamed. It can happen for a number of reasons. You may simply have bumped your elbow or spent too many hours on your knees in the garden. Or the problem may be caused by infection or gout.

The first signs of bursitis are usually pain and swelling. "For example, with bursitis over the elbow, there is often obvious swelling, the flesh is soft, and it feels like there's fluid inside," says Morris B. Mellion, M.D., who is clinical associate professor at the University of Nebraska Medical Center and medical director of the Sports Medicine Center, both in Omaha.

But that joint pain might also be a symptom of arthritis, which is a condition that demands long-term treatment. So the first thing you should do is visit a doctor to find out which *-itis* is causing you problems.

If it's bursitis, here are some ways to give your doctor's advice a healing boost.

Rest is best. Some people might use a splint or a sling to immobilize the area, says Steven F. Habusta, D.O., of Parkwood Orthopedics in Toledo. But for the most part, the affected area just needs time to rest. When the pain is gone and the bursae are no longer inflamed, then slowly resume your regular activities.

Find relief with nonprescription medications. "There are things you can buy without a prescription to relieve bursitis," says James Richards, M.D., an

When to See the Doctor

Though painful, bursitis may subside after you give your body some tender loving care. But if the bursitis is due to infection or gout, you have a problem that requires a doctor's care.

"Septic bursitis, due to infection, can spread or become severe," says Morris B. Mellion, M.D., who is clinical associate professor at the University of Nebraska Medical Center and medical director of the Sports Medicine Center, both in Omaha. "If it does, surgical drainage may be needed. But in its early stages, septic bursitis should respond well to antibiotics." If bursitis is caused by gouty arthritis, it can also be treated with medication.

How can you tell if your bursitis is due to infection or gout? "The bursa is tender, warm and red," says Dr. Mellion. "But sometimes those signs *won't* be present, even though you have an infection there." So rather than trying to diagnose it yourself, you should get a doctor's advice when you have a flare-up of bursitis.

orthopedic surgeon with Matthews Orthopedic Clinic in Orlando, Florida. "Aspirin, or anything with ibuprofen in it (such as Advil), will decrease the swelling and hopefully the pain."

However, says Dr. Habusta, painkillers aren't always painless. He has three cautions. First, don't use aspirin and ibuprofen *together;* they don't work well in combination. Second, some adults are allergic to aspirin. Third, children should avoid aspirin, which in those under age 12 can cause Reye's syndrome, a potential killer.

Try ice. "Ice reduces inflammation and pain by decreasing swelling," says Dr. Habusta. "You can use ice on a regular basis—there is no such thing as too much!

"But if the skin gets too cold, it could 'burn' and blister. To avoid that, place a terry cloth towel between the ice pack and the treatment site."

Warm up the compresses. Warm compresses might make bursitis feel better, says Dr. Richards. Place a damp, hot (but not too hot to handle—you don't want to burn the skin) towel on the area and leave it on as long as it feels comfortable.

Go for a cold/warm combo. The other option is to alternate ice and heat applications. Dr. Richards recommends cooling the area with ice for 15 minutes, then applying a warm compress for 15 minutes.

Wrap it up. "An elastic bandage around a knee or another affected area might not make bursitis go away, but it may make it feel better," adds Dr. Richards.

Eliminate the cause. "You might have to cut out the activity that is causing the bursitis for a while," says Dr. Richards. "If you've been bowling, or painting, or doing anything else that uses the same joints over and over and you have pain in those areas, it's best to stop the activity until you're feeling better."

Limber up. "A great number of Americans think that building muscles is the best way to protect against problems such as bursitis," says Dr. Richards. "But that is not necessarily true. Staying limber through stretching is a better way to help you stay comfortable through your entire life."

Relax in a spa. "Anything that reduces the inflammation of the bursae will help bursitis," says Dr. Richards. "Soaking in a Jacuzzi or whirlpool will do this." So if you have access to either of these, give it a try.

Caffeine Dependency

There's more brewing in that Mr. Coffee machine than Colombian supreme beans. Seems you can't read the morning paper in peace while enjoying the old morning cup of joe without running across some controversy about caffeine.

But despite headlines alleging that caffeine raises cholesterol, impairs fertility or causes some other dire problem, caffeine continues to be the world's most widely used beverage—and drug. With good reason: Caffeine almost instantly makes you feel alert and helps you think more clearly by triggering a release of adrenaline.

As with any other drug, failing to get that regular dose can lead to discomfort. Caffeine withdrawal is very common, but most people don't recognize it when it's happening to them. "Most people who are heavy caffeine drinkers will experience some withdrawal symptoms if they try to go cold turkey," says Roland Griffiths, M.D., professor of biological and behavioral psychiatry and professor of neuroscience at Johns Hopkins University School of Medicine in Baltimore and a caffeine researcher. "The most common are headache and lethargy or fatigue, but some people report nausea and vomiting, depression and even flulike symptoms." Symptoms usually last a week, peaking on the first or second day you go without caffeine. If you want to quit the caffeine habit, here's how to make the going easier.

Don't go cold turkey. Even "light" coffee drinkers can have withdrawal symptoms. "It's best if you *gradually* give up caffeine over the course of several weeks, rather than giving it up abruptly," says John Hughes, M.D., director of the Human Behavior Pharmacology Laboratory at the University of Vermont in Burlington. "I recommend a 10 to 30 percent reduction every few days. So if you drink 3 cups of coffee a day, drink 2 or 2½ for three or four days, then decrease by another ½ cup a few days later and so forth. Give yourself plenty of time."

Drink more decaf. "Simply switching to decaf, as some people do, isn't the answer, because even though you're still drinking coffee, it's *caffeine* withdrawal that causes the problems," advises Dr. Griffiths. "But it is a good idea to begin substituting more decaf for some of that caffeinated coffee you usually drink.

"For instance, if you drink six cups of coffee a day, it's a good idea to make every other cup decaffeinated. Then the following week, have two cups of caffeinated and four cups of decaf. Then one cup of caffeinated and five cups of decaf, until you eventually wean yourself off caffeine."

Give up the drug, not the ritual. Just because you're giving up coffee doesn't mean you have to give up the coffee break. "You will probably be more aware of your withdrawal symptoms if you completely forgo your regular coffee break when you're trying to give up coffee," says Manfred Kroger, Ph.D., professor of food science at Pennsylvania State University in University Park. "Our bodies and psyches seem to value these rituals in which we consume caffeine—whether it's reading the morning newspaper at home or taking a break at work. So I advise that you continue these routines, but substitute decaffeinated coffee or juice for the caffeinated coffee, tea or cola you're trying to quit."

Be wary of pain relievers. *Don't* blindly reach for a headache remedy when caffeine withdrawal gives you a headache. "Products such as Excedrin and Anacin are *loaded* with caffeine—containing from 100 to 150 milligrams per dose," says Dr. Hughes. (By comparison, a cup of coffee averages about 85 milligrams.) There are several pain-relief products available in drugstores that are caffeine-free, however. Read labels carefully.

Shun the sources of "hidden caffeine." Besides pain relievers, other sources of caffeine include some soft drinks like Mountain Dew and colas, which contain anywhere from 33 to 67 milligrams per can; chocolate, which has about 15 milligrams per ounce; nonherbal teas, with nearly 50 milligrams per cup; and weight-control and "no doze" products that contain upward of 200 milligrams per tablet. Even cold remedies and decongestants have a small amount of caffeine, says Dr. Hughes.

Canker Sores

Along with Zsa Zsa's *real* age and the location(s) of Jimmy Hoffa's grave, the mystery of the canker sore continues to baffle the experts. For some reason, those little white ulcers with red borders visit the mouths of some people quite frequently—while others get them rarely. And while some may have canker sores for just a few days, other people have them for weeks.

No one's really sure what causes these pesky and painful ulcers on the tongue or gums or inside the cheeks (although a predisposition for them seems to be hereditary). Luckily, doctors do have some answers on how you can cut short the usual 10- to 15-day life span of these annoying, although nonthreatening, lesions—or avoid them altogether.

Make yogurt a daily ritual. "Eat at least four tablespoons of unflavored yogurt every day and you'll prevent canker sores," says Jerome Z. Litt, M.D., assistant clinical professor of dermatology at Case Western Reserve University School of Medicine in Cleveland. He adds that it's unclear why the yogurt works, but for some people it can be very effective.

See the difference with vitamin C. "Vitamin C is very effective at preventing or healing canker sores, particularly for people who are under a lot of stress, consume a lot of alcohol or smoke," says David Garber, D.M.D., clinical professor of periodontics and prosthodontics at the Medical College of Georgia in Augusta. And that's worth noting, since these are the very people most at risk for canker sores. Five hundred milligrams a day is sometimes recommended for a vitamin C supplement—but check with your doctor first. To introduce more vitamin C to your daily diet, go for broccoli, cantaloupe, red bell peppers and cranberry juice. (Once you have a sore, however, the acidic juice may be more pain than gain.)

Squeeze on some vitamin E. Vitamin C isn't the only nutrient that can help heal canker sores. Craig Zunka, D.D.S., a dentist in Fort Royal, Virginia, and chairman of the board of the Holistic Dental Association, says squeezing the oil from a vitamin E capsule onto your canker sore can bring relief.

Put some sore relief in your diet. Several studies show that one in seven people with canker sores is deficient in folate, iron and vitamin B, and doctors believe that upping these nutrients can help prevent sores or quicken recovery from them. Peas, beans and lentils are excellent folate sources; lean beef, tofu and fortified cereals are high in iron; and meats and seafood are high in B vitamins.

Gargle with peroxide. "A solution of three parts water and one part hydrogen peroxide changes the pH of your saliva and makes for a harsh environment for the bacteria causing canker sores," says Palm Harbor, Florida, dentist Paul Caputo, D.D.S. "Mixing this solution and gargling or swishing it around your mouth several times a day is very helpful when you have a canker sore. But don't swallow it."

Baste it with Orabase-B. This over-the-counter remedy gets thumbs-up from all our experts as the best relief money can buy at your neighborhood drugstore. "It's a sticky substance you put directly on the sore to stop the pain and promote healing," says Dr. Caputo.

Another over-the-counter product that comes highly recomended is Zilactin, a medicated gel. And for those preferring a liquid form, there's Zilactol, says Dr. Garber.

Avoid sharp or spicy foods. And we mean that in both a culinary *and* a literal sense. "Many people know that you should avoid foods that are spicy or salty when you have a canker sore, because those foods increase the pain," says D'Anne Kleinsmith, M.D., a cosmetic dermatologist at William Beaumont Hospital near Detroit. "But you should also avoid foods with sharp *edges,* such as potato chips. Anything with rough edges can puncture the skin and cause canker sores."

Besides spices and salt, it's best to avoid or limit citrus fruits and strawberries, cheeses, coffee, nuts and chocolate if you're prone to canker sores.

Bag your pain with a tea bag. Rubbing a wet tea bag directly on the sore is another helpful home treatment, says Dr. Litt. Black tea contains tannin, an astringent with powerful pain-relieving qualities. "If you're into herbal teas, drink chamomile tea, which cools canker sore pain and other mild skin irritations," says Varro E. Tyler, Ph.D., professor of pharmacognosy at Purdue University in West Lafayette, Indiana.

Ice it. Old cures are often the best, and there are few older (or better) than simply applying ice to the sore to help reduce pain and swelling.

Mylanta may be your healer. Swish a tablespoon of the antacid Mylanta or milk of magnesia around your mouth to coat the sore, advises Robert Goepp, D.D.S., Ph.D., professor of oral pathology at the University of Chicago Medical Center. But only use this technique if you are sure your ulcer is not infected. If you coat an infected ulcer, the coating will protect the bacteria causing the infection. An infected ulcer is usually marked by a red ring around its base and a grayish yellow color, Dr. Goepp says.

Carpal Tunnel Syndrome

Yes, the computer has certainly expanded our horizons and given us the ability to perform lightninglike calculations. But along with every computer comes a keyboard—and human fingers that hit the keys with the speed of raindrops in a thunderstorm.

Unfortunately, the human wrist wasn't made for this kind of frantic activity. Hands that carry out repetitive tasks at the computer keyboard (or anywhere else, for that matter) may begin sending up protests of pain. This wrist pain is the screaming ouch of a disorder called carpal tunnel syndrome.

Carpal tunnel syndrome is like a traffic jam in the wrist, resulting from too much crowding in too little space. Nestled among the bones and tendons of the wrist area is a major median nerve that leads from the arm into the fingers. This is the nerve that "signals" some of the small muscles in the hand and also provides sensation to the thumb and first three fingers.

Crowded in next to that nerve, inside the "carpal tunnel," are several tendons. When the tendons are overworked, they become inflamed and swell, and the median nerve is literally crushed within the carpal tunnel.

As the tendons swell and the tunnel size shrinks, the median nerve gets crushed like a piece of soft spaghetti. No wonder it hurts!

Although often caused by the repetitive movements of keyboard operation or typing, hammering or other hand-intensive job chores, carpal tunnel syndrome can result from just about anything in which your hands are used frequently and for long periods. A good start toward stopping the pain is to eliminate the cause (if you know it). And here are some other approaches.

Stretch your hands. To keep pain at bay, start off each activity with a series of hand-stretching exercises. "Anything that extends the range of motion in your fingers and wrist will help," says Janna Jacobs, president of the American Physical Therapy Association's Section on Hand Rehabilitation. "Open and close your fingers, bend your wrists in both directions—do various things to exercise your hands for about 10 or 15 minutes before beginning the activity."

Watch out for bad vibes. Although electric tools do quick work, they're also a bad influence on your wrist. "True, there may be less force placed on your wrist, but the vibrations of an electric knife or other power tools could require a tighter grip to steady them and lead to another disorder called

When to See the Doctor

You need a doctor's examination to confirm that you have carpal tunnel syndrome. But how can you tell whether you should see the doctor?

"It may be normal to have your hand fall asleep sometimes or ache when you use it excessively," says Peter C. Amadio, M.D., associate professor of orthopedics at Mayo Medical School in Rochester, Minnesota. "And if the pain and numbness go away after you rest it, you're probably fine. But if you notice a constant problem or severe pain, numbness or tingling at night, and if it's not improving, then you might want to see your doctor."

Symptoms of carpal tunnel syndrome include:
- Numbness, tingling or a "pins and needles" feeling in the thumb, index and middle fingers, particularly after you use your hands.
- Trouble using your fingers or thumb, as demonstrated by dropping things or losing dexterity.

hand-arm vibration syndrome," says occupational medicine specialist Thomas Hales, M.D., of the National Institute for Occupational Safety and Health in Denver. When buying tools like a power painter or chain saw, look for those with special "vibration control" mechanisms.

Fatten tool handles. Placing foam rubber over the handles of brooms, rakes and other tools—or simply wrapping handles in foam tape to fatten them— makes them easier to hold, decreasing or eliminating pain. "If handles are too small, they can press directly on the tendons and median nerve in the palm," says David Rempel, M.D., an ergonomist and expert in occupational medicine at the University of California, San Francisco. But don't make handles too big, either—that also hurts wrists.

Sharpen your knives. Simple household chores such as cutting meat or clipping hedges can cause big-time pain for those with carpal tunnel syndrome. "Keeping your tools sharp or well lubricated reduces the amount of pressure needed to use them," says Peter C. Amadio, M.D., associate professor of orthopedics at the Mayo Medical School in Rochester, Minnesota.

Write with a light touch. "Using pencils with soft lead or pens with easy-flow ink also helps a lot," says Dr. Amadio. "And the fatter and rounder the pen or pencil, the easier it is to use."

"B" aware of vitamin deficiencies. Why do some people who use their hands and fingers a great deal develop carpal tunnel syndrome while others don't? Some studies suggest that it may be partly the result of a borderline B-vitamin deficiency, specifically vitamin B_6. Although excessive doses of vitamin B_6 supplements may cause nerve damage, a low dose is safe. "Studies suggest that 100 milligrams a day of vitamin B_6 can significantly reduce the debilitating and crippling symptoms of carpal tunnel syndrome," says Hans Fisher, Ph.D., professor of nutrition at Rutgers University in New Brunswick, New Jersey.

Wear a wrist splint to bed. All of our experts recommend wearing a wrist splint whenever possible and especially at night. Splints are available at most drugstores without a prescription. "Carpal tunnel pain is usually worse at night, when body fluids collect in wrists and other body parts," according to Steven Barrer, Jr., M.D., a clinical assistant professor of neurosurgery at the Medical College of Pennsylvania in Philadelphia who has written numerous articles on carpal tunnel syndrome. "In fact, loss of sleep due to the pain of carpal tunnel syndrome is probably the most bothersome symptom of the disease."

Another problem: Many people inadvertently curl their wrists while sleeping, putting pressure on the median nerve and causing pain. "A wrist splint immobilizes your wrist," says Jacobs. In fact, you should wear a wrist splint whenever you're not doing a "hands-on" activity. (Wearing one *during* such activities may reduce range of motion too much.)

Take frequent breaks from "hands-on" activity. "If your carpal tunnel syndrome is related to your job, taking a five-minute break from the offending chore every hour or so will make a big difference in your condition," suggests Dr. Barrer. "Even a few minutes' rest can often relieve the pain you feel. Of course, if possible, try to completely avoid the activity causing the trouble."

Pack on an ice pack. You may find that the pain lessens when you put an ice pack on your wrist, according to Dr. Barrer. "If you use an ice pack (a bag of frozen vegetables works fine), wrap it in a dish towel and hold it between your wrists for 10 or 15 minutes, then remove it for about the same amount of time, and repeat. This will prevent a freeze burn."

Or warm your wrists with a heating pad. Others find relief by holding a heating pad or warm compress between their wrists to relax muscles, adds Dr. Barrer. "The best thing to do is try both and see what works for you," he says. "For some, it's heat; for others, it's cold."

Cataracts

A cataract is a painless clouding of the normally clear lens of the eye. Left untreated, it can cause blindness. But this clouding has a silver lining: Surgery can restore lost sight in most cases.

While many people over age 60 do have some clouding of the eye lens and therefore some degree of cataracts, there are ways to help prevent cataracts from forming or getting worse at any age. Here's how to help make sure your lenses stay clear.

Drink your orange juice. "Our research shows there's a lower risk of developing cataracts in people who consume a lot of vitamin C in their diets," says Allen Taylor, Ph.D., director of the Lens Nutrition and Aging Division of the U.S. Department of Agriculture Human Nutrition Research Center on Aging at Tufts University in Boston. "We're still trying to find out exactly how much is needed for protection against cataracts, but we know it's at least two times the Recommended Dietary Allowance." That amounts to 1 cup of orange juice, two oranges or 1½ cups of strawberries.

Get your beta-carotene and vitamin E. "Vitamin E and beta-carotene also seem to offer some protection," adds Dr. Taylor. He recommends yellow and orange vegetables such as carrots, squash and sweet potatoes as excellent sources of beta-carotene. Foods high in vitamin E include almonds, fortified cereals, peanut butter and sunflower seeds.

Wear sunglasses or a hat. "The most credible evidence shows that the *best* way to prevent cataracts is to protect your eyes from the sun's ultraviolet rays," says Merrill M. Knopf, M.D., an ophthalmologist in Long Beach, California, and an officer of the California Association of Ophthalmology. "Be sure to wear sunglasses or a hat when you're outdoors. And there's no need to spend $100 or more for a pair of designer sunglasses, since all sunglasses sold in the United States offer UV protection. Putting a sticker on them to say that is simply a way to drive up the price. The kind sold at your drugstore will do as well as those sold by your eye doctor."

Look away when the microwave's in use. Even small doses of radiation make you more prone to developing cataracts, so limiting exposure to radiation sources—such as microwave ovens and x-ray machines—is recommended. "I know that all manufacturers say their ovens are safe, and maybe they are, but I make a point of turning my head away from my microwave oven and closing my eyes while it's in use," says Dr. Knopf. "I do the same when I'm at my dentist's office getting x-rays."

Control your vices. Occasional drinking won't affect you, but prolonged, problem drinking will. "Alcoholics are especially prone to developing cataracts, because alcoholism interferes with the nutritional pathway of food to the lens, making cataract formation more likely," says Dr. Knopf. Even in alcoholics who have good diets, essential nutrients intended for the eye are diverted.

Remember: Smoke gets to your eyes. Researchers at Johns Hopkins University in Baltimore report that cigarette smokers are more likely than nonsmokers to develop cataracts. That's because toxic substances in smoke damage the lens nucleus, causing cataracts. The good news is that by quitting smoking, you *halve* your risk of developing cataracts (compared with those who continue to smoke).

Take pain relievers. British researchers report that people who take aspirin, ibuprofen (Advil) and acetaminophen (Tylenol) are *half* as likely to develop cataracts as other folks. That's because cataract formation is related to blood sugar (one reason why people with diabetes are more susceptible to cataract formation), and there's some evidence that aspirin and aspirin-like products reduce the rate at which your body uses glucose.

Cavities

One crummy little tooth. Less than ½ square inch of your entire body, a mere pittance of your total being. But when a cavity hits deep, with its pounding and throbbing and aching and wild reactions to anything as cold as ice cream, your being can be totally in the pits.

Sometimes it's so bad that you actually *want* to sit with your mouth open, staring at the ceiling, while some guy grinds into your tooth with a high-speed drill. So you know we're talking *pain!*

Since remedying already formed cavities is no do-it-yourself job (unless you're incredibly adept with power tools), you can help avoid this double whammy of torment by practicing that old dental hygiene adage: An ounce of prevention cures a lot of pounding.

How? You already know the importance of brushing and flossing daily. "Hey, we get tired of saying it as much as you get tired of hearing it," says David S. Halpern, D.M.D., a dentist in Columbia, Maryland, who is spokesdentist for the Academy of General Dentistry. "But doing a good job of brushing and flossing *every* day is the best way to prevent cavities and keep your teeth healthy." But there are a few other secrets.

Use a straw. Cola, fruit juice and other sugared or acidic drinks can decay teeth, causing cavities. But you can minimize their damage by "bypassing" teeth and drinking these beverages with a straw, says Dr. Halpern. "Decay is

89

formed when teeth are literally bathed in these drinks, but when you use a straw, the drinks go directly to the back of your throat and have *much* less chance of affecting your teeth."

Drink water—even when you're not thirsty. "If you can't brush and floss after eating, swish some water around your mouth," adds Dr. Halpern. "This helps flush food and debris away from teeth and dilutes some of the bacteria from your mouth that cause cavities." If you can disrupt this bacteria activity, you can nip cavity-forming decay in the bud.

Don't milk that bottle. Kids who fall asleep with milk in their mouths are risking "baby bottle syndrome"—severe decay that affects children's primary teeth. "Just as the baby is falling asleep, replace the milk with a bottle of water to avoid this," says Dr. Halpern.

Change your toothbrush often. Some people keep the same toothbrush for years, which does practically *nothing* to help prevent cavities. "When the bristles get frayed and wear out, the toothbrush doesn't do an efficient job of cleaning," says Wistar Paist, D.M.D., a dentist in Allentown, Pennsylvania. "Once the bristles start curving or leaning over, it's time to toss it and get a new one. Certainly don't keep the same brush more than three months."

Brush up on good brush buying. Some toothbrushes are better than others, according to the American Dental Association (ADA), which puts the label "professionally recognized" on about 45 toothbrushes. Studies show that curved-bristle brushes (called Collis-Curve toothbrushes) improve plaque removal 63 percent compared with traditional straight-bristle brushes. (They're available at some health food stores.) And brushes with soft, round-ended, polished bristles are less likely to cause gum damage than those with ordinary bristles. Also, a brush with a curved head may be more effective than a straight-handled toothbrush: "I think that's because most people find curved brushes are easier to use," says Dr. Paist. So look for these characteristics—and the ADA label—next time you go brush shopping.

Time your snacks. Even more important than *what* you eat is *when* you eat it in relation to brushing and flossing your teeth. "The decaying process starts the moment sugar enters your mouth and lasts for about 20 minutes afterward," says Barry Dale, D.M.D., an Englewood, New Jersey, cosmetic dentist who is also assistant clinical professor at Mount Sinai Medical Center in New York City.

Wax: An Emergency Fix-It

Losing a filling can be quite a loss. When raw nerve endings are suddenly exposed, just breathing is painful, let alone consuming hot or cold foods and drinks. So how can you pamper your sensitive tooth until the dentist can do his handiwork?

"You can temporarily replace a lost filling with a piece of wax from a birthday candle, which will relieve the pain until you can see your dentist," says Wistar Paist, D.M.D., a dentist in Allentown, Pennsylvania. "If you cover the exposed area, it won't be as sensitive to hot and cold. Wax is great because it's soft and goes in easily, but you can use any soft, easily moldable item. *Don't* use bubble gum."

Adds Dr. Halpern: "Believe it or not, if you ate a pound of chocolate and immediately brushed and flossed, you'd have less of a problem than if you had just one chocolate kiss and then went to bed without brushing."

Say "cheese" for a healthy smile. Studies by Ralph Burgess, D.D.S., head of preventive dentistry at the University of Toronto Dental School, revealed that topping off a meal with a piece of aged cheese also helps take the bite out of tooth decay. "The chewiness and taste stimulate saliva tremendously, which washes away the sugars from food," says Dr. Burgess. "And the high levels of calcium and phosphate in the cheese form a kind of protective barrier in the plaque. (The acids that cause tooth decay also reduce the calcium and phosphate in your teeth; eating cheese helps prevent this loss.) Cheddar works best, but a few bites of any kind of hard aged cheese will do." (Other aged cheeses include Gouda, provolone, Edam and Gruyère—not processed or American.)

Chew some sugarless gum. Chew a stick of sugarless gum for about 20 minutes immediately after eating and you'll actually help prevent cavities. That's because sugarless gum is made with xylitol, a natural sweetener (also found in fruits and vegetables) that helps knock out microorganisms that form plaque and encourage cavities. "The gum mixes up bacteria before they have a chance to organize; once the bacteria get organized in one place, they can do a lot of damage," says Dr. Halpern. "The gum also stimulates saliva flow, which helps flush away food debris." But note that he specifies *sugarless* gum, which doesn't add sugar—a main ingredient in the bad-guy bacteria.

Clean your teeth with toothpicks. A blunt-tipped toothpick, used carefully, is an excellent way to dislodge food *before* it can form into harmful, decaying bacteria, says Dr. Halpern.

Take antacids if you need them. "People who bring up a lot of acid from stomach problems such as gastritis need to take Tums or another antacid to counter the acidic environment in their stomachs," says Dr. Halpern. "That's because these acids can erode the enamel of their teeth—usually the backs of their front teeth—making them more susceptible to decay and increasing tooth sensitivity."

Chafing

N ow here's a condition that really rubs you the wrong way. You buy a wash-and-wear outfit to make your life a little easier, or you decide to get your body into shape with a new exercise program—and what happens? Your skin gets all irritated and sore.

Mild chafing happens to everyone, and usually just applying baby powder or talc to the problem area will help keep your skin happy. Another easy prevention technique is to wear a soft fabric like cotton rather than a more abrasive synthetic blend or a rough wool. But if your hide can't seem to hide from chafing, here's what to do.

Zap it with zinc. "Zinc oxide, the white paste that lifeguards put on their noses, is wonderful for treating chafing—it's simple and inexpensive," says dermatologist John F. Romano, M.D., clinical assistant professor of medicine at The New York Hospital-Cornell Medical Center in New York City. "Just apply a thin layer on the area where you tend to chafe. If you have trouble removing the zinc oxide because that area is hairy, apply a little olive oil or mineral oil and wipe it off."

Smear on petroleum jelly. Another simple and inexpensive remedy is petroleum jelly. "It's best to apply the jelly before you exercise," says D'Anne Kleinsmith, M.D., a cosmetic dermatologist at William Beaumont Hospital near Detroit. The petroleum jelly protects the area from friction.

And there might be some areas that need special attention. "Runners frequently complain that their nipples get chafed by a shirt in the up-and-down motion. I advise my patients to spread some petroleum jelly over their nipples before running," says Dr. Kleinsmith. For even more protection, cover each nipple with a small adhesive bandage.

Put away the panty hose. Women who are prone to chafing should definitely avoid wearing panty hose, according to Dr. Kleinsmith. "Panty hose don't allow the skin in your upper thighs to breathe," she says.

Men: Switch to boxers. Men who get chafing around the waist, crotch and upper thighs might want to try wearing boxer shorts. Tighter-fitting jockey underwear is more likely to cause chafing around the waist and thighs.

Wash before you wear. Be sure to wash any new clothes before you wear them, says Richard H. Strauss, M.D., a sports medicine doctor at Ohio State University College of Medicine in Columbus. Washing sometimes softens fabric enough to lessen abrasion. It also removes dyes and sizing (chemicals used to add crispness and luster to new clothes) that can irritate skin in some people, says Dr. Romano. Washing is especially important when you wear dyed exercise clothes, Dr. Romano points out. The skin absorbs dye as you sweat—and that's something you want to avoid.

Wrap it up. People who are overweight or who have big thighs are more likely to have chafing, but there's a way to find relief. Wrap elastic bandages around the portions of the legs that rub, suggests Tom Barringer, M.D., a family physician in Charlotte, North Carolina, who is a fitness runner. For any vigorous exercise, wrap elastic bandages around each thigh or wear cycling-style shorts, which come down farther on the thigh and are tighter than regular shorts. That will shield the skin on the inside of your thighs. But be sure the elastic bandage is secure, so it does not move across the skin.

Don't forget skin folds. Applying an over-the-counter cream like Micatin, mixed with a 1 percent hydrocortisone cream, *in between* skin folds can also help overweight people cure chafing. "Skin folds are prime areas for chafing because they're moist and there's a lot of friction from movement," says

Nicholas J. Lowe, M.D., clinical professor of dermatology at the University of California, Los Angeles, School of Medicine and director of the Skin Research Foundation of California in Santa Monica.

Chapped Lips

As if squeezing down chimney after chimney with a 46-inch waist isn't impressive enough, what's truly amazing about Santa is how he manages to grin merrily all winter long. After all, when the rest of us try to crack a smile during the Yule season, we literally *crack* a smile—courtesy of chapped lips.

Unlike your skin, lips lack the natural oils needed to protect against drying winter winds and the low humidity of indoor heating. And lips are easily burned by the sun's rays (which do double damage when reflecting off snow) because they contain no melanin, the pigment in the rest of the skin that causes freckles and suntan. But here's how to give the kiss-off to chapped lips and smile without wincing through those dry winter months.

When to See the Doctor

If your chapped lips do not respond to treatment, they should be evaluated by a dermatologist. Persistent chapping may indicate chronic overexposure to sunlight and could be a sign of premalignant or malignant activity, says Nelson Lee Novick, M.D., associate clinical professor of dermatology at Mount Sinai School of Medicine in New York City. A biopsy of the lips may be necessary.

Cracking at the corners of the mouth that does not heal may indicate a yeast or bacterial infection. Such cracking can spread to the lips or cheeks and should be treated by a dermatologist to prevent serious complications.

Forgot Your Lip Balm? Try This Treatment!

Credit it to our nose for news, but here's one of the more unusual and effective remedies we sniffed out. When you don't have lip balm, try this.

"Put your finger on the side of your nose and then rub your finger around your lips," suggests dermatologist Joseph Bark, M.D., past chairman of the Department of Dermatology at St. Joseph's Hospital in Lexington, Kentucky. When your finger rubs your nose, he points out, "it picks up a little of the oil that's naturally there, and it's the kind of oil the lips are looking for anyway."

Don't lick the problem. Since chapped lips are *dry* lips, the obvious answer is to simply lick your lips to keep them moist, right?

Wrong: "This is one of the very *worst* things people can do," says Ronald Sherman, M.D., a dermatologist and member of the attending staff at Mount Sinai Medical Center in New York City. "It only *increases* chapping. When the moisture from licking your lips evaporates, so does some of the moisture from your lips." Another problem is that lip lickers tend to also be lip biters, and biting your lips removes the protective layer of skin.

Water your dry cells. Drinking additional fluids in the winter is a natural and easy way to keep your lips from chapping. "I recommend several ounces of water every few hours," says Diana Bihova, M.D., clinical assistant professor of dermatology at New York University Medical Center in New York City. "As you age, the ability of your cells to retain moisture decreases, so your dryness problem may actually increase each winter. Another way to help counter wintertime dry lips is to humidify the air in your home and office."

Be wise to vitamin B. "Nutritional deficiencies—such as the lack of B-complex vitamins and iron—can play a part in scaling of the lips and cracking at the corners of the mouth," says Nelson Lee Novick, M.D., associate clinical professor of dermatology at Mount Sinai School of Medicine in New York City. "So make sure you're okay on that front with a multivitamin/mineral supplement."

Apply lip balm frequently. "You should apply lip balm every hour or two—both to prevent chapped lips and to treat them once you get them," says John

F. Romano, M.D., a dermatologist and clinical assistant professor of medicine at The New York Hospital–Cornell Medical Center in New York City.

Using petroleum jelly is fine, but if you go with a commercial product specifically made for chapped lips, "make sure you use one that contains sunscreen with an SPF (sun protection factor) of at least 15," adds Nicholas J. Lowe, M.D., clinical professor of dermatology at the University of California, Los Angeles, School of Medicine and director of the Skin Research Foundation of California in Santa Monica.

Give toothpaste the brush-off. "Allergy and sensitivity to flavoring agents in toothpaste, candy, chewing gum and mouthwash can cause chapped lips in some people," says Thomas Goodman, Jr., M.D., assistant professor of dermatology at the University of Tennessee Center for Health Sciences in Memphis. "Cinnamon-flavored products and some tartar control toothpastes can be especially irritating. I tell my patients to avoid them."

Charley Horse

This out-of-the-blue leg cramp is as intense as a kick from a palomino. "You'll be lying in bed or even asleep when you get this terrible knot— usually in the calf but sometimes in the thigh or the arch of your foot," says Steven Subotnick, D.P.M., a sports podiatrist in Hayward, California, and author of *Sports and Exercise Injuries*.

What causes a charley horse? It can be the result of sore muscles, a mineral deficiency or hormonal imbalance or even a process known as calcification, in which blood gets trapped in a muscle and hardens. No matter the cause, here's how to get fast relief.

Rub for relief. A little kneading may be all you need to pull in the reins on a charley horse. Always rub *with* the muscle, not across it. So for a charley horse in your calf, start behind the knee and rub toward the heel.

Stretch for success. If you get an exercise-related charley horse, it's best treated with a good stretch. If you should develop a charley horse in your thigh, here is a good method to treat it. Stand on the "good" leg and grasp the

Leg Cramps or Charley Horse: What's the Difference?

When your calf tightens up and the ache begins, you probably don't waste time wondering whether it's a leg cramp or a charley horse. But there is a difference. Leg cramps, especially in the elderly, often result when not enough blood gets to the muscles. A charley horse is likely to be caused by *too much* blood getting to the muscle (though there may be other causes as well).

Also, cramps and charley horses attack in different ways. "Leg cramps usually occur while you're walking and will come more gradually, building as you use the muscle more," says Steven Subotnick, D.P.M., a sports podiatrist in Hayward, California, and author of *Sports and Exercise Injuries.* "After a rest, the cramps will usually go away."

A charley horse, on the other hand, "comes more suddenly and isn't necessarily related to physical activity or using the muscle," says Dr. Subotnick.

So if you're just lying in bed and you suddenly feel that telltale tightening in your calf, it's probably a charley horse rather than a cramp.

ankle of the leg that has the charley horse from behind. "Then slowly pull the ankle of the injured leg up toward your buttocks and hold it for 10 to 15 seconds," advises Craig Hersh, M.D., a sports injuries specialist at the Sports Medicine Center in Fort Lee, New Jersey. "Doing that provides a nice stretch."

Avoid heat. While many muscle aches are best treated with a warm compress or heating pad, heat treatment is *not* recommended initially for a charley horse. Applying warmth can cause swelling or bring more blood to the muscle, which could increase the likelihood of calcification, adds Dr. Hersh.

Let gravity help. As with any type of leg cramp, encouraging blood flow away from the limbs and *toward* the heart can bring quicker relief and less throbbing. "Elevate the area you're rubbing, so gravity works with you," suggests Ed Moore, the massage therapist for the 1984 U.S. Olympic Cycling Team.

Take vitamin E and see. For frequent nighttime charley horses, a vitamin supplement may prevent recurrences. "If you get a charley horse at night, usually while you're lying in bed, then it may be a circulatory problem, which can be cured by taking a vitamin E supplement," says Dr. Subotnick. "If you're a woman going through menopause, taking 1,200 international units of vitamin E every day for two weeks will probably end the problem." Prolonged high dosages of vitamin E are not recommended, says Dr. Subotnick. After 14 days, he advises, reduce your vitmain E intake to 400 international units daily. And he says those *not* going through menopause should start with 600 international units and decrease to 400 international units after two weeks.

Or take more magnesium. If vitamin E doesn't bring relief, then perhaps you need to compensate for a mineral deficiency or hormonal imbalance. "If you get a steady kind of pain, then you probably need more magnesium in your diet, " says Dr. Subotnick. Good sources of magnesium include many kinds of fish (halibut and mackerel are tops), rice bran, tofu and spinach. And next time you have the munchies, try some dried pumpkin seeds: You get a lot of magnesium in a few quick bites.

Cheek Bites

Maybe it was that high-back chair that threw you off—or maybe the tuna casserole. More likely, it was just a momentary lapse in your chewing coordination that caused the inside of your cheek to meet the ravaging power of your choppers.

Yow! Cheek bite! That blasted curse of dysfunctional diners!

But here's how to soothe the pain and get your inner cheek in shape for chowing down again.

Wash out your mouth. Gargle with 2 percent hydrogen peroxide, a popular over-the-counter antiseptic. "It helps keep your mouth sterile to prevent infection," says Las Vegas orthopedic surgeon Michael Rask, M.D., chairman of the American Academy of Neurological and Orthopedic Surgeons and the American Board of Ringside Medicine and Surgery. He suggests that you dilute the peroxide first by mixing it with an equal amount of water and "gargle no more than once a day for no more than one week." If you gargle *more* frequently with peroxide, you can irritate gums and harm tissues within the mouth.

Put ice on the bite. "There's not a lot you can do for a cheek bite, other than relieve some of the pain with ice," says D'Anne Kleinsmith, M.D., a cosmetic dermatologist at William Beaumont Hospital near Detroit. "I suggest holding a piece of ice against the bite with your tongue."

Apply gentle pressure. "If the bite is bleeding slightly, hold a piece of gauze or even your finger against it to stop the bleeding," says Robert Duresa, D.D.S., a Chicago dentist and team dentist for the Chicago Blackhawks professional hockey team. But Dr. Duresa warns that you may need stitches if the bleeding is severe or continuous.

Take a tab of acidophilus. Acidophilus is a type of "helpful" bacteria that can fight *harmful* bacteria and help prevent infection, says Dr. Rask. He recommends taking it in the form of chewable lozenges or capsules. Two capsules twice a day should help lesions clear up.

Brush your tongue, too. "Brushing thoroughly—including your tongue—is another good way to keep your mouth sterile and help prevent infection," adds Dr. Rask.

Chickenpox

With its trademark red bumps that later turn crusty, chickenpox is not the prettiest disease around. And since its victims are usually kids—often not the easiest patients to deal with—you're likely to hear plenty of complaints.

But there's no need to let chickenpox ruffle your feathers. From a medical standpoint, your kids and you should fly through this sick time with a minimum of fuss.

The Aspirin Danger

*D*on't give children aspirin to treat the pain and fever that accompany chickenpox, because aspirin has been associated with Reye's syndrome, a life-threatening neurological disorder. While its cause is unknown, Reye's syndrome is associated with the use of aspirin by children who have viral infections, most often chickenpox or influenza.

Better: Use Tylenol or another acetaminophen preparation for fever, says Edgar O. Ledbetter, M.D., former chairman of the Department of Pediatrics at Texas Tech University in Lubbock.

"In an otherwise healthy child, chickenpox is such a mild disease that it's really hardest on parents who have to miss a week of work to stay home with the child," says George Sterne, M.D., clinical professor of pediatrics at Tulane University in New Orleans. "Sure, the child may be miserable, but he's usually not that *sick*. For a single parent or a dual-income family, chickenpox is usually hardest on the parents because of the financial problems resulting from missed work."

In contrast to measles and mumps, which can be avoided with vaccines, there's currently no prevention generally available for chickenpox, which is caused by a virus in the herpes family. (A new vaccine is being developed, however.) And since chickenpox gets passed around at school more frequently than stolen test answers, just about *everyone* gets it sometime in his life (although it's most common between ages five and nine).

"Generally, the older you are, the worse the case," says Dr. Sterne. It's hardest on adults who have never had it before; they are much more likely than kids to suffer rare complications such as pneumonia or encephalitis. It can also cause permanent skin damage in those of all ages who have ongoing skin problems, such as eczema or psoriasis. And anyone taking cancer drugs or cortisone must alert his doctor *immediately* at the first sign of chickenpox infection.

But for most of the kids who get it, there's more itching than health risk with this inevitable ailment. If your tot has the unquenchable urge to scratch, here's how to make the going a little easier.

Head for the kitchen cabinet . . . then the bath. "The best home remedy to relieve the itching from chickenpox is to mix 1 cup of white kitchen vinegar, ½ cup of baking soda and one to two capfuls of Alpha Keri body oil in a bath," says Marian H. Putnam, M.D., a pediatrician in Boston and clinical instructor of pediatrics at Boston University School of Medicine. "After a good soak of 15 to 20 minutes, leave the bathtub and then apply Dyprotex cream, an over-the-counter product that is sold as pads or in lotion form. This relieves itching better than some of the other anti-itch formulas, and since it doesn't crust like those other drying agents, there's less chance of scarring."

You can also soak a washcloth in the bath and just apply it to the face to soothe the itching, according to Dr. Putnam.

File nails daily. "Kids will tear themselves up trying to scratch themselves, so I recommend you get a few emery boards and file their nails down, literally on a daily basis," says Dr. Sterne. "Most people simply cut the nails, but doing that doesn't give you as smooth an edge."

Wash 'em, too. "It's a good idea to scrub a child's nails with soap and water or even a gentle brush once or twice a day in order to prevent secondary infection," says Edgar O. Ledbetter, M.D., former chairman of the Department of Pediatrics at Texas Tech University in Lubbock.

Nix the itch with oatmeal baths. Doctors recommend colloidal baths using preparations such as colloidal oatmeal to treat itchy skin. "I recommend twice-daily colloidal baths for patients with chickenpox, because colloidal oatmeal

The Chickenpox Treatment

Chickenpox *can* be a severe medical problem for teenagers or adults—or for those of any age with compromised immune systems or skin conditions or those who take certain medications. Be sure to see the doctor if you have been exposed and see early signs that you may have the virus.

Symptoms usually begin with a slight fever and malaise a day or so before the characteristic rash starts to appear. The prescription drug acyclovir may be recommended, but "the key with acyclovir is to start taking it at the *earliest* indication of the rash, as the drug is not effective after 24 hours from onset of the rash," says Henry M. Feder, Jr., M.D., a professor of family medicine and pediatrics at the University of Connecticut Health Center in Farmington who headed several studies on the drug. "The sooner you start taking the drug, the better it works."

is nonirritating and soothing and has a slight anti-inflammatory effect," says Lawrence Charles Parish, M.D., a Philadelphia dermatologist. (Colloidal oatmeal, such as Aveeno, can be purchased in any drugstore. It is simply raw oatmeal that's been ground to a fine powder.)

Keep cool. English researchers speculated in the *British Medical Journal* that keeping patients cooler than usual might result in milder cases with fewer pockmarks. This is still in the theory stage, but Dr. Sterne has a possible explanation: "When people are warmer, they do tend to itch more, and the rashes are more prominent," he says. (And you'll note that more pockmarks appear on "warm" areas of the body, such as the armpits and groin.)

Forget steroid creams. Probably the biggest and most dangerous mistake people make in treating chickenpox is reaching for relief with an over-the-counter anti-itch cream. "Never put on a steroid cream like Cortaid, because using it may cause an additional bacterial infection," according to Henry M. Feder, Jr., M.D., professor of family medicine and pediatrics at the University of Connecticut Health Center in Farmington. "Besides that, it can make the pox a lot worse."

Try to limit exposure. While it's practically guaranteed that an infected family member will pass chickenpox to others who haven't previously been exposed, limiting contact with the "contagious" child can make for a milder case. "There's a trend that the more time you spend around the person who initially has it, the longer and worse your case will be," says Dr. Feder.

Chipped Tooth

Maybe it was the way you landed when you scored that winning goal. Or the way you clenched your teeth the last time the stock market tumbled. It might even have been the left hook you received during that barroom brawl. However you chipped your tooth, the story of what happened is no doubt priceless.

Still, that little chip can lower the value of your million-dollar smile. And if that chipped condition is close to a major knockout, you'll want to visit your dentist soon to make sure those pearly whites don't depreciate even more. (If there is throbbing pain or swelling, seek professional help immediately.)

Often, however, the little chipper is just an annoyance: It feels rough against your tongue. And every time tongue meets tooth, you wish the surface action were smooth again. If you can't see your dentist right away, here's what you can do to smooth the rough edges.

File it carefully. A plain emery board, available at any drugstore, can be used to file the jagged edge, says Douglas Brown, D.D.S., a dentist in Wyomissing, Pennsylvania. "Of course, you have to be careful not to file too much—only a couple of strokes would be enough to smooth the tooth's broken edge so that it's not sharp to your tongue." Dr. Brown recommends that you do the filing in front of a mirror, so you can see what you're doing.

Give it a quick fix. "A product called Dentemp, sold at any drugstore, is specially made for situations where you chipped a back tooth or lost a filling and can't get to the dentist right away," says Allen R. Crawford, Jr., D.M.D., a dentist in Macungie, Pennsylvania. "It instantly makes the tooth feel smooth, so you don't cut yourself."

Dentemp also acts as an insulator against hot and cold. That's important, because the nerve in a chipped tooth can transmit a lot of pain when you bite into very hot or cold foods.

Cholesterol Control

You may have noticed that *beef* and *eggs* have become four-letter words. It's all because of cholesterol, a substance that's gotten a reputation for breaking more hearts than a high school prom queen.

But cholesterol isn't entirely bad. The human body actually needs it—and produces it—to help protect nerves and build new cells and hormones. In fact, our bodies get all the cholesterol they need by making it on their own. The trouble starts when we *add* to the cholesterol our bodies produce, which can happen when we eat the all-American diet of cheeseburgers, steaks, pizza, ice cream or any food that is or includes an animal product.

Excess cholesterol settles along arterial walls, and that excess can clog arteries and restrict blood flow, leading to angina pain, heart attack or stroke. (Cholesterol is also a leading cause of gallstones.)

If your doctor has determined that you have high levels of cholesterol in your blood, you probably have been told the importance of limiting or eliminating it—which means reducing or avoiding its only dietary sources: meat, eggs, dairy products and the foods that contain them. But here are some other ways to control your cholesterol with diet.

Stock up on vitamin E. Scientists have discovered that we have both good (high-density lipoprotein, or HDL) and bad (low-density lipoprotein, or LDL) cholesterol running through our bloodstream. Consuming 400 international units of vitamin E each day may help keep the bad cholesterol from oxidizing—an internal "rusting" process that causes the cholesterol to harden into arterial plaque, which in turn causes heart disease. Vitamin E also raises the level of good cholesterol.

"Taking vitamin E supplements helps prevent the cholesterol in your body from plaquing, so it does less damage," says Karen E. Burke, M.D., Ph.D., a

Understanding Cholesterol Lingo

If all this talk about good and bad cholesterol is confusing, take heart. Here's how to understand it.

Serum cholesterol is the amount of this fatty substance in your bloodstream. Your serum cholesterol is what your doctor measures in a cholesterol test. A reading *under* 200 is desirable; a reading *over* 240 may be dangerous and is cause for concern.

Dietary cholesterol is what you eat. For instance, an egg has 213 milligrams; an apple has none. The American Heart Association recommends that you eat no more than 300 milligrams a day.

Low-density lipoprotein (LDL) is the bad cholesterol that clogs arteries. The lower your LDL, the better.

High-density lipoprotein (HDL) is the good cholesterol that scours artery walls and helps remove harmful LDL. The higher your HDL, the better.

dermatologist and dermatologic surgeon in New York City who has studied the various effects of vitamin E. Vitamin E is found in vegetable oils, nuts and grains, but it would be very difficult to obtain 400 international units daily from diet alone. Be sure to check with your doctor, though, before beginning a supplement program.

Eat breakfast *every* morning. Breakfast skippers tend to have higher cholesterol levels than those who start off their mornings with a bellyful, according to studies. One reason may be that breakfast skippers make up for missing the morning feast by munching on unhealthy snacks later on, suggests John L. Stanton, Ph.D., professor of food marketing at St. Joseph's University in Philadelphia.

Research also shows that those who eat ready-to-eat cereal for breakfast have lower cholesterol levels than those choosing other morning entrées.

Nibble throughout the day. One way to lower your cholesterol is simply to change how often you eat. Research has shown that large meals trigger the release of large amounts of insulin, according to David Jenkins, M.D., Ph.D., director of the Clinical Nutrition and Risk Factor Modification Center at St. Michael's Hospital at the University of Toronto. Insulin release in turn stimulates the production of an enzyme that increases cholesterol production by the liver.

Having smaller, more frequent meals (but *not* increasing overall calories) may limit insulin release and play a role in cholesterol control and heart disease prevention, speculates Dr. Jenkins.

Add vitamin C to your menu. Other vitamins and minerals also have a beneficial effect on cholesterol. Research by Paul Jacques, Sc.D., an epidemiologist at the U.S. Department of Agriculture Human Nutrition Research Center on Aging at Tufts University in Boston, shows that people with diets high in vitamin C tend to have higher HDL levels. Vitamin C is especially beneficial when you get it from fruits and vegetables that also have a cholesterol-lowering fiber called pectin. Pectin surrounds cholesterol and helps transport it out of your digestive system before it gets into your blood. Vitamin C–rich, pectin-rich foods include citrus fruits, tomatoes, potatoes, strawberries, apples and spinach.

Go heavy on garlic. Vampires aren't the only thing garlic keeps away. In large doses—at least seven cloves daily—this food can significantly reduce cholesterol. Of course, that's probably more garlic than most people eat in a month. To get a similar benefit, try odorless garlic pills. When people with moderately high cholesterol took four capsules a day of an odorless liquid garlic extract called Kyolic, their cholesterol levels initially rose but then fell an average of 44 points after six months, according to a research study headed by Benjamin Lau, M.D., Ph.D., at Loma Linda University School of Medicine in Loma Linda, California. You can find garlic pills at most health food stores.

Don't depend on decaf. Decaffeinated coffee actually *raises* LDL levels more than regular brew, so it's the *worst* beverage selection if you have high cholesterol, according to Dr. Jenkins. It may be because the beans used for decaf are stronger than "regular" beans. Frequent coffee drinkers (those who drink it daily) typically have a 7 percent cholesterol increase, as shown in a study at Stanford University in Stanford, California.

Gravitate toward grapes. There's a cholesterol-lowering compound in virtually all products containing grape skin, including wine, according to pomologist Leroy Creasy, Ph.D., of Cornell University College of Agriculture and Life Sciences in Ithaca, New York. You can take advantage of these cholesterol-clobbering qualities by drinking grape juice or simply eating grapes.

Reach for grapefruit. In a study conducted by James Cerda, M.D., a gastroenterologist and professor of medicine at the University of Florida Health Science Center in Gainesville, people who ate at least 1½ cups of grapefruit sections every day lowered their cholesterol over 7 percent in two months. Grapefruit is among the fruits that contain cholesterol-lowering pectin.

Cook up some beans. Lima beans, kidney beans, navy beans, soybeans and other legumes can all help lower your cholesterol, according to James W. Anderson, M.D., an expert in cholesterol research who is professor of medicine and clinical nutrition at the University of Kentucky College of Medicine in Lexington. The reason these high-fiber legumes are so effective is because they, too, contain pectin. The more of these beans you can eat, the greater the benefits.

In one study, Dr. Anderson asked men to eat 1½ cups of cooked beans a day. The result? Their cholesterol plummeted 20 percent in just three weeks. You probably won't go for much, but the more beans, the better—and high-fiber diets have many other benefits besides. Look for a cookbook or two that have great recipes with beans, and try to get more in your diet.

Munch a couple of carrots. Bugs Bunny's favorite entrée is a boon to arteries, because carrots have plenty of cholesterol-lowering pectin. "It may be possible for people with high cholesterol to lower it 10 to 20 percent just by eating two carrots a day," says Peter D. Hoagland, Ph.D., a researcher at the U.S. Department of Agriculture Eastern Regional Research Center in Philadelphia.

Chronic Fatigue Syndrome

If the flu makes you feel as though you've been hit by a car, then chronic fatigue syndrome (CFS) is like getting socked by the entire General Motors assembly line. Flulike symptoms are typical of CFS—a low-grade fever, sore throat, assorted aches and pains and the kind of dead-on-your-feet fatigue that makes a slug look industrious.

But *unlike* real flu, this so-called yuppie flu just won't go away—not in days, weeks or even months; it's so bad that many people can't get out of bed, let alone hold jobs.

Doctors aren't sure what causes CFS, nor do they agree on how best to treat it. Some consider CFS a sleep disorder, since its victims often sleep *twice* as long as other people yet still feel severely fatigued. Others think it results from stress, since CFS often strikes young high achievers who lead stressful lives but otherwise are in good health. And researchers wonder why 80 percent of CFS patients are women, most of them between the ages of 25 and 45.

While the search for some concrete answers continues, here are some of the things doctors say you should do if you're diagnosed as having CFS.

Try to stay active. Some experts heartily encourage CFS patients to exercise *lightly* each day. "It's important to stay active, even if a 50-yard walk up and down the block is you all can do comfortably," says James F. Jones, M.D., immunologist at the National Jewish Center for Immunology and Respiratory Medicine in Denver.

Jay A. Goldstein, M.D., director of the Chronic Fatigue Syndrome Institute in Anaheim Hills, California, suspects that exercise plays a key role in preventing CFS. "It's been documented that people who were in good physical condition before they got sick don't get as sick from CFS as those who weren't exercisers, and they rebound quicker."

107

When to See the Doctor

Do not try to diagnose chronic fatigue syndrome (CFS) yourself, recommends Walter Gunn, Ph.D., former principal investigator for CFS studies at the Centers for Disease Control and Prevention in Atlanta. Dr. Gunn notes that fatigue is frequently a symptom of other conditions, such as certain cancers, diabetes, anemia and other serious illnesses that may be treatable. These illnesses need to be ruled out by a reputable physician before a diagnosis of CFS can be made.

But don't overexert yourself. "While exercise is important, you don't want to exercise to the point where you'll wind up in bed for a week afterward because you overexerted yourself," says Dr. Goldstein. "I tell people that they should exercise until they begin to perspire."

Get *mucho* magnesium. Some doctors and researchers have concluded that CFS sufferers may have abnormally low levels of magnesium in their blood. "I've noticed that about *half* of my CFS patients are also magnesium-deficient," says Allan Magaziner, D.O., a family practitioner in Cherry Hill, New Jersey, who specializes in nutritional therapy and preventive medicine. Good food sources of magnesium include dark green, leafy vegetables, peas, nuts and whole grains such as brown rice and soybeans.

Junk the junk food in your diet. "Another thing I've noticed is that many of my CFS patients eat way too much sugar, white flour and processed foods," adds Dr. Magaziner, who has treated more than 200 CFS patients. He recommends to his patients that they stick with well-balanced, "home-cooked" meals with plenty of fresh vegetables.

Make up for missing nutrients. Several vitamins and minerals that may be missing from processed foods can benefit CFS patients. "I tell all my patients to take a multivitamin, even if they are eating fairly good diets. It certainly can't hurt," says Dr. Goldstein.

Pay *special* attention to allergies. "Allergies in CFS patients can sometimes be very pronounced, since the immune system is activated to fight whatever is causing this illness," says James Kornish, a CFS researcher at Brigham and Women's Hospital in Boston. "If you know you are allergic to something, be careful to avoid it." And Dr. Goldstein advises against drinking red wine or eating aged cheeses, since these foods can trigger migrainelike headaches in CFS patients.

Have a *good* night's sleep. CFS patients have a greater need for sleep, and while they may get *more* sleep, it's not always good quality. "You aren't going to get better if you don't sleep well," says Dr. Goldstein. (See page 310 for tips on how to get better sleep.)

Talk it out with loved ones. "It helps when family members and significant others can understand the illness, so they don't think the person is lazy or crazy," says Dr. Goldstein. "Many CFS patients feel very unsupported because they can't work and their families think they're just being lazy. Many marriages and friendships have broken up over this disease." Dr. Goldstein points out that conflict in relationships can add to stress, and additional stress only makes symptoms worse.

Cold Hands and Feet

Everyone expects to feel chilly when Jack Frost starts nipping. But if you feel a severe chill just from opening your refrigerator door or walking into an air-conditioned room, it's a good bet you have Raynaud's disease.

Actually, *disease* is too big a word for this baffling ailment. Everyone gets cold hands and feet sometimes, especially during winter. The big difference is that those with Raynaud's lose some blood circulation in their outer extremities at the *slightest* change in temperature. The fingers and toes turn white or take on a bluish tinge as they get colder. They may feel painful or numb. When they warm again, they become red as the blood returns and may throb with pain for a few minutes to several hours, depending on the severity of the reaction.

Raynaud's may be the result of overactive blood vessels, disorders of the connective tissue or emotional upsets. But whatever the cause, those feel-

When to See the Doctor

Raynaud's disease is usually a mild condition that doesn't require a doctor's care, according to experts. In advanced stages, however, it can weaken the fingers and dangerously damage your sense of touch. And in some cases, the symptoms may be a sign of nerve damage or another disease. So if you notice that your fingers feel weaker or the condition worsens, be sure to seek professional care.

ings of chilliness or numbness are truly uncomfortable. So here are some ways to give your blood flow a little nudge and to get your extremity temp closer to normal.

Become a swinger. You can warm your hands with a simple arm-swinging exercise, says Donald McIntyre, M.D., a dermatologist in Rutland, Vermont. Pretend you're a softball pitcher, but keep your fingers, wrist and elbow straight while swinging your arm in windmill fashion. The recommended speed is about 80 twirls per minute, but *any* windmill speed will boost blood flow to those tingling digits.

Get heavy into herring. Fish rich in omega-3 fatty acids—such as mackerel, herring, salmon and anchovies—help reduce the painful blood vessel spasms that cause the shutdown of blood flow. So eat plenty of these cold-water fish to ease the pain of Raynaud's or other circulatory problems due to cold weather or emotional stress. *An added bonus:* These fish also help cut triglycerides, a factor that contributes to heart disease.

Iron up. Fact number one: A woman's core body temperature is one or two degrees lower than a man's. Fact number two: Women are more likely to have cold hands and feet (whether due to Raynaud's or not). One reason for the lower average body temperature is that many women are iron-deficient, according to Henry C. Lukaski, Ph.D., a supervisory research physiologist at the U. S. Department of Agriculture Human Nutrition Research Center in Grand Forks, North Dakota. Lack of iron can alter your thyroid hormone metabolism, which regulates body heat generation. Women who are aware of this try to consume the recommended 18 milligrams of iron a day, but even so, iron stores are depleted during menstruation.

If your body iron is low, greater iron consumption translates into more body heat, which is a good way to counteract cold hands and feet. So look for good sources of absorbable iron, such as clams, tofu, Cream of Wheat cereal, poultry, fish, lean red meat, lentils and green leafy vegetables. (With vegetables and legumes, make sure you drink plenty of orange juice, because vitamin C increases the body's ability to absorb the type of iron in these foods.)

Give your feet a powder. Dampness leads to chilliness, so try to keep chilly parts dry. "Absorbent foot powders are excellent for helping keep feet dry," says Marc A. Brenner, D.P.M., past president of the American Society of Podiatric

---

Dress for Success

There's no secret about the best way to keep warm in cold weather. Go for great covering, and never mind glamour. Among the most important items:

Wear a hat. You lose more body heat from the top of your head than anywhere else, so cover your noggin with a warm hat, advises John Abruzzo, M.D., director of the Division of Rheumatology and professor of medicine at Thomas Jefferson University in Philadelphia. Wool is best, but any fabric is better than nothing.

Go synthetic. The best way to keep warm is by dressing in layers. The inner layers should be synthetic or "blend" fabrics that transport perspiration away from the body. (Cotton or wool blends are also good, but avoid 100 percent cotton and other threads that absorb perspiration.) Wool is a good choice for outer layers because it traps heat. The outermost layer should be of a wind-resistant, water-repellent but breathable material. And wear loose-fitting garments, because tight clothes can cut circulation.

Choose mittens over gloves. Experienced skiers know that mittens are warmer because they trap the heat from the entire hand better than gloves, which cover each finger individually.

Cover your feet with blends. All-cotton socks can soak up perspiration and chill your feet, so wear polypropylene or polyester blend socks, which help transport moisture away from your skin.

Dermatology. He recommends using foot powder on a regular basis, even sprinkling it between the toes.

Train yourself with a warm soak. It may sound obvious, but placing your hands in warm water before venturing into the cold weather helps keep blood flowing to your fingertips. Murray Hamlet, D.V.M., director of the Plans and Operations Division at the U.S. Army Research Institute of Environmental Medicine in Natick, Massachusetts, devised this exercise for troops in Alaska: Place your hands in a container of water heated to 104° to 107°F (hot water from the tap) for two to five minutes while you're sitting in a comfortable room. Then go to a cold area—preferably someplace outdoors—and place your hands in 104° to 107° water for ten minutes. Then repeat the two- to five-minute indoor hot soak again.

While the cold environment normally makes your peripheral blood vessels constrict, the sensation of the warm water makes them open. When you repeatedly get the blood vessels to open despite the cold, you are effectively "training" your hands to counter the constriction reflex. After 50 treatments, Dr. Hamlet says, most people can go into the cold without losing circulation in their hands.

Scorn cigarettes—even their secondhand smoke. Cigarette smoke adds to circulation problems by narrowing the blood vessels of the fingers and toes and therefore decreasing blood flow, according to Jay D. Coffman, M.D., chief of peripheral vascular medicine at Boston University Hospital. These effects can be especially hard on people with Raynaud's. In fact, if you have Raynaud's, it's even a good idea to stay away from *other* people who are smoking.

Watch what (and how much) you drink. Dehydration aggravates chills by reducing your blood volume, so be sure to drink *at least* eight ounces of water, cider, herbal tea or broth before venturing outdoors—and as much when you return indoors. But stay away from coffee and other caffeinated products, because they constrict blood vessels and can interfere with your circulation. And forget about hot toddies—alcohol's "warming" effect is only temporary and actually *lowers* your body temperature.

Colds

The ancient Greeks thought leech-induced bleeding was the answer. More recently, Mom's answer was her chicken soup. And guess what? While we *still* spend more than $1 billion each year on cold remedies—nothing to sneeze at—we have yet to find a single way to make the common cold less common.

The good news is that the older you get, the less likely you are to fall victim to any of the 200 different viruses that can cause a cold. Children typically get six to ten colds a year, because their immunity hasn't matured; adults usually get two to four.

While scientists are currently working on high-tech ways to stop cold viruses from spreading, here are some ways to cut down your risk—or at least reduce the time you spend suffering from America's most frequent health complaint.

Drink vitamin C–rich juice. Orange, tomato, grapefruit or pineapple juice can help you get over a cold—but you need to drink at least five glasses a day. "Studies show it takes that much vitamin C (about 500 milligrams) to reduce sneezes and coughs in cold sufferers," says Jeffrey Jahre, M.D., clinical assistant professor of medicine at Temple University School of Medicine in Philadelphia and chief of the Infectious Diseases Section at St. Luke's Medical Center in Bethlehem, Pennsylvania. If that amount seems like a bit much to swallow, you can take vitamin C supplements. But don't go overboard: Larger doses of vitamin C can cause stomach upset in some people.

Serve a steamy bowl of comfort. Any hot liquid helps cut through congestion, but chicken soup is probably best of all, according to Frederick Ruben, M.D., professor of medicine at the University of Pittsburgh and spokesperson for the American Lung Association. No study has shown *why* chicken soup seems to work so well, but it's certain that the soup is protein-rich, tasty and a comforting way to get nutrients if you're not up to eating. "People who wouldn't drink hot water will readily eat chicken soup," says Dr. Ruben.

Keep a glass of water on your nightstand. "Taking sips of water during the night is another way to moisten the nose and help breathing," says Dr. Ruben. It also helps combat the dehydration that can result from fighting a cold.

Try a ginger brew. "For chills, I have patients drink tea made with a tea-spoon of ground ginger in boiling water," says Charles Lo, M.D., a physician in Chicago and Oak Park, Illinois.

Eat south of the border. Break up congestion with a bowl of chili or other spicy foods containing horseradish, hot pepper sauce, hot mustard or curry, suggests Irwin Ziment, M.D., chief of medicine at Olive View Medical Center in Los Angeles. Hot Mexican or Indian foods are good congestion busters. As a rule of thumb, says Dr. Ziment, "if it makes your eyes water, it will also make your nose run."

Pump your legs. A daily 45-minute walk can help speed recovery from colds, according to studies conducted by David Nieman, Ph.D., a health researcher at Appalachian State University in Boone, North Carolina. "A daily walk helps shake up and spread out the natural killer cells—the Marine Corps of your immune system—making them more vigilant," says Dr. Nieman. But don't push yourself. Exhaustive exercise can actually impair the immune system. If you pace yourself so that you can comfortably talk while you walk, you're going at the right speed, according to Dr. Nieman.

Don't bother with antihistamines. Over-the-counter cold medicines that contain antihistamines do little more than make you sleepy. "New findings show that histamine is not produced when you have a cold," says Dr. Ruben, so the drugs designed to fight it won't help.

For headache, be selective. New evidence from Johns Hopkins University School of Hygiene and Public Health in Baltimore has shown that aspirin and acetaminophen (Tylenol) actually increase nasal blockage and reduce the level of virus-fighting antibodies. If you have a headache, ibuprofen (Advil) may be the better choice, says Dr. Ruben. If your child has a headache along with a cold, ask your doctor about child-size doses of ibuprofen. (Never give children aspirin without consulting a doctor, because it can contribute to Reye's syndrome, a life-threatening neurological condition.)

Snort salt water. For a stuffy nose, nasal sprays are safer and better than oral decongestants, says Herbert Patrick, M.D., assistant professor of medicine and medical director of the Respiratory Care Department at Jefferson Medical College of Thomas Jefferson University in Philadelphia. But if you use them longer than three days, your nose will become stuffier than ever. So after you've used a nasal spray for a couple of days, switch to a commercial saline solution such as Ayr. Or make your own saline solution: Dissolve a teaspoon of salt in a pint of water, then use a nosedropper to drop it in your nose. Gently blow your nose on a tissue.

Sit in a sauna. There's no sure way to prevent a cold, but the Swedes may be on the right track. According to Dr. Jahre, researchers found that if you indulge in a sauna twice a week or more, you're less likely to catch a cold. Possibly, he says, the high temperature may block the cold viruses from reproducing.

Make your home tropical. "It's not the cold weather but the lack of humidity that is a major issue in catching colds," says Dr. Patrick. Overheated homes and offices are the perfect setup for a cold, he adds. "When our nose and tonsils are dry, they cannot trap germs efficiently. It becomes difficult to sneeze and cough, so it's difficult to expel germs from the body." Turning down the thermostat and turning on a room humidifier keeps virus-laden mucus flowing out of your body, according to Dr. Patrick.

Chill out. In a study involving more than 400 people, researchers at Carnegie Mellon University in Pittsburgh and Britain's Common Cold Unit found that people who reported high levels of psychological stress were twice as likely to develop a cold as those reporting low stress levels. "We can only speculate that a change in stress hormones wears down the immune system," says Sheldon Cohen, Ph.D., professor of psychology at the university and the study's author. This study is a first step in understanding a complex issue, he says. Whether stress has an actual impact on colds is still unknown. Still, using stress management on a daily basis can't hurt, and it may help defend you against a season of sniffles.

Cold Sores

C old sores (also known as fever blisters) are uninvited guests. You may be free of them for months or even years . . . until one day when they drop in on you, usually at the *worst* possible time. Their stay may be merely inconvenient or downright painful, but it's never pleasant. And once you get them, they stay a *lot* longer than a weekend. In fact, once you have the herpes simplex virus—which is what causes cold sores—you never permanently get rid of it.

It's the virus that gives you a blister, usually on the outside of your lips or mouth or on your nose, cheeks or fingers. The blister may ooze and form a yellow crust. It can also sting or itch. And often it lingers for a week or ten days. But here's how to ease cold sore pain and make that blister disappear faster.

Smear yourself with sunscreen. Sunlight triggers one of every four cases of cold sores. New research shows that applying an SPF (sun protection factor) 15 sunscreen to your lips and other susceptible areas before venturing outdoors may be all you need to prevent recurring cases. In studies, researchers at the National Institutes of Health in Bethesda, Maryland, and the University of California Hospital in Los Angeles found that patients prone to cold sores who applied sunscreen prior to ultraviolet light exposure got *total* protection. Those who didn't apply sunscreen got their usual number of new outbreaks.

Replace your toothbrush. Your trusty toothbrush can harbor the herpes virus for days, reinfecting you again and again after the cold sore first heals. So toss your toothbrush as soon as you notice the beginning of a blister, advises Richard T. Glass, D.D.S., Ph.D., chairman of the Department of Oral Pathology at the Colleges of Dentistry and Medicine at the University of Oklahoma in Oklahoma City. Use the new toothbrush until the sore has healed completely, then replace that one.

Try milk. A compress of *whole* milk placed directly on the cold sore can ease pain and speed the healing process, says Jerome Z. Litt, M.D., assistant clinical professor of dermatology at Case Western Reserve University School of Medicine in Cleveland. Allow the milk to sit at room temperature for 10 to 15 minutes before placing the compress on your skin. Be sure to rinse your skin afterward, because the milk can become sour smelling. *Note:* Whole milk, with its extra protein, works—other kinds don't have the same healing effect.

Watch what you eat. The herpes simplex virus needs the amino acid arginine for its metabolism. So if you're prone to cold sores, limit your intake of arginine-rich foods such as chocolate, cola, peas, cereals, peanuts, gelatin, cashews and beer, advises D'Anne Kleinsmith, M.D., a cosmetic dermatologist at William Beaumont Hospital near Detroit. Of course, during an outbreak, *eliminate* these foods altogether.

Lick it with lysine. People who get more than three cold sores a year are advised to supplement their diets with between 2,000 and 3,000 milligrams daily of lysine, an amino acid that counteracts arginine, says Mark A. McCune, M.D., chief of dermatology at Humana Hospital in Overland Park, Kansas. Lysine is sold at most health food stores and some drugstores.

Try the direct method. Applying ice or an over-the-counter product containing zinc oxide directly to the cold sore can speed healing. Gauze soaked in Domeboro astringent solution and applied to the cold sore helps dry it up. "Witch hazel also works by drying out the blister, but it hurts and may not be quite as effective," says Dr. Kleinsmith.

Colic

I s that cute, cuddly new baby driving everyone wild with howls, screams and shrieks of discomfort? Welcome to the wacky, nerve-racking presence of a colicky kid. When the pediatrician says a baby has *colic*, he's using a term that describes frequent attacks of abdominal pain that may originate in the infant's intestines.

Though a baby with colic may cry to the point of exhaustion, the pain may be as upsetting to parents as to the child. The cause of colic is not definitely known, but sometimes the attacks are associated with hunger or swallowing air. Occasionally the attacks end when the baby passes gas or has a bowel movement.

Colic tends to be worst when a child is three weeks to three months old. It usually ends spontaneously, without any special help from parents, within five months. But during that time, here are some ways to encourage a colicky baby to simmer down.

Try a hum drum. Try anything that creates a low-level humming in the background: Running a vacuum cleaner, a dishwasher or another appliance can help calm Kid Colic.

Get a fish tank. "Some parents got an aquarium filter and put it in their baby's room," says pediatrician Ronald G. Barr, M.D., director of Child Development at Montreal Children's Hospital in Quebec. "The sound of the bubbles going through the filter helped quiet their colicky baby."

Put baby next to the washer. "For years, parents have been taking their colicky babies for a drive to soothe them—and it really works," adds Dr. Barr. But he points out that *any* movement that's soothing can help. So here's a variation.

Put your baby in his infant seat, fasten him securely, and place the seat next to the washing machine or dryer while it's in operation, suggests Helen

---

Is It Colic—Or a Protein Reaction?

Sometimes a baby who seems to be colicky is actually having an allergic reaction to protein, says pediatrician Ronald G. Barr, M.D., director of Child Development at Montreal Children's Hospital in Quebec. Protein is contained in formula as well as in breast milk, so a baby may have a reaction even if he is fed formula. According to Dr. Barr, only 3 to 5 percent of babies have this allergy, so it's relatively rare.

To find out whether this is the problem, your pediatrician may want you to switch the baby to a protein-treated formula: The protein is "broken down" chemically, so allergic babies won't react. If there is no change in symptoms, you can always go back to regular formula or return to breast milk (if you've been expressing milk during the formula trial).

To Feed or Not to Feed?

In the past, some doctors have suggested that babies should not be fed during a colic attack. But a growing number of doctors believe that food is the *best* thing for a colicky baby. "There's a lot of debate, but I think you should feel free to feed the baby as frequently as you wish," says pediatrician Ronald G. Barr, M.D., director of Child Development at Montreal Children's Hospital in Quebec. "When a baby is fed, he's not crying because he's eating, and in cultures where babies are fed three or four times an hour, there is little colic. So I suggest trying to *feed* your baby during a colic attack."

Neville, R.N., a pediatric nurse at Kaiser Permanente Hospital in Oakland, California. For this to work, the seat must be touching the appliance, so the baby can feel the vibrations.

Use some pressure tactics. Take a hot water bottle and place it in the baby's crib. Then put a towel over the bottle and place the baby so that his head and feet drape over the bottle and his belly is on it.

For some babies, "the warmth and pressure of the hot water bottle appear to help a lot," says Birt Harvey, M.D., professor of pediatrics at Stanford University School of Medicine in Stanford, California.

Schedule baby's playtime. Keeping a log of your child's episodes will help you recognize the times when baby is more agitated. "You can schedule specific playtimes to keep the baby happy, so he'll be less likely to have crying fits," says Becky Luttkus, head instructor at the National Academy of Nannies of Denver.

"Keeping a calendar can also help you discover a pattern as well as aid your physician with data he might need," says Dr. Barr.

Give plenty of TLC. Snuggling is good medicine for crying babies, whether the sobs are caused by colic or something else. "Anything you can do to keep the baby calm and happy certainly helps," says Dr. Barr, who has studied the effects of snuggling on crying infants.

One of the best ways to soothe your child is to pick him up, hold him and cuddle him.

Colitis

I f you have been diagnosed with chronic colitis, you are already familiar with some of its unpleasant symptoms—diarrhea, abdominal pain and rectal bleeding.

Colitis is one of a group of conditions known collectively as inflammatory bowel disease. Ulcerative colitis causes open sores in the large intestine and almost always results in bloody, watery stools. Plain colitis, which is less severe, doesn't involve ulcers and tends to be confined to the upper part of the large intestine.

Although having a chronic inflammatory condition like colitis is no picnic, there is encouraging light on your health horizon. With good care, proper diet and a less stressful approach to life, you may be able to ease some of the discomfort of colitis and keep it under control. But flare-ups do happen. And when the symptoms start up again, the first thing you'll be looking for is some fast-track roads to relief.

Here are some routes top doctors recommend—and some detours around future problems.

Supernourish yourself. "During colitis flare-ups, you may feel too rotten to eat well, so it's important to eat a high-quality diet the rest of the time," says Joel Mason, M.D., a nutritionist and gastroenterologist with the U.S. Department of Agriculture Human Nutrition Research Center on Aging at Tufts University in Boston. "You want to build an adequate store of nutrients in your body."

Be your own diet detective. Since each individual case of colitis is so different, you need to be on the lookout for specific foods that your body may not tolerate well, says Stephen McClave, M.D., a gastroenterologist and associate professor of medicine at the University of Louisville School of Medicine in Louisville, Kentucky. If a specific food causes trouble on multiple occasions, avoid it. But if it happens only once, retest. If you find that cabbage makes your symptoms worse, for example, don't avoid all leafy vegetables.

Tell it to Dear Diary. Recording your foods, moods and flare-ups can help, says James Scala, Ph.D., a nutritional biochemist and lecturer at Georgetown University School of Medicine in Washington, D.C. "Keep track not just of what you ate or drank but also where, when, why and how you felt at the time. If you can relate the onset of a flare-up to a food or an emotional experience, you'll be able to manage your illness more effectively in the future."

Try pectin protection. Fiber may be an important dietary help for colitis sufferers, says Danny Jacobs, M.D., a surgeon at Brigham and Women's Hospital and assistant professor of surgery at Harvard Medical School, both in Boston. And pectin, the soluble fiber found in apples and other fruits and vegetables, is particularly pleasing to the colon. "Apples are a marvelous source of pectin," he says, "and as long as you don't eat the seeds (or peels), there's no limit to how many you can consume."

But phase out fiber during flare-ups. "If you're having a flare-up, use a very low-fiber diet," says Dr. Mason. "You want to pass as little undigested residue through the bowel as possible. But as soon as the flare-up is over, return to a normal or high-fiber diet."

When to See the Doctor

The fact is, colitis can get out of control. That's why you need to see your doctor during an acute flare-up, says Joel Mason, M.D., a nutritionist and gastroenterologist with the U.S. Department of Agriculture Human Nutrition Research Center on Aging at Tufts University in Boston. "Self-medicating is not a good idea. The antidiarrheal medications Imodium and Lomotil can be very harmful if used inappropriately," he says.

Dr. Mason also recommends a regular screening for colon cancer if you've had chronic ulcerative colitis for more than seven years, because the disease does increase your risk. "If a cancer is detected very early, it increases the likelihood that you can be adequately treated and even cured," he says.

Fix friendly fruits. Dr. Scala offers these suggestions for taking the trouble out of fruit by reducing the amount of fiber. Be sure to peel all fruits (even grapes!), he advises. And if you're eating a citrus fruit, cut it into sections, removing all white, fibrous material. Dr. Scala also recommends eating canned fruit that's preserved in juice rather than sugar syrup. And be sure to avoid dried fruit.

Supplement your strategy. Since colitis can attack your nutritional status, multivitamin/mineral supplements are important, says Dr. Scala. "Take a multivitamin/mineral supplement that provides twice the Recommended Dietary Allowance of key nutrients," he recommends. "For about seven cents a day, it's worth it."

Fuel yourself with folate. People with ulcerative colitis should consider taking a daily multivitamin/mineral supplement that contains at least 400 micrograms of folate, recommends Dr. Mason. This is particularly true for those individuals who use sulfasalazine (Azulfidine), the most commonly prescribed drug for controlling colitis. The drug tends to inhibit your body's ability to use this B vitamin, he says. If more than 400 micrograms of folate is taken per day, however, it should be done under the supervision of a physician.

De-stress for less distress. After food intolerance, emotional stress is the biggest challenge for colitis sufferers, says Dr. Scala. To reduce stress, he calls for "a regular exercise program. Exercise will dissipate the effects of stress better than anything." In addition, Dr. Scala recommends stress counseling.

Lighten up on lactose. Inability to digest lactose, the sugar in milk, can be a factor in colitis, says Dr. McClave. "A lot of us teeter on the edge of milk intolerance, and a bowel disease like colitis can tip the balance." By avoiding all milk products, you may be able to reduce your symptoms.

Avoid crunchy veggies. You need to take the crunch out of carrots, asparagus, zucchini, squash and other popular vegetables, says Dr. Scala. The best way is to cook them until they are very tender, he says. Pressure cooking is especially effective.

Check your medicine chest. Ulcerative colitis patients need to be cautious about using nonsteroidal anti-inflammatory drugs, warns Gary R. Gibson, M.D., assistant professor of medicine at Northeastern Ohio University College of Medicine in Warren. Over-the-counter ibuprofen (Advil), aspirin and a dozen prescription drugs (including Naprosyn, Voltaren and Feldene) can erode the lining of the small intestine and colon. Be sure to check with your doctor before taking any of these medications.

Conception Problems

The one thing that can be more frustrating than being a parent is trying to become one with no success. For one in seven couples, conceiving a child can be a long and difficult process—it can take at least one year and sometimes requires several.

Some "trying" couples are infertile because of physical problems. But most couples are simply "underfertile"—they are physically able to conceive but have to nudge the stork just a bit more than usual. Here's what experts recommend for them.

Take cough syrup. "Before we had high-tech measures, a lot of doctors would recommend that women take cough syrup containing guaifenesin about four times a day around the time of ovulation," according to Arthur L. Wisot, M.D., a fertility specialist who is affiliated with the Center for Advanced Reproductive Care in Redondo Beach, California. "And that's still sound advice, because guaifenesin thins the cervical mucus, making it easier for sperm to swim through to meet the egg."

Don't lubricate with commercial products. When intercourse needs a helping hand, couples sometimes use a commercial lubricant like K-Y jelly. But that can hurt your chances of conceiving. That's because these products can impair sperm, making them less able to reach the egg, says John Willems, M.D., associate clinical professor of obstetrics/gynecology at the University of California, San Diego, and a researcher at the Scripps Clinic and Research Foundation in La Jolla. "A woman's natural lubricants should be all you need."

But egg white may help. If you need a lubricant during intercourse, try using egg white instead of a pharmaceutical lubricant, suggests Andrew

123

Toledo, M.D., a fertility specialist and reproductive endocrinologist who is assistant clinical professor of medicine in the Department of Gynecology and Obstetrics at Emory University in Atlanta. Because the egg white lubricant is pure protein—as are sperm—it makes a better "carrier" than lubricants made from nonprotein substances.

If dryness is a problem, Dr. Toledo recommends using the egg white lubricant during the days when a woman is fertile and a regular lubricant the rest of the time. But don't use egg white if you're allergic to it, and be sure to separate the white from the yolk before applying it to either the penis or the vagina.

Take more vitamin C. Studies by researchers at the University of Texas Medical Branch at Galveston show that large doses of vitamin C can *reverse* some cases of male infertility. The team there, headed by Earl B. Dawson, Ph.D., reported that men who increased their vitamin C intake to 1,000 milligrams daily (the Recommended Dietary Allowance is 60 milligrams) showed increased sperm count, motility and longevity.

Stub out cigarettes. Smokers' alert: Women who smoke have more difficulty getting pregnant, according to studies by researchers at the National Institute of Environmental Health Sciences in Research Triangle Park, North Carolina. "But we don't yet understand the biological reason why," says Allen Wilcox, M.D., Ph.D., chief of the Epidemiology Branch at the institute. So if you smoke, you may better your chances of conception by giving it up.

Practice clean living. Smoking isn't the only vice that hurts your chances of conceiving. Studies at the National Institute of Environmental Health Sciences showed that women who drink just one cup of coffee daily may *halve* their chances of becoming pregnant each menstrual cycle (compared with those who don't get any caffeine). "Cutting out caffeine seems to help some women, but not others. It may be worth a try," says Dr. Wilcox.

And there are other factors to consider as well. "You need to get your act together—don't use drugs, stop drinking, and avoid all unnecessary medications," says Dr. Wisot. To add to their healthy lifestyle, he also recommends that women start taking prenatal vitamins.

Wear boxer shorts. For some men, fashionable underwear styles may be the shortcut to fatherhood. Tight-fitting jockey shorts pull the testicles close to the body, and body heat impairs sperm, according to Dr. Wisot. He recommends wearing looser-fitting boxer shorts.

Don't soak in a hot tub, guys. High-temperature water can also lower sperm count and motility, says Dr. Wisot, so the man who wants to be Dad should stay away from hot tubs.

Go missionary. Although sexual position usually has no bearing on conception, "the missionary position assures better contact of the semen with the cervix—and may make the difference in marginal cases," says Dr. Wisot.

Keep a calendar. Most fertility specialists say that you and your partner should try to conceive for at least one year before assuming you have a conception problem.

"Generally, if a woman has an average 28-day cycle, she will begin ovulating on the 14th day," says Dr. Wisot. "If she's on an irregular cycle, ovulation usually occurs 14 days before her next expected menstrual cycle." Keeping track on a calendar for a few months is a good way to see your pattern.

Get help from a kit. "There are several ovulation kits that you can buy over the counter that help tell a woman when she's ovulating," adds Dr. Wisot. "Starting on the 16th or 17th day before your period, you should test your urine each evening with these kits. When you get a positive test, have intercourse the next day."

Go for the gold the second time around. Probably the biggest mistake couples make is assuming that a man's first ejaculation is his best. Actually, a woman is more likely to get pregnant when a man ejaculates two days before she starts ovulation and then they wait until she *is* ovulating before they try to conceive. "Usually that second specimen is better, both in sperm count and motility," says Dr. Wisot.

Constipation

D o you take *War and Peace* into the bathroom instead of *Reader's Digest*? If so, you're probably constipated.

Constipation actually has two forms. Some people have to strain to move their bowels every time they want to go. But others just feel the urge too seldom.

How often is often enough? Routines vary. But if you have to go fewer than three times per week and each time it's a strain, there's a mighty good chance you're constipated. Here's how to get things moving again.

Lotion the motion with fiber. "Go on a high-fiber diet," says Edward P. Donatelle, M.D., professor emeritus of the Department of Family Practice and Community Medicine at the University of Kansas School of Medicine in Wichita. Soluble fiber, found in grains, legumes and fruits, is particularly effective. Oatmeal, rice, wheat germ, corn bran, prunes, raisins, apricots, figs and an apple a day are all good sources, Dr. Donatelle says.

Try a natural laxative. For a concentrated constipation buster, go for a fiber supplement that will budge that balky bowel. One of the best is psyllium, which is sold in health food stores. Marvin M. Schuster, M.D., chief of the Department of Digestive Diseases at Francis Scott Key Medical Center in Baltimore, recommends one teaspoon of psyllium with meals. Add the teaspoonful to a glass of water or juice and stir thoroughly before drinking. (You can also make a "paste" of one teaspoon of psyllium moistened with water, but be sure to drink at least a full glass of juice or water afterward.) Another alternative: Metamucil, a bowel regulator that contains psyllium and is sold in most drugstores and some supermarkets.

Use fluids to fuel the fiber. "Drink plenty of fluids," suggests John Sutherland, M.D., clinical professor of family practice at the University of Iowa College of Medicine in Iowa City and director of the Waterloo Family

When to See the Doctor

Although constipation is usually not a serious problem, there are times when you should seek a doctor's advice. If you've had symptoms for more than three weeks and home remedies don't help—even with lots of fluid, fiber and exercise—be sure to see your doctor.

You should also consult your doctor if there is blood in your stool. Although rare, constipation can sometimes signal a serious intestinal disease or disorder, including cancer, according to gastroenterologist Nicholas Talley, M.D., Ph.D., associate professor of medicine at the Mayo Clinic in Rochester, Minnesota.

Practice Residency Program in Waterloo. Fluid expands and softens the fiber you're eating, allowing it to form bulk in the colon. That bulking action in turn triggers the urge to move your bowels.

"Ordinarily you need to drink about a gallon of fluid a day—the more, the better," Dr. Sutherland says.

Avoid milk and cheese. If you have a problem with constipation, try avoiding milk products temporarily, says Dr. Donatelle. Both milk and cheese contain casein, an insoluble protein that tends to plug up the intestinal tract.

Get your body moving and your bowels will, too. "Exercise can help that lazy bowel to function better," according to gastroenterologist Nicholas Talley, M.D., Ph.D., associate professor of medicine at the Mayo Clinic in Rochester, Minnesota. "Aerobic exercise such as walking, running and swimming is best." If you're a walker, for instance, go for a brisk 20- to 30-minute arm-swinging stroll every day.

Listen when your body talks. "Sometimes people who are constipated ignore 'the urge' and wait until later. This can aggravate the problem," says Dr. Sutherland. When your body tells you it's time to go, head for the bathroom as soon as possible.

Get into training. You can actually train your bowels to get on a regular schedule, says Vera Loening-Baucke, M.D., a pediatrician at the University of Iowa Hospitals and Clinics in Iowa City. Her advice: Sit on the toilet for about

Be Selective about Laxatives

Many over-the-counter products are sold as laxatives, but not all laxatives are recommended by doctors. In fact, heavy use of some laxatives can be counterproductive and even risky, according to Ronald L. Hoffman, M.D., director of the Hoffman Center for Holistic Medicine in New York City.

Heavy use of some laxatives can give you diarrhea, according to Dr. Hoffman. And many are habit-forming: If you always rely on a laxative to prompt bowel movements, your body may begin to need it to trigger the action. Laxatives containing castor oil can damage your intestinal lining, and those that have mineral oil can interfere with your ability to absorb certain vitamins and minerals, according to Dr. Hoffman.

Safest are the natural or vegetable laxative products, high-fiber bulking agents such as Metamucil, Citrucel or Perdiem that are sold in most drugstores. "If you can't tolerate a high-fiber diet, these bulking agents are very safe, helpful supplements," according to gastroenterologist Nicholas Talley, M.D., Ph.D., associate professor of medicine at the Mayo Clinic in Rochester, Minnesota.

Dr. Talley recommends taking the cautious approach with bulking agents. Follow the directions on the package, increasing the dosage slowly if needed.

ten minutes after the same meal every day. The key is to stay relaxed. Eventually, says Dr. Loening-Baucke, your body will catch on.

Reach for the rhubarb. "When it's in season in early summer, fresh rhubarb is a delicious and powerful antidote to constipation," says Ronald L. Hoffman, M.D., director of the Hoffman Center for Holistic Medicine in New York City. It contains a good amount of fiber, which helps keep things moving. For a rhubarb juice refresher that will get your tract on track, try this cooling recipe: Chop three stalks of rhubarb (remove the leaves, which are toxic) and mix with one cup of apple juice, ¼ of a peeled lemon and one teaspoon of honey. Put all the ingredients in a blender or food processor and puree until smooth.

Some advice: Try a small amount of rhubarb juice at first and see how your body responds. It can be as powerful and quick-acting as prune juice. Also, depending on how you like the taste, you might want to mix it with other juices. Caution: Rhubarb should be avoided by people with a history of calcium kidney stones.

Watch out for water robbers. Coffee, tea and alcohol are all diuretics that can leave you somewhat dehydrated, says Dr. Hoffman. Since you need fluids in your system to aid bowel movements, you're more likely to have constipation if you drink these beverages. When you *do* have them, go for moderation and help compensate by drinking plenty of water, Dr. Hoffman suggests.

Give a high-fiber cookie to the kid in you. When you need a break from bran cereals, don't give up on fiber. Instead, try a fiber cookie supplement like Fiberall or Fibermed wafers, says Arnold Wald, M.D., head of the Gastroenterology Division at Montefiore University Hospital in Pittsburgh. "Be sure to take them with plenty of fluids—at least a six- to eight-ounce glass with each," he suggests.

Review your Rx. Medicines that can contribute to constipation include prescription antidepressants and painkillers as well as some over-the-counter remedies such as iron supplements and aluminum-containing antacids. Dr. Hoffman recommends that you check with your doctor if you suspect your medication is causing your constipation.

Contact Lens Problems

The *disposable* contact lens has joined the Q-Tip as a personal care item with a very short life. But don't think disposable contact lenses (or any other type) are worry-free just because they're so convenient. Eye doctors say *any* lens can become contaminated and cause eye damage. Here's how to see your way to eye health.

To be safe, avoid sleeping with lenses in. Even if you have contact lenses that are labeled "extended wear," it doesn't mean you should leave them in every night. According to a study at the Massachusetts Eye and Ear Infirmary and

Harvard Medical School in Boston, you raise your risk of ulceration 5 percent for each night you sleep with extended-wear lenses in. The reason: Continuously worn contacts rub away the cornea (the covering of the eyeball). This causes tiny rips that invite infection and may lead to vision loss. Also, covering the cornea for extended periods blocks out oxygen, providing an ideal breeding ground for harmful bacteria.

"My recommendation is to never sleep wearing any lenses, period," says Mitchell H. Friedlaender, M.D., director of the Cornea Service at the Scripps Clinic and Research Foundation in La Jolla, California.

Clean and disinfect any time you remove lenses. Whenever you take out your lenses, they must be cleaned as well as disinfected, says Joseph P. Shovlin, O.D., an optometrist at the Northeastern Eye Institute, with headquarters in Scranton, Pennsylvania, and chairman of the Contact Lens Section of the American Optometric Association. And if you wear the disposable kind, be sure to throw them away at the time prescribed by your doctor.

Clean the lens case, too. Scrub the case with hot water every other day with a toothbrush that's used only for that purpose, says Dr. Friedlaender.

Never use homemade saline solutions. Use a fresh solution each day, and use only commercial contact lens preparations. That's because homemade salt solutions might harbor a microorganism that can scar the cornea and cause partial or complete blindness, according to studies at the Centers for Disease Control and Prevention in Atlanta. And since tap water, distilled water and mineral water are not sterile, they may harbor infection-causing impurities, says Dr. Friedlaender. "Don't use them with contacts."

As for generic hydrogen peroxide, it may contain irritating additives, says Thomas Gossel, Ph.D., R.Ph., professor of pharmacology and toxicology and associate dean at Ohio Northern University College of Pharmacy in Ada.

Stick with one lens-care regimen. A disinfecting/cleaning regimen is always specified for your lens type, says Dr. Gossel, and that shouldn't be changed. If you switch from chemical to heat, for example, chemicals might be "baked into" soft lenses, and that could irritate your eyes. Whatever the recommended procedure, be sure to stick with it!

Never lick your lenses. Saliva is teeming with bacteria. "If you give your lenses a spit bath, you might as well rub your lenses on the floor," according to Dr. Friedlaender.

Makeup first, lenses second. Use water-based, not oil-based, cosmetics, says Dr. Friedlaender, and apply makeup and hair spray before you put in your lenses. Around the eyes, use water-resistant mascara and apply to lash tips only, he adds.

Take out your lenses before swimming. The risk of wearing hard lenses in a pool or tub is that they may float out if your eyes get wet. With soft lenses, impurities in the water might be absorbed, which could cause infection, according to Paul Vinger, M.D., assistant clinical professor of ophthalmology at Harvard University in Cambridge, Massachusetts. "If you need to see underwater, get prescription goggles."

Switch to glasses before that big cleaning job. Remove contacts when using volatile household cleaners, which may be absorbed by the lenses, advises Scott MacRae, M.D., associate professor of ophthalmology at Oregon Health Sciences University in Portland and chairman of the Public Health Committee of the American Academy of Ophthalmology. "Volatile" cleaners include any cleaner containing ammonia or another strong-smelling chemical.

Remove your contacts if your eyes turn red. If your eyes become irritated, remove your contacts, says Dr. Shovlin. If the irritation doesn't go away after two to three hours, contact your eye-care practitioner. Tears, discharge, redness around the eyes and a change in vision are all indications of eye irritation.

Corns and Calluses

The average Joe or Josephine takes as many as 10,000 steps a day, most of them on hard surfaces. Multiply that by 365 days a year, and then multiply *that* by 75 or so years, and you've taken enough footsteps to walk around the world—*several* times over.

The only problem is that most of this traveling is done in shoes designed for fashion rather than function. The very same footwear that protects your feet from the hard realities of glass-littered streets and pebble-pocked lawns is an

131

Achilles' heel to your toes. The friction shoes cause, as you may be uncomfortably aware, can leave you with corns and calluses.

These ugly bumps and lumps of thickened and hardened dead skin cells produce discomfort that can range from minor to extreme. So here are some treatments for the next time corns or calluses crop up.

Support your arches. "People with high arches are particularly susceptible to corns," says dermatologist Joseph Bark, M.D., past chairman of the Department of Dermatology at St. Joseph's Hospital in Lexington, Kentucky. How do you find out whether the shape of your arches is a contributing factor? "Check for corns on three pressure points on your feet that carry your weight: on the ball of the foot, right below the smallest toe and on your heel," Dr. Bark suggests. If this is your problem, try store-bought arch supports.

Be a beachcomber. "Walking barefoot on the beach can get rid of your calluses," says Robert Diamond, D.P.M., a Pennsylvania podiatrist affiliated with Muhlenberg Hospital Center in Bethlehem and Allentown Osteopathic Hospital. "The sand acts as a natural pumice stone and files them down."

When to See the Doctor

Corns and calluses may require the attention of a doctor if they are very painful. And you should also consult a doctor if you have numbness or reduced sensation in your feet.

"Should pumice stones, moleskin and pads fail to eliminate pain, medical attention is recommended," says Robert Diamond, D.P.M., a Pennsylvania podiatrist affiliated with Muhlenberg Hospital Center in Bethlehem and Allentown Osteopathic Hospital. For some people, surgery may be necessary, according to Dr. Diamond.

If you have reduced feeling in your feet, however, you may have a medical problem such as diabetes or possibly poor circulation. If you have a serious cut or injury on your foot, you might not feel it—and you could wind up with a dangerous infection.

If you are diabetic or have poor circulation in your feet, Dr. Diamond recommends that you see a doctor any time you have corns or calluses. Those with diabetes, he notes, should not try any home remedies.

Avoid "Medicated" Corn Pads

One of the most popular store-bought remedies for corns is among the worst, says podiatrist Robert Diamond, D.P.M., a Pennsylvania podiatrist affiliated with Muhlenberg Hospital Center in Bethlehem and Allentown Osteopathic Hospital.

"Medicated corn pads cause more problems than they're worth," says Dr. Diamond. "The 'medication' is salicylic acid, which turns the corn white and blister-free, so it can peel off. But what happens frequently is that the acid is so strong it goes through the corn and eats at the toe, causing an ulcer in the toe."

Bag 'em with aspirin. One way to soften hard calluses is to crush five or six aspirin tablets into a powder, then add ½ teaspoon each of lemon juice and water. Apply this paste to all hard-skin areas. Wrap your entire foot with a warm towel, then cover with a plastic bag, suggests Suzanne M. Levine, D.P.M., adjunct clinical instructor at New York College of Podiatric Medicine and clinical assistant podiatrist at Wycoff Heights Medical Center, both in New York City. After sitting still for at least ten minutes, remove the coverings and file the callus with a pumice stone. *Caution:* Don't try this remedy if you are allergic or sensitive to aspirin.

Soak your feet in Epsom salts. To relieve pain, Dr. Levine recommends soaking your feet in Epsom salts and warm water. Soaking twice a day, for ten minutes each time, should provide some relief.

For footwear, think round. "Many women who wear pointy-toed shoes get corns on the fourth or smallest toe," says Dr. Bark. "Even if you don't get corns there, you're much better off with round-toed shoes or any style shoes with a large toe box." If corns are a recurring problem, he recommends getting a pair of open-toed shoes or sandals and wearing them as often as possible. With no friction on the toes, there's less discomfort—and you're less likely to develop *new* corns.

Lay on the low-cost lotion. There are many products that can help soften corns and calluses. Lotions and bath oils that contain lanolin, glycerin or urea start at around $2 in most drugstores. "Fruit acid moisturizers such as LactiCare are also very effective when you apply them heavily," says Dr. Bark.

Pump up the padding. Place "horseshoe" moleskin or foam pads *around* a corn if it continues to hurt when you walk. Be cautious with these pads, though, as they can pressure the surrounding area too much when you're walking. "And if you wear nylons, which can be very irritating, even putting a bandage over the corn helps reduce the friction," says Dr. Diamond.

Go for the insole. "Wearing a Spenco insole to give you more padding is a good idea," says Dr. Diamond. The insole helps protect against calluses on the sole of the foot.

Coughing

Whether caused by a tickle in the throat, an affinity for cigarettes or a problem with allergies, a cough is one of those things you can always do without. But sometimes, if you don't know what's causing the hack attack, you don't know how to get rid of it.

For a clue to the cause of the cough, note at what point in the day it occurs, suggests Gailen D. Marshall, Jr., M.D., Ph.D., assistant professor and director of the Allergy and Clinical Immunology Division at the University of Texas Medical School at Houston. If you cough in the morning, it may be because of asthma. If you cough at night while lying on your back, postnasal drip probably is to blame. Sinus infections also produce coughs that become worse at night, especially in children, according to Howard J. Silk, M.D., assistant professor of pediatrics at the Medical College of Georgia in Augusta and a physician at the Atlanta Allergy Clinic.

But some coughs are *very* uncomplicated. A tickle in the throat can cause coughing. Or you may get a cough during a brief encounter with a mild cold.

You'll want to see a doctor if a cough continues more than a few days or if it develops into continuous hacking or wheezing. But if all you've got is a now-and-then case of coughing, here are some remedies to try.

Lounge with a lozenge. Cough drops will help thin phlegm as well as soothe scratchy membranes in your throat, according to Alexander C. Chester, M.D., clinical professor of medicine at Georgetown University Medical Center in Washington, D.C. While some cough drops just soothe, nothing more, the best kinds have eucalyptus to reduce nasal swelling and decongest your nose, according to Dr. Chester.

Water your cough. Drink plenty of water while you've got that troublesome tickle, Dr. Chester says. Keeping the body hydrated will help thin the mucus.

Nurture your nostrils. "Oftentimes coughing is a response to some nasal irritation," Dr. Chester says. For relief, he suggests you try any of the same methods you might use to treat congestion—taking hot showers, carefully inhaling the steam from a boiling pot of water or using saline nasal sprays and vaporizers.

But stay away from cough syrup. Don't reach for over-the-counter cough suppressants, advises Horst R. Konrad, M.D., chairman of the Division of

When to See the Doctor

Any time you have a fever along with a cough, you should see a doctor, according to Alexander C. Chester, M.D., clinical professor of medicine at Georgetown University Medical Center in Washington, D.C.

You should also call the doctor when:

- Your cough does not go away after one week.
- You see any signs of blood when you cough up phlegm.
- You develop a hacking cough when you already have another illness.
- You are short of breath, yet continue to cough frequently.
- You have very thick phlegm that doesn't come up easily when you cough.

While many coughs are harmless, some indicate you have an underlying condition, advises Horst R. Konrad, M.D., chairman of the Division of Otolaryngology/Head and Neck Surgery at Southern Illinois University School of Medicine in Springfield. Sometimes a cough is a sign of bronchitis, a bacterial infection, pneumonia or asthma. In rare cases, it indicates a tumor.

Otolaryngology/Head and Neck Surgery at Southern Illinois University School of Medicine in Springfield. Nonprescription cough syrups thin the secretions that cause a cough, but that's not all beneficial. In the process of thinning, the syrups also seem to increase the amount of mucus, according to Dr. Konrad.

Don't make it milk. If you continue to have a cough when you don't feel sick or congested, try staying away from all milk products, Dr. Chester says. A milk allergy often can manifest itself as a cough.

Up with phlegm. Hacking up phlegm, what's called a productive cough, is your body's way of getting rid of mucky mucus—so don't swallow it. Spit the phlegm into a tissue—and throw the tissue away.

Cracked Skin

D ry, itchy skin is bad enough, but when eczema gets an attitude or psoriasis gets super serious, you may make the transition from considerable discomfort to full-fledged torture. Your skin can crack, leaving painful slits that bring agony with even the most basic body movements such as stretching.

Doctors call these cracks skin fissures. You will probably call them something a little more colorful. Hands and feet are the most likely spots for cracked skin, but there are other vulnerable places, too.

"Sometimes the feet are so dry that they crack, particularly on the heel and between the toes—and these cracks are like little portholes for infection," says Houston podiatrist William Van Pelt, D.P.M., former president of the American Academy of Podiatric Sports Medicine. "Women who wear open-backed heels and slides are particularly prone."

Here's how to take the fire out of painful fissures.

Give yourself a good soak. "The best way to treat very dry skin is to hydrate it every night," says Dr. Van Pelt. "Each skin cell is like a little sponge, so each night before going to bed, I recommend soaking your feet or whatever part of

Cracked Lips? Maybe It's Your Toothpaste

Brushing twice daily with a tartar control toothpaste may be a good way to fight plaque, but that toothpaste apparently doesn't do much good for your lips. Regular use of these toothpastes can leave skin cracked and cause an itchy rash around the mouth, according to research conducted by Bruce E. Beacham, M.D., associate professor of dermatology at the University of Maryland School of Medicine in Baltimore.

The reason: Tartar control toothpastes contain compounds that can irritate mucous membranes and other tissues, especially if you have atopic dermatitis or sensitive skin. In Dr. Beacham's research, however, he found that cracked lips and the accompanying rash *don't* occur when tartar control brands are used less often than once a day. So if you use the toothpaste every other day or so, you'll help prevent your lips from cracking.

your body is especially dry in warm water for about 20 minutes. During this soak, the skin cells will absorb water. Then pat yourself dry."

Seal up with a lube job. After soaking, seal in the moisture by applying a coating of a petroleum jelly product such as Vaseline, adds Dr. Van Pelt. "It works much better than commercially sold moisturizers, which don't have the same 'sealing' effect," he says. For foot care, he suggests, "after you apply Vaseline, put on a pair of socks and go to bed." If it's your hands that need attention, put on light cotton gloves at night after you give them the Vaseline treatment.

"Glue" the cracks. Although it doesn't cure skin fissures, you can lessen the pain by applying Super Glue to the slits, says Rodney Basler, M.D., a dermatologist and assistant professor of internal medicine at the University of Nebraska Medical Center in Omaha. "A little dab of Super Glue takes the air away from the nerve endings and seals the slits." He says this procedure is perfectly safe on slits and minor paper cuts but shouldn't be tried on deep wounds.

Croup

Parenthood has its nightmares, but few terrors can compare with this: You wake up to the sound of Junior struggling for breath with a cough so deep that it sounds like the barking of a St. Bernard. He gasps and sputters for a lungful of air—only to spill it out with the most shrill cry ever to punish a set of eardrums. Yes, it *does* sound awful—but as many parents have learned, to their relief, this terrible sound is usually nothing worse than quite common croup.

Croup is an inflammation of the voice box and windpipe that usually strikes children between three months and five years of age. "It usually occurs at night, because breathing becomes more shallow and the muscles in the neck don't work as well when you're asleep," says Karen Wendelberger, M.D., a pediatrician at Children's Hospital of Wisconsin in Milwaukee. It won't go away in the wink of an eye, whatever you do. But you can help *ease* your child's hacking. Here's how.

Bring vapors to the child. "Since a narrow airway doesn't get enough secretions, probably the best thing you can do is add humidity to your surroundings with a cool-mist vaporizer," says Leonard Rappaport, M.D., assistant professor of pediatrics at Harvard Medical School and senior associate in medicine at Children's Hospital in Boston. "Place it with the vaporizer blowing in your child's face, so when he's asleep, he's literally getting wet. If croup is bad during the day, run the vaporizer during the day as well." A cool-mist vaporizer can be purchased at most department stores and drugstores.

Or bring the child to the vapors. If you don't have a cool-mist vaporizer, take the child into the bathroom, close the door, and run a hot shower. That will produce enough steam to give short-term relief.

Calm Junior with extra TLC. When they're sick and unhappy, babies cry—but crying and getting agitated will further swell the airways. "Doing anything

When to See the Doctor

Sometimes those crouplike sounds can signal something far more serious: epiglottitis, an inflammation of the lidlike cartilage that covers the windpipe. You should suspect epiglottitis, says Birt Harvey, M.D., professor of pediatrics at Stanford University School of Medicine in Stanford, California, if your child is between two and six years of age and has any of the following symptoms.

• High fever
• Forward-leaning posture when sitting
• Drooling
• Difficulty swallowing, with a very sore throat

Seek immediate medical attention, so the airway can be kept open and treatment can be started immediately.

to soothe the child and keep him calm and happy will certainly help," says Birt Harvey, M.D., professor of pediatrics at Stanford University School of Medicine in Stanford, California. He recommends "holding, rocking, cuddling and talking—anything that will help soothe the child."

Adds Dr. Rappaport: "The calmer the child is, the more likely he'll breathe normally."

Go outdoors. "If it's a cool night, exposing your child to the cool night air can help add humidity and moisture," adds Dr. Harvey. "Just make sure to keep your child bundled up."

Ban the milk bottle. Milk and other dairy products cause more phlegm, just adding to congestion. "Eliminating milk won't cure croup, but avoiding it will make it easier for your child to breathe," says Dr. Wendelberger. "Instead of milk, try giving a child with croup clear liquids like water or apple juice, especially before bedtime."

Hold baby's head high. Keeping your child upright helps make breathing easier, adds Dr. Harvey.

Cuts and Scrapes

No offense to Mom's healing kisses, but you might need more than tender loving care to help you handle everyday scrapes and cuts. Here's some practical medicine for you—and for Kid Katastrophe, with his always-scraped knee.

Give the wound a hold. "The first thing you should do to any cut or scrape is apply pressure on it, so you stop the bleeding," says Las Vegas orthopedic surgeon Michael Rask, M.D., chairman of the American Academy of Neurological and Orthopedic Surgeons and the American Board of Ringside Medicine and Surgery. If possible, wrap a *clean*, absorbent cloth or towel around the wound and press your hand against it. If no such compress is available, press

When to See the Doctor

Although self-treatment is the Rx for most cuts and scrapes, doctors advise that you should seek emergency medical treatment when:

- Blood is spurting and it's bright red in color. This suggests you may have punctured an artery.
- The wound is large and deep enough to see "inside." This suggests you may need stitches.
- You can't wash out all the debris. If bacteria-laden dirt is inside the cut, there's a good probability of infection.
- The wound is on your face, your genitals or another area where you don't want a permanent scar.
- The wound develops redness, streaks or weeping pus that extends more than a finger's width beyond the cut.

Take the Boo-Hoo out of Boo-Boos

To remove adhesive strips without stripping your skin, use nail scissors to separate the gauze part in the center from the adhesive, says Nelson Lee Novick, M.D., associate clinical professor of dermatology at Mount Sinai School of Medicine in New York City. Lift off the gauze center, then gently pull the adhesive strips from your skin on either side.

If the scab is stuck to the bandage, however, soak the area in a mixture of warm water and salt—about a teaspoon of salt for each gallon of water. The dressing will eventually free itself.

To remove bandages from areas with hair, pull in the direction of hair growth. But first wet down your skin in the shower or use cotton balls or a swab soaked in plain tap water to moisten the adhesive before pulling.

the wound with your fingers for at least 60 seconds—releasing the pressure as soon as bleeding has been reduced. Then elevate the wounded area above the level of your heart to slow down blood flow.

Put on some cold. Once bleeding is controlled, apply an ice pack wrapped in a towel to constrict blood vessels and *stop* bleeding, adds Dr. Rask. But leave the cold pack on for *only* 15 minutes, or until the area begins to feel numb. Clean the wound. After 10 minutes, reapply the ice pack for another 15 minutes. You can repeat this 15-on, 10-off procedure a number of times.

Take your time to clean it. When you wash out the wound, do it thoroughly. You can use soap and water, hydrogen peroxide, a drugstore-bought antibacterial agent or even contact lens saline solution. "The secret here is to wash it thoroughly, for no less than a minute or two," says Robert D. Aranosian, D.O., trauma director at Pontiac Osteopathic Hospital in Pontiac, Michigan, and past president of the American College of Osteopathic Emergency Physicians. "If you're not cleaning the wound for at least 60 seconds, you're not cleaning it well enough."

Go undercover the first day. After washing the cut or scrape, apply an over-the-counter antibacterial ointment and cover the wound with a bandage for at least 24 hours. "The bandage should be loosely tented over the wound, not applied tightly like tape," says Nelson Lee Novick, M.D., associate clinical professor of dermatology at Mount Sinai School of Medicine in New York City. "You want to protect it from dirt while minimizing external irritation."

Read ointment labels. In picking an antibacterial ointment—which helps prevent infection and shorten healing time—look for the active ingredients bacitracin or polymyxin B, contained in over-the-counter products such as Polysporin. Dr. Novick also recommends plain Aquaphor ointment, which doesn't have antibacterial qualities "but can often be just as effective."

Give it air. You want to keep the bandage on if the cut will be exposed to anything that might infect it. And you also need a bandage if the wound would rub against other areas. "But if it's a minor wound and it won't be exposed to anything that will infect it, remove the bandage and let the wound heal in the open air," says Dr. Aranosian.

Keep cleaning. Whether you bandage or not, you must continue to clean the wound daily. But after the initial cleaning, forget the soap and water. "Soap is notoriously drying on your skin, and water is also a drying agent," according to Dr. Novick. "You want to keep the wound as moist as possible, so the wound heals with less crusting." (With less crusting, you aren't as likely to get a "dented mark" or scar where the wound is.) Instead of using soap and water, Dr. Novick recommends that you clean the area with plain tap water and apply an antibiotic ointment every day.

Cysts

Sometimes unpleasant things just happen without any reason. You get caught in a downpour without an umbrella. You get a flat tire on the way to the airport. You spill ketchup on your suit a few minutes before an important meeting. Or you get a cyst.

In a world of random events, getting a cyst is right up there with the least of the least explainable. Doctors don't know for certain how or why they develop.

Cysts are permanent little lumps, usually harmless and almost always painless, that can appear anywhere on your body but especially around the head, neck and back. The surface of a cyst is smooth, but underneath there's some problem that causes the swelling—a buildup of the body's natural oil (sebum), layers of impacted hair follicles or layers of accumulated skin scales.

Usually it's no big deal. You might see an enlarged, dark pore on the surface, and sometimes there's a bit of oozing. With doctor-prescribed medications and some surgical procedures, a cyst can be treated or removed. But as long as the cyst is not infected and doesn't burst, you can usually just live with it. In fact, the leading advice from dermatologists is:

Let it be. "If the cyst is small and unobtrusive, if it doesn't hurt or itch and if it isn't red or tender, then you can just leave it alone," says Jack L. Lesher, Jr., M.D., associate professor of dermatology at the Medical College of Georgia in Augusta. A hands-off policy is best for any cyst. Don't touch, pick, paw, squeeze or manipulate it in any way. If the cyst is in a position where it can easily be bumped or scratched, shield it with a gauze pad or some moleskin.

Apply warm compresses. Is the cyst red, oozing its contents or just plain sore? Place a washcloth soaked in warm (not hot) water over the irritated cyst several times a day, says Loretta S. Davis, M.D., assistant professor of dermatology at the Medical College of Georgia. "This will increase the blood circulation to the area, quieting down an angry cyst."

Wash and dress a ruptured cyst. "If a cyst should rupture and drain, you run the risk of developing a severe infection," according to dermatologist Joseph

When to See the Doctor

Any unusual growth or mark on your skin that you're not sure about should be checked by your doctor. It could be cancerous. And even a benign cyst can warrant special medical attention.

"If a cyst appears to be growing, if it hurts or itches or if it's swollen and oozing profusely, it may be showing signs of serious infection," says Jack L. Lesher, Jr., M.D., associate professor of dermatology at the Medical College of Georgia in Augusta. "You'll need to see a dermatologist to have the cyst surgically removed or treated with antibiotics."

There's also a chance of severe infection after a cyst bursts or ruptures, so be sure to see the doctor if this occurs.

Bark, M.D., past chairman of the Department of Dermatology at St. Joseph's Hospital in Lexington, Kentucky. "Wash it with soap and water, dab on some hydrogen peroxide with a cotton ball, and apply an antibacterial ointment such as Polysporin. Cover the area with a bandage or gauze pad to keep dirt off it until a doctor can check it out."

Never, ever remove a cyst yourself. "Bathroom surgery is the worst thing you can do for a cyst," says Dr. Davis. "If you squeeze it, some of the contents will probably be forced deeper into the skin. Your body will view it as foreign material and react with an extreme inflammation. Infection may also occur. You'll succeed only in turning a quiet cyst into an angry one, as well as in leaving a scar."

Dandruff

Everyone has dandruff—at least *some* dandruff—and that includes bald people. That's because every human scalp sheds dead cells, which "flake" off as new ones are pushed up from deeper skin layers. When these flakes become obvious on our hair and clothing, we call them dandruff. Perfectly natural stuff—but too often, we're made to feel as though this "problem" falls somewhere between global warming and playing high-stakes poker with someone named Ace.

In reality, there's nothing unusual about dandruff, and it definitely *doesn't* mean you're going bald. But here's how to remedy this nuisance if you're itching for some answers.

Bag the mousse. "A lot of times, what we call dandruff is not really a scalp problem at all but rather the result of using hair sprays, styling gels and mousse," says Nelson Lee Novick, M.D., associate clinical professor of dermatology at Mount Sinai School of Medicine in New York City. "Some of these products cause the flakiness that we think of as dandruff—particularly hair sprays when they're used to excess."

Hit the showers. If you ignore dandruff or the flakiness associated with the use of hair cosmetics, you allow scale to build, resulting in itchiness and possible infection, says Maria Hordinsky, M.D., associate professor of dermatology at the University of Minnesota Medical School in Minneapolis and the director of the Center for Hair Diseases at the University of Minnesota. Most experts say that shampooing often—daily, if necessary—with a specially medicated "dandruff" shampoo is the best way to control this problem.

Take five to do it right. What you may not know about that special shampoo is *how* to use it. "You've got to leave the shampoo on the scalp for a full five minutes," says Thomas Goodman, Jr., M.D., assistant professor of dermatology at the University of Tennessee Center for Health Sciences in Memphis. "If you leave it on for less time, you're undermining the shampoo's effectiveness."

Spread some oil. "Massaging some heated pure virgin olive oil into the scalp and then vigorously brushing with a natural-bristle hairbrush helps loosen dandruff scales," says Markus Bluestein, a St. Louis hair stylist and makeup consultant. "It's also an excellent way to treat a dry scalp—the cause of much of the flaky, 'snowy' dandruff. You should microwave the oil until it's warm to the touch and apply it no more than twice a week. Each time, leave it on for about 20 minutes and then wash it out with a good shampoo."

Beat the tar out of it. If your scalp is oily rather than dry, you'll see "chunkier" dandruff that looks greasy and has a yellowish tint. Go with a tar-based shampoo such as Ionil T or Neutrogena's T/Gel. If you have blond or graying hair, however, stay away from tar shampoos, because they can give your hair a brownish tint, warns Patricia Farris, M.D., a dermatologist and

When to See the Doctor

Severe dandruff is actually a disease known as seborrheic dermatitis that requires prescription medications. See a doctor if you have:
- Scalp irritation or persistent itchiness.
- Thick scale despite regular use of dandruff shampoos.
- Yellowish crusting.
- Red patches, especially along the neckline.

clinical assistant professor at Tulane University School of Medicine in New Orleans.

Invest extra thyme. A potion made with thyme is believed to have medicinal powers that help dandruff when the solution is rinsed into the hair after shampooing, says New York City hair stylist Louis Gignac, owner of Louis-Guy D Salon and author of *Everything You Need to Know to Have Great-Looking Hair.* Boil four heaping tablespoons of dried thyme in two cups of water for ten minutes. Strain it and allow the brew to cool. Then pour half over your just-shampooed hair while it's still damp. Massage in gently and *don't* rinse. (Store the rest in the refrigerator for another treatment.)

Dark Circles under the Eyes

D ark circles under your eyes might reveal a couple of "dark truths" about your personal health. They usually occur when you're overtired or developing an illness or an allergy. They can also result from losing a lot of weight. But the discolorations—the result of engorged blood vessels around your eyes—are themselves medically harmless. In fact, sometimes they're not even an indication of physical problems. "They may be frightening, but probably the best thing you can do is to stop worrying about them," says Merrill M. Knopf, M.D., an ophthalmologist in Long Beach, California, and an officer of the California Association of Ophthalmology.

And they tend to run in families, so you're more likely to get them if your parents or grandparents had them. While you can't do anything about the inheritance factor, you might be able to try a few tactics to make those dark circles a bit lighter.

Give them the washcloth treatment. "Applying a cold compress helps constrict blood vessels and turns tissue white, so the 'darkness' doesn't show as much," says Eric Donnenfeld, M.D., associate professor of ophthalmology at North Shore University Hospital/Cornell Medical College in Manhasset, New York. He advises regularly applying a washcloth wrung out in cold water for 10 to 15 minutes, or longer when dark circles are more noticeable.

Address those allergies. In children especially, the sudden onset of dark circles means allergies. "Simply removing the offending allergen will usually solve the problem and get rid of the dark circles," says Dr. Knopf. The most common allergens are pet dander, house dust, pollen and foods such as wheat, milk and chocolate. (Because detection and elimination of these allergens is a complicated process, you should take your child to an allergist if the condition persists.)

Cover them up. Many cosmetics will cover up dark circles. "There's a product called Clinique Continuous Cover that hides dark circles under the eyes," says Dr. Knopf. Dermablend, a product used to cover black eyes, is also very effective at hiding dark circles.

Denture Problems

A lot has changed since George Washington chewed over America's early problems with wooden teeth. But some things never change—like the problems caused by a new set of dentures: slipping, sore gums, excess saliva (or not enough of it) and difficulty chewing or talking.

True, the nation's 23 million denture wearers have it a lot easier than their whittle-toothed forefathers, thanks to advances in denture technology. "But most people don't realize how long it takes to *really* get used to a new set of dentures," says Frank Wiebelt, D.D.S., associate professor and chairman of the Department of Removable Prosthodontics at the College of Dentistry at the University of Oklahoma Health Sciences Center in Oklahoma City. "For most people, it takes between four and six weeks."

During that time, a new set of choppers may need a hopperful of early adjustments, which can lead to plenty of frustrations. But before you let frustrations get the upper hand and you toss those new dentures across your neighborhood river, try these problem solvers that the Father of Our Country never knew.

Steam your vegetables. "You tend to bite your cheek or tongue when you get a new set of dentures—particularly your first set," says Dr. Wiebelt. To avoid

When to See the Doctor

Occasionally dentures may cause problems that can't be treated at home.

"You should see a dentist immediately if you have prolonged gum bleeding," says Frank Wiebelt, D.D.S., associate professor and chairman of the Department of Removable Prosthodontics at the College of Dentistry at the University of Oklahoma Health Sciences Center in Oklahoma City. Other reasons to see a dentist:

• You get a swelling around the mouth that extends up under the eye.
• You get swelling in the throat that makes swallowing difficult.
• Lumps, bumps or sores appear in the mouth.

These may be signs of gum disease, infection or other conditions that will require medical treatment, according to Dr. Wiebelt.

this, chew slowly. Also, stay away from raw vegetables or anything else that's crunchy or difficult to chew. "It's funny, because one of the first things my patients want to eat when they get new dentures is a steak and a salad, and both are among the most difficult things to eat," he says. "A steak is very tough. And believe it or not, lettuce is also difficult to chew. So eat your vegetables, but eat them steamed, and try to avoid anything that's tough for the first two weeks or so."

Read out loud. New dentures can make talking difficult for the first week or so. One of the best ways to overcome this problem is to read out loud, advises Jerry F. Taintor, D.D.S., an endodontist in Memphis, Tennessee. As you're reading, listen to your pronunciation and your diction and correct what doesn't sound right.

"Keep in mind that you're probably more aware of any changes in speech than anyone else is. But any time you speak out loud—whether reading or just talking to yourself in the car—you help yourself accommodate more quickly," says Dr. Wiebelt.

Videotape yourself. A videotape can help you, suggests George A. Murrell, D.D.S., a prosthodontist in Manhattan Beach, California. A videotape allows you to see what others see when you're talking. And a dentist can use the pictures to determine any problems in jaw or lip movements.

Massage your gums. To relieve sore gums associated with new dentures, massage your gums several times a day, following this routine recommended by Richard Shepard, D.D.S., a dentist in Durango, Colorado. Place your thumb and index finger over your gum, with your index finger on the outside. Massage each section of sore gum by squeezing and rubbing with your thumb and finger. This will promote circulation and give your gums a healthy firmness.

Drink a lot of water. New denture wearers often suffer from either dry mouth or excessive saliva. Either way, frequent sips of water will solve the problem, says Dr. Wiebelt. "Excessive saliva results because the mouth can't tell the difference between the dentures and food in the early going. By sipping water, you wash away the excessive saliva that can cause a gagging or sick feeling." Sucking on hard candy also helps dry mouth, but sipping water is better, especially for people who are overweight, have diabetes or suffer from serious tooth decay.

Don't use adhesives. If you're having trouble with dentures slipping, don't reach for a denture adhesive. If you continually add denture creams and powder, a layer builds up between gums and dentures, which can cause the gum and bone to shrink over time, says Dr. Wiebelt. "The best thing to do is just wait

Are Your Dentures the Right Fit?

It takes more than a month for most people to adjust to new dentures. But don't wait that long if you notice any of these symptoms, which can indicate a problem in the fit of your set.
- Teeth don't meet properly. "When you close your mouth, the top and bottom dentures should meet at both sides of your mouth," says Frank Wiebelt, D.D.S., associate professor and chairman of the Department of Removable Prosthodontics at the College of Dentistry at the University of Oklahoma Health Sciences Center in Oklahoma City. "If they meet only on one side, that's one sign the fit is wrong."
- The denture "teeth" are too long, resulting in problems with closing your mouth. (Your dentist can simply file down the teeth that are too long.)
- Dentures continually cut into your gums or cheeks.

Cleaning Your Dentures

The best way to clean dentures and keep your breath fresh is to brush your dentures *nightly* with regular hand soap and lukewarm water, using a soft-bristle toothbrush. "If you're going to use toothpastes, don't use any brand advertised as a whitener. Those toothpastes are too abrasive for the denture surface," says Frank Wiebelt, D.D.S., associate professor and chairman of the Department of Removable Prosthodontics at the College of Dentistry at the University of Oklahoma Health Sciences Center in Oklahoma City.

Other tips:

Wear your glasses. If you wear glasses for reading or close work, put them on when you're cleaning your dentures. And make sure you have plenty of light. Your eyesight and lighting conditions should be optimal for a good cleaning. Dentures won't be cleaned properly through "feeling."

Clean dentures over a filled sink. That way, if you drop your dentures, the water will break the fall and prevent chipping. Alternatively, clean them over a thick towel.

Brush your gums and tongue. Even though you have dentures instead of a full set of teeth, brushing is important, because bacteria still invade the gums and tongue. Brush with a soft-bristle brush to remove bacteria and keep breath fresh. Toothpaste is optional. Rinse with salty water.

it out, because slipping problems usually end in a week or so. If they last longer, there's probably a problem with the fit, and you should see your dentist." If you *must* use adhesives, be sure to clean your dentures and your gums thoroughly each night to remove all the adhesive.

Depression

Depression used to be such a depressing subject that people often felt compelled to fake a smile and keep their anxious, sad feelings inside. Not anymore. Ever since researchers started to discover the mix of psychological and physical causes for this problem, depression has seemed much less mysterious and forbidding. People are acknowledging it, and talking about it, out in the open.

There's even something called healthy depression, according to Ellen McGrath, Ph.D., former chairperson of the American Psychological Association's National Task Force on Women and Depression. Dr. McGrath is the author of *When Feeling Bad Is Good*, which discusses in more detail the concepts of healthy and unhealthy depression and offers strategies for action.

"*Healthy depression* is defined as realistic feelings of pain, sadness and disappointment, accompanied at times by guilt, anger and/or anxiety, that stem from a negative experience such as trauma, loss and unfair treatment," Dr. McGrath explains. People experiencing healthy depression can still function, although usually not as well as they would otherwise.

Unhealthy depression involves being unable to function in one or more areas of life, such as work or relationships, due to the depth of bad feelings. "These bad feelings can be caused by changes in body chemistry, genetic vulnerability and/or too many painful psychological experiences that you are unable to resolve," says Dr. McGrath.

You can take healthy depression as a signal that it's time to make some changes and take some actions in your life, according to Dr. McGrath. While unhealthy depression will benefit from the same approach, it first requires professional help—the sooner, the better.

There are countless ways to tackle depression, from exercise to drugs to support groups. Often it's a combination of things—getting organized, learning new behaviors, becoming more self-aware—that finally breaks depression's hold.

The following tips can help you deal with life's normal ups and downs and perhaps help you bounce back faster from the downs.

Take the high road. Or the low road—it doesn't matter. Just get out there and *move*. "I tell my patients 'The odds are good to excellent that if you exercise, you will be virtually depression-free in three to five weeks,'" says psychologist Keith Johnsgard, Ph.D., professor emeritus of psychology at San Jose State University in San Jose, California, and author of *The Exercise Prescription for Depression and Anxiety*.

Studies are clear on this. The less active you are, the more likely you'll be depressed. "And a dozen or so studies show that all but the most severely depressed people who begin to exercise do as well as those who get standard psychotherapy," Dr. Johnsgard says. His exercise Rx: an hour a day of brisk walking.

What if you're too bummed out to boogie? "Get a family member or friend to come and drag you around the block a few times," he says.

Stay up to watch the sunrise. Some studies show that approximately 60 percent of depressed people who deprive themselves of a night's sleep may help thwart their symptoms, but the effects last only until the next time they sleep, says Ronald Salomon, M.D., assistant professor of psychiatry at Yale University

When to See the Doctor

Experts at the National Institute for Mental Health in Bethesda, Maryland, suggest that anyone who experiences four or more of the following symptoms of depression for more than two weeks should seek professional help.

- Persistent sad, anxious or "empty" feelings
- Feelings of hopelessness and/or pessimism
- Feelings of guilt, worthlessness and/or helplessness
- Loss of interest or pleasure in ordinary activities, including sex
- Sleep disturbances (including insomnia, early-morning waking and/or oversleeping)
- Eating disturbances (changes in appetite and/or weight loss or gain)
- Decreased energy, fatigue and/or a feeling of being "slowed down"
- Thoughts of death or suicide, or suicide attempts
- Restlessness and/or irritability
- Difficulty in concentrating, remembering and/or making decisions

School of Medicine in New Haven, Connecticut. And if you use sleep deprivation for more than a night or two in one week, the mood-enhancing effects may drop off significantly, he says.

Cultivate friends. "Being able to develop and maintain intimate, supportive relationships with other people is the survival skill of the 1990s," according to Dr. McGrath. "These relationships are critical to our health."

Realize that it takes time and effort to build these special relationships—then get to work! "Do everything and anything you can to develop the skills it takes to have quality relationships," she says. That includes learning communication skills, improving self-esteem and taking the time to be with people, Dr. McGrath says.

Know that action equals power. "Talking about your fears and anger can be helpful, but for women, it isn't enough to avert depression," says Dr. McGrath. "Taking some positive action, on the other hand, creates its own energy, which leads to a feeling of power and control." She suggests ritual actions—burning a list of worries, for instance—and real actions—such as getting organized, getting enough sleep or delegating household chores—as ways to convert uncomfortable feelings into positive action.

Tell your internal critic to take a hike. Do you have a little (or a big) voice inside you that insists nothing you do is right? That you're never going to get what you want?

"Rather than trying to get it to go away, which it never does, change your response to it," suggests Michael D. Yapko, Ph.D., a clinical psychologist in San Diego and author of *Free Yourself from Depression*. "Rather than just believing what it tells you, say to yourself 'Okay, I understand that there is this critical voice, but I don't have to listen to it.'"

People with high self-esteem also have this critical voice, Dr. Yapko says. "But they know to ignore it or at least respond to it as though what it's saying isn't true."

Don't take things so personally. "Because I don't return your phone call, you decide that I must be angry with you. That's personalizing," Dr. Yapko explains.

The problem with personalizing is that it's not a very objective way to look at things. "You jump to the first plausible conclusion, but is that the true explanation?" he asks.

A key strategy for jettisoning this kind of faulty negative thinking is to generate multiple explanations for important things that happen. "Consider a variety of possibilities and look for facts. That, at least, puts you in reality," he says.

Avoid all-or-none thinking. Do you get a C on an exam and feel like a failure? Do you miss out on a promotion at work and feel like a loser? If so, you tend to see things in black and white, with little or no gray in between. Few things in life are so extreme.

"Depressed people tend to have a low frustration tolerance," Dr. Yapko says. "They want immediate answers and immediate clarity. Typically, that's the way they've learned to be. And that's why they get depressed, because life choices are rarely clear and often ambiguous."

Learning to recognize and live with life's uncertainties is a key strategy for avoiding depression.

Get to know yourself better. "People often get depressed when they aren't doing what they want to be doing," Dr. Yapko says. "They may want to play, for example, but feel they must always work." Fortunately, everyday life gives you the opportunity to ask yourself important, self-defining questions, he says. "Who are you? What do you want out of life? What are the things that really matter to you? What things do you need to include in your life that are uniquely you? Make sure you build those things into your life."

Do a medicine chest shakedown. "Many drugs can cause depression," says Arthur Jacknowitz, Pharm.D., professor and chairman of clinical pharmacy at West Virginia University School of Pharmacy in Morgantown. The most likely culprits are high blood pressure medications, anti-arrhythmic drugs, prednisone and similar corticosteroids, glaucoma medications, sedatives such as Xanax and Valium, oral contraceptives and some over-the-counter drugs containing antihistamines.

"Symptoms of drug-related depression may not surface right away," explains Dr. Jacknowitz. "So even if you've been taking a medication for six months to a year and then begin to experience the blues, it could still be your medication." Discuss the problem with your doctor, he suggests. It may be possible to taper off the use of the drug or to switch to another.

Diabetes

W ho'd think you can be *too* sweet? Well, it's possible. If you have diabetes, all that extra sugar (or glucose) floating around in your bloodstream can lead to trouble—nerve damage, vision loss, infections, poor circulation, kidney and heart problems, you name it. That's why it's so important to get blood sugar down to a normal level.

Normally the food we eat is converted into glucose and used or stored by the body with little problem. Circulating insulin hormone stimulates the uptake of sugar by the body's cells. But with diabetes, something goes awry. The pancreas, which is the organ responsible for producing insulin, becomes irresponsible. It either stops producing the hormone completely (Type I diabetes) or else produces too much, which leads to insulin resistance (Type II diabetes). Either way, concentration of sugar in the blood shoots sky-high.

People with Type I, or insulin-dependent, diabetes need daily insulin injections. Those with Type II, or non-insulin-dependent, diabetes—the most common form of the disease—usually don't need insulin injections. But 25 percent of them take drugs to improve sugar metabolism.

Treating Type II diabetes with drugs *does* reduce blood sugar, it's true. But in many cases, doctors are electing to treat Type II patients with diet and exercise. They find that this lifestyle approach does more than just reduce blood sugar.

"It does a *lot* more," says James Barnard, Ph.D., professor of physiological science at the University of California, Los Angeles, and consultant to the Pritikin Longevity Center in Santa Monica. "The same regimen that puts diabetes on hold has a favorable impact on high cholesterol, high blood pressure and obesity." Those three, along with high blood sugar, are what doctors call the deadly quartet.

Here's what doctors are recommending to treat diabetes with diet and exercise. To determine what's appropriate for your individual situation, it's important that you check with your doctor before making changes.

Peel off some pounds. Most people with Type II diabetes are 30 to 60 pounds overweight, and for them, losing weight is often the *only* thing they

155

have to do to get their diabetes under control, Dr. Barnard says. Several studies point out that it's not necessary to reach your normal weight to see a big drop in blood glucose, he adds. "Ten pounds may make a difference."

But don't go to extremes. Fad diets, fasting and skipping meals don't work. Decreasing dietary fat is the best approach if you're overweight. One way is to decrease total fat to no more than 50 grams daily, says Christine Beebe, R.D., director of the diabetes program at St. James Hospital in Chicago Heights, Illinois, and chairman of the Council on Nutritional Science and Metabolism for the American Diabetes Association.

Get moving. "Spend 45 minutes to one hour taking a good brisk walk every day," Dr. Barnard says. "It helps normalize body weight, and it helps correct insulin resistance, which is the main problem in Type II diabetes."

Stay regular as clockwork. "If you take insulin or insulin-stimulating drugs, as some people with Type II diabetes do, exercising at the same time three to six days a week for the same amount of time can be helpful," says Beebe. "That makes it easier to control your blood sugar."

If you *don't* exercise every day, pay particular attention on the days that you do. "You may need to cut your insulin dose 30 to 50 percent," Beebe says.

Change flab to firm. Muscle building and weight training can play an important role in diabetes control. "Having more muscle and less fat improves insulin sensitivity, so less insulin is needed to respond to sugar in the blood," says Bruce W. Craig, Ph.D., associate director of exercise science at Ball State University in Muncie, Indiana. "It means people with diabetes may be able to reduce their insulin intake and still handle the sugar in their blood—their glucose—effectively." Once you get your doctor's okay, join a health club that has weight-training equipment. Ask the club for professional instruction before you begin.

Cut the fat. At the Pritikin Longevity Center, the diet is carefully designed to cut out fat. Meals at the center are super low in fat, with less than 10 percent of calories from fat, 10 to 15 percent from protein and 75 to 80 percent from carbohydrates (such as veggies and fruits). What does that look like on your plate? Grains and beans, vegetables, fruits, nonfat milk and an occasional piece of fish or fowl. The good part is that except for the meat, you get to eat as much as you want. Adds Dr. Barnard: "Any reduction in fat is going to help your diabetes and your overall health."

When to See the Doctor

If you have diabetes, you should work closely with your doctor, because regular checkups are a must.

So if you're planning to start exercising, or if you want to change your diet, it's important that your doctor be involved from the start.

And because diet and exercise can have an immediate and profound impact on glucose metabolism and insulin levels, if you're taking insulin or insulin-stimulating drugs, your doctor should advise you regarding your dosage. "People may need to reduce their dosage within a day or two of starting to exercise to avoid low blood sugar," according to James Barnard, Ph.D., professor of physiological science at the University of California, Los Angeles, and consultant to the Pritikin Longevity Center in Santa Monica.

And cut the sugar. "This is becoming a real problem, because many low-fat or fat-free foods now on the market have a lot of refined sugar added to make them taste good. People with diabetes need to avoid most refined sugar," according to Dr. Barnard. "It really causes problems for them." His advice: Skip the sugar and satisfy your sweet tooth with fruit. Read the labels and buy low-fat foods sweetened with artificial sweeteners.

Be especially particular about breakfast. "There's some evidence that those with diabetes have a harder time with carbohydrates in the morning, when insulin resistance is greatest," Beebe says. Reducing carbohydrates and adding protein might be your best bet. Try skim milk and oatmeal, for example, or an occasional poached egg with a slice of whole wheat toast, or cottage cheese and crackers. Check your blood glucose before lunch to see how you're doing. The next day you can adjust your food intake further, if necessary.

Treat booze like fat. Alcohol is high in empty calories. "We recommend that people keep their alcohol consumption down to fewer than three drinks a week," Dr. Barnard says.

Chrome-plate your diet. Make sure you're getting enough chromium, a trace mineral that helps normalize blood sugar levels—high *or* low (it gives

157

insulin a boost). In fact, in some cases, chromium may help *prevent* Type II diabetes.

Studies show that the typical American does not get nearly enough chromium in his diet, even when calorie intake is fairly high, says Richard A. Anderson, Ph.D., a biochemist at the U.S. Department of Agriculture Human Nutrition Research Center in Beltsville, Maryland. "Regardless of how you cut the cards, you're not getting enough chromium in your diet," he says. "Even diets designed by dietitians don't provide nearly enough chromium."

His suggestion: Take a chromium supplement in addition to a balanced multivitamin/mineral supplement. "In our studies, we use 200 micrograms a day, and that works very well," says Dr. Anderson. But check with your doctor before taking any supplemental dose.

Honor the East when you eat. Laboratory tests show that cinnamon and turmeric (the golden spice used in curry dishes) *triple* the ability of insulin to metabolize glucose, says Dr. Anderson. "There's a long history of spices being used in the treatment of diabetes, especially in India, Pakistan and China," he says. If cooking is your thing, get a couple of oriental cookbooks that have tasty recipes using these spices. And look for curry dishes when you dine out.

Diaper Rash

Whether your child consists of snips, snails and puppy dogs' tails or sugar, spice and everything nice, it all seems to come out the other end as one disgusting, irritating mess that turns baby's soft, sweet bottom into something that resembles a swamp. And from this mire—as surely as babies cry and backsides itch—comes diaper rash.

The good news about diaper rash is that half the time, it clears up within one day. The bad news? If your child's latest case is the long, lingering kind, it could keep Junior's backside looking red, irritated and nasty for many days. But here's how to rush away that rash and prevent it from returning.

Use "gel" disposable diapers. If you go the disposable route, choose diapers with the newer absorbent gelling material. "These diapers pull wetness away

Wipe Out Soap and Baby Wipes

Two of the most widely used products to clean baby bottoms and protect them from diaper rash cause the biggest pains in that area—both literally and figuratively.

"Commercially sold baby wipes contain alcohol, which aggravates diaper rash and causes a lot of pain," says Becky Luttkus, head instructor at the National Academy of Nannies in Denver. "Besides the pain they cause, some wipes actually promote diaper rash because of chemicals they contain."

Soap is another no-no for those with diaper rash. It is too harsh on the sensitive skin and also causes pain in the area. "Instead, you should rinse off the baby's bottom with plain, cool water," adds Luttkus. "Baths should be free of soap if your baby has a problem with diaper rash."

from the skin better than other types of diapers, and they also keep the skin's pH level more acidic, resulting in less diaper rash," says Alfred T. Lane, M.D., associate professor of dermatology and pediatrics at Stanford University School of Medicine in Stanford, California. Most major brands of disposable diapers have this gelling material.

Rinse cloth diapers with vinegar. If you have reusable cloth diapers, rinse them in vinegar during the wash to change the pH and help reduce diaper rash. "Just add ¼ cup of plain white kitchen vinegar to each load of diapers during the final rinse cycle of your wash," suggests Becky Luttkus, head instructor at the National Academy of Nannies in Denver. Also, don't use fabric softeners when washing diapers, because the softeners put a coating on the diapers that keeps them from absorbing as well, adds Luttkus.

Apply warm cornstarch. Store-bought "baby" (talcum) powders do *nothing* to treat diaper rash, according to studies by British researchers. "What may be tried instead is to take cornstarch, spread it out across a baking pan and warm it in an oven at 150°F for about ten minutes, so it's really dry. Test the temperature first. Then lightly dust it onto the baby's bottom," suggests Birt Harvey, M.D., professor of pediatrics at Stanford University School of Medicine. The cornstarch is as "smooth" as baby powder, yet it is less expensive and appears to be more effective.

159

Blow-dry that bottom. Keeping the infected area clean and dry promotes healing, but a towel can be too abrasive for the baby's battered bottom. "You can dry the baby just as effectively using a hair dryer set on the low (or cool) setting. Use the dryer for about three minutes," says Luttkus.

Don't fasten diapers. "Probably the best thing you can do is leave diapers off as much as possible, so the skin can air out. But since that isn't always advisable, try to place the diaper under the baby when he's lying on his stomach. You can do this during naps and other times when he's still," says Dr. Harvey.

Use paper instead of plastic. If your baby has excess leakage—which can contribute to diaper rash—place a paper towel between his skin and the diaper, advises Luttkus. The paper towel helps stop leakage, but without blocking air circulation. The disadvantage of a plastic diaper cover is that it "seals in" the moisture.

Breastfeed your baby. Various studies show that babies who are initially breastfed have a much lower incidence and severity of diaper rash than infants fed baby formula. In fact, the effects due to dietary influences are evident even after the infants are weaned, says John L. Hammons, Ph.D., a staff chemist at Procter & Gamble Company in Cincinnati who conducted one such study.

Diarrhea

As they say in football, the best offense is a good defense. And diarrhea is your body's best *offensive* defense. Whether its much-ballyhooed revenge can be blamed on Montezuma, the blue plate special, a disagreeable antibiotic, a sneaky viral infection or even stress, diarrhea is the body's painful way of saying "No, thanks!"

Sure, diarrhea lacks a certain something in elegance, but it sure makes up for it in effectiveness. A couple of trips to the toilet (okay, so maybe *more* than just a couple) and you're usually back on your feet.

Although it typically takes nature anywhere from two to four days to run this course, here's how to help take the kick out of the "runs."

Be clear on your diet. Most folks know that liquids are the suggested nourishment for the first 24 hours when diarrhea hits. But don't assume that any old liquid will do. "You should take only clear liquids: If you *can't* see through it, stay away from it," says William B. Ruderman, M.D., chairman of the Department of Gastroenterology at the Cleveland Clinic–Florida in Fort Lauderdale and an expert on diarrhea. "That means you *should* consume soda, tea, bouillon and apple juice. Sports drinks like Gatorade are especially good, because they replace sugars and electrolytes (potassium and sodium). But *avoid* acidic citrus juices, such as orange and grapefruit, and *especially* tomato juice." Exceptions? Beer doesn't qualify, even though you can see through it. Nor do wine, clear alcohol and mixed drinks. In fact, too much beer, wine or any other kind of alcohol can cause diarrhea.

Food-wise, the best choices after the initial 24 hours include "translucent" foods like chicken broth and Jell-O. Whatever you choose to eat at this time should be bland and easily digested.

Get cultured with yogurt. One of the few exceptions to the clear cuisine rule is yogurt, whose active cultures contain "good" bacteria your bowel loses to the "bad" bacteria that prompted the diarrhea. "Yogurt is especially effective when the diarrhea is caused by food poisoning (like traveler's diarrhea)," says Manfred Kroger, Ph.D., professor of food science at Pennsylvania State University in University Park. "And it's also effective when diarrhea is the result of

---

When to See the Doctor

See your doctor if your diarrhea symptoms include any of the following.
- A sustained fever of over 101°F
- Abdominal pain more severe than the "churning stomach" sensation normally associated with diarrhea
- No progress or a worsened condition after three or four days
- Blood, pus or mucus in your stool
- Inability to keep liquids down, lasting for more than 24 hours—or other signs of dehydration such as constant, extreme thirst, tongue dryness, sunken eyeballs and cracked or dry lips

Although these may be symptoms of minor ailments, all require a doctor's attention for diagnosis.

stress or antibiotic or radiation treatment. Basically, yogurt's active cultures help Mother Nature speed up the process of replacing the beneficial benign bacteria, and it makes you feel a lot better faster." If yogurt isn't your thing, any acidophilus or fermented dairy product will do. Check the supermarket's dairy case.

Exercise your sweet tooth. A spoonful of sugar helps your body hold on to whatever you're drinking. "Glucose aids the absorption of water by the gut, so if you have sugar in whatever you're taking, you can absorb it more easily," says Dr. Ruderman. "If you're drinking tea or apple juice, add a teaspoonful of sugar to aid in absorption. If you're drinking soda, stick with regular sugared types and stay away from 'diet' varieties." (If you *do* drink soda, he adds, open the cap and let the soda go flat before you imbibe.)

Avoiding Traveler's Diarrhea

Sure, you want to "experience" a foreign country—but only to a point. So here's how travelers can stay one step ahead of the "runs" while abroad, according to William B. Ruderman, M.D., chairman of the Department of Gastroenterology at the Cleveland Clinic–Florida in Fort Lauderdale and an expert on diarrhea.

- "When traveling abroad, drink *only* bottled or canned beverages— including water. Just because you're staying in a fancy hotel, don't assume the water is safe. The hotel gets its water from the same city water supply as everyone else."
- Don't use ice in your drinks. "People think they're safe drinking bottled sodas, but then they use ice, get diarrhea and wonder what happened. It may not be as refreshing, but you're better off with a warm soda."
- Don't eat any food that is unpeeled or raw. "If you're having any local fruit, peel it—even if it's an apple or a pear. And make sure everything you eat is cooked thoroughly."
- Don't assume you're A-OK when traveling in the U.S.A. "I would be suspicious of the water supply in every camping area in the country that's in a backwoods, mountainous area. Take your own water supply."

Forget about high fiber—for now. Now's *not* the time for oat bran and other high-fiber foods or complex carbohydrates. "It's unwise to stress your system with a lot of nonabsorbable fiber," adds Dr. Ruderman. "When you have diarrhea, the blander, the better." That means choose white toast, *not* wheat. And go for light foods such as cooked carrots, applesauce, baked chicken (without the skin) and other things that don't cause gas. Avoid pasta, corn, oats and most fruits, particularly prunes, pears and apples. Also, have some bananas: Diarrhea can cause potassium depletion, and bananas are high in potassium.

Be anti-antacid. Yesterday's heartburn often becomes today's diarrhea, especially when you treat it with over-the-counter medications. "Antacids are the most common cause of drug-related diarrhea," says Harris Clearfield, M.D., professor of medicine and director of the Division of Gastroenterology at Hahnemann University Hospital in Philadelphia. "Maalox and Mylanta both have magnesium hydroxide in them, which acts exactly like milk of magnesia, making these antacids a common cause of diarrhea." Meanwhile, antacids with aluminum hydroxide, such as Riopan and Amphojel, can cause constipation. (True, this is the opposite effect, but it's just as unwanted.)

Keep drinking. "The more you drink, the better you'll be," says Dr. Ruderman. "Even if you're not thirsty, it's important to take in a lot of fluids, because diarrhea can cause dehydration." His advice? At *least* 6 to 8 ounces every two hours. "You should drink between two and three liters a day," Dr. Ruderman adds. That's the equivalent of 1½ 32-ounce bottles of soda.

Note: Drink even more if you haven't urinated in the past six hours, feel thirsty or experience sunken eyeballs. And drink a *lot* if your tongue feels very dry or your lips become dry and start to crack.

Don't assume you'll be in the pink with the pink stuff. If you think diarrhea is the result of something you ate and you also have a fever, *don't* take Pepto-Bismol. "Antidiarrheals such as Pepto-Bismol can *prolong* salmonella (food poisoning)," says Dr. Ruderman. The medication slows down "gut motility"—that is, the speed at which the food moves through your system—so the bad stuff stays in your body longer. (However, if you have familiar traveler's diarrhea, *without* fever, Pepto-Bismol may help.)

Diverticulosis

I t's okay to *act* refined at the dinner table, but when you *eat* that way, don't expect your colon to always keep its good manners.

Living off refined or overly processed foods and other low-fiber fare puts so much pressure on colon walls (as you try to pass hard, dry stools) that they may develop tiny pouches called diverticula. This results in gas, cramping, severe indigestion and even diarrhea or constipation as these pouches become inflamed.

In a worst-case scenario, feces can get stuck in the pouches, causing internal bleeding and serious infection. This condition, called diverticul*itis,* occurs in only about 5 percent of cases and usually requires surgery. But there's a minor form of this problem called diverticul*osis* that's far more common than the version requiring surgery. Many people have learned after seeing their doctor that they can treat diverticulosis themselves. And here's how.

Feast on fiber. "A high-fiber diet is *the* answer for treating diverticulosis," says gastroenterologist Alex Aslan, M.D., a staff physician at North Bay Medical Center in Fairfield, California. "That helps normalize the stool and reduce the pressure on your colon that's causing the problem in the first place."

To get more fiber, limit consumption of processed foods. Instead, always try to eat more whole-grain breads, grains and cereals, beans, fruits and vegetables.

You can also benefit from taking a psyllium product such as Metamucil each day. Psyllium is a natural high-fiber ingredient that can help speed movement in the intestines. Just follow the directions on the package.

Be sure to increase your fiber intake slowly, says Stephen B. Hanauer, M.D., professor of medicine in the Section of Gastroenterology at the University of Chicago Medical Center. And don't give up if you develop some gas symptoms—that's a normal introduction to a high-fiber diet.

When to See the Doctor

More than half of all people over age 60 have diverticulosis, and most in this age group never need serious medical attention, according to doctors. However, you may be developing the more serious (and potentially life-threatening) diverticulitis if you notice fever and severe pain in the lower left portion of your abdominal region.

This might indicate a mild infection that can be handled with antibiotics and rest or a more serious problem or internal bleeding that may require surgery. Either way, only your doctor can tell.

Wet your whistle. While most doctors recommend that everyone should drink no less than six glasses of water a day, it's especially important if you have diverticulosis. Liquids are an important partner to fiber in softening stools and combating constipation, which is associated with diverticulosis, says Samuel Klein, M.D., associate professor of medicine in the Division of Gastroenterology and in the Division of Human Nutrition at the University of Texas Medical School at Galveston.

Don't smoke. "Besides being the single worst thing you can do to your overall health, smoking is terrible for your intestines," says Dr. Hanauer. "What smoking does is increase motility in your intestines, but the nicotine decreases the blood supply. This causes or increases your cramps."

Coffee, no; alcohol, yes, but . . . You should also limit or avoid coffee, since caffeine can cause diarrhea, while chemicals in coffee beans may cause cramping, adds Dr. Aslan. But alcohol in small quantities—no more than two drinks daily—may actually *help* by relaxing colon spasms, says Marvin M. Schuster, M.D., chief of the Department of Digestive Diseases at Francis Scott Key Medical Center in Baltimore.

Hit the road. "Running stimulates bowel activity and is very useful to anyone who is irregular," says Dr. Hanauer. Other forms of aerobic activity such as swimming, cycling and fast walking also help by improving blood flow through the colon.

Avoid seeds. Foods such as nuts and popcorn contain seeds or other hard particles that could become lodged in the diverticula and cause inflammation, Dr. Klein says. In fact, some experts recommend that you avoid any small, hard particle that can become lodged in the pouches, including poppy and sesame seeds.

Dizziness

You're woozy and wobbly, and the room's spinning faster than a Las Vegas slot machine. The last time you felt like this, you were riding the killer coaster on Coney Island.

But what does it mean if you get that kind of dizzy feeling when you're simply rolling over in bed? Or just walking across the room?

There's no easy answer. Dizziness is one of the leading complaints heard by doctors (second only to backache), and it has many causes. Among them: certain medications, fainting, dehydration and a range of more serious health problems.

Doctors carefully distinguish between *vertigo,* which means a spinning sensation; *disequilibrium,* which is the sensation of being off balance; and *dizziness,* which can include light-headedness, a swimming sensation, vertigo or disequilibrium.

The merry-go-round feeling of vertigo indicates an inner ear problem and may have many causes, including head injury, viral infection or Meniere's disease (excessive pressure in the inner ear fluid). The inner ear relays messages to the balance center in your brain, and when those messages are incorrect, your brain reads "TILT!" Sometimes an inner ear problem causes you to feel off balance when you stand or walk.

If you experience occasional dizzy spells and your doctor has ruled out a serious medical condition, here are some tactics that can't do any harm and may help you stop the merry-go-round.

Focus on a fixed point. If you suddenly feel dizzy, stand still and focus on something stationary, such as a window frame. "Focusing on a fixed point across the room gives your brain more visual information about balance and helps the dizziness pass quickly," says Dennis O'Leary, Ph.D., professor of otolaryngology/head and neck surgery at the University of Southern California and director of the University of Southern California Hospital Balance Center, both in Los Angeles. If you have a dizzy spell when traveling in a car or on a boat, focus on the distant scenery or the horizon.

Rise s-l-o-w-l-y. Many people feel dizzy when they get out of bed too suddenly, says Susan Herdman, Ph.D., associate professor of otolaryngology/head and neck surgery at Johns Hopkins University in Baltimore. Getting up too quickly results in a temporary drop in blood pressure and a decrease in the blood flow to the brain. The solution is simple. "Don't bound out of bed," says Dr. Herdman. "Instead, sit on the edge of the bed for a minute to normalize blood pressure, then slowly stand."

Remember to drink up in summer. When you perspire excessively in hot weather or during exercise, your blood pressure may drop, and you lose important minerals, according to Dr. Herdman. So try to drink at least 8 to 12 ounces of water on hot days. If you're exercising, drink water before and after exercise as well.

Breathe slowly and steadily. If you sometimes hold your breath or hyperventilate (breathe too rapidly) when you're stressed or exercising, your body

When to See the Doctor

A mild dizzy spell now and then is probably harmless. But if dizziness comes on suddenly and is accompanied by chest pains, a rapid heartbeat, blurred vision or numbness, see a doctor immediately, advises Michael Weintraub, M.D., clinical professor of neurology at New York Medical College in Valhalla. "This kind of dizziness could signal a heart attack or stroke," he says.

Also be sure to see the doctor if you experience deafness or hear ringing in your ear after an attack of dizziness. This could be symptom of Meniere's disease, a disorder of the inner ear, according to Dr. Weintraub. Other symptoms of Meniere's disease include nausea and vomiting, jerky eye movements and a feeling of pressure or pain in one or both ears.

Safety Tips for the Dizziness-Prone

Do you have frequent dizzy spells? If so, you may be tempted to spend a lot of safe, snug hours in your favorite armchair rather than risk an off-balance experience. But staying active is essential, because frequent activity helps "retrain your brain" to reduce the dizzy response, according to Dennis O'Leary, Ph.D., professor of otolaryngology/head and neck surgery at the University of Southern California and director of the University of Southern California Hospital Balance Center, both in Los Angeles. With continued movement, in fact, some people find that their dizziness and unsteadiness will decrease dramatically and even disappear, he says.

Here are some precautions to take while you stay on the move.

Get rid of thick carpets. If you have trouble maintaining balance, think about safety when you furnish your home. Choose low-pile carpets or bare wood, says Dr. O'Leary.

Make sure pathways are well lighted. And get rid of toys, scatter rugs and any other objects that may cause you to slip.

Ask someone else to climb ladders. "Don't put yourself in situations where you could easily lose your balance and fall," says Dr. O'Leary.

Try for dizzy-free driving. If riding in a car tends to make you feel dizzy, fix your eyes on the car ahead of you and try not to notice other cars whizzing by, suggests Dr. Leary. He also recommends that you avoid glancing out the side windows. And as a passenger, you're less likely to feel dizzy if you avoid reading in the car.

expels more carbon dioxide than usual. The result: dizziness. To slow down your breathing, concentrate on pushing your belly out when you inhale and pulling it in as you exhale. And while you're doing that, keep your shoulders still. With slower, deeper breathing, the carbon dioxide balance is restored, and dizziness disappears.

Take a second look at medications. "Dizziness can be an uncomfortable side effect of many common drugs, including antihistamines and blood pressure medications," according to Dr. Herdman. But be sure to ask your doctor before you change your dosage of prescription medications.

Avoid iced tea and piña coladas. Caffeine and alcohol can cause problems for dizziness-prone people, says Dr. Herdman.

Don't go for diet drinks, either. "For some people, consuming foods made with aspartame (NutraSweet) inhibits the uptake of substances that affect the central nervous system as well as the balance center," according to Michael Weintraub, M.D., clinical professor of neurology at New York Medical College in Valhalla. So check labels before you buy.

Nix salty nuts and sweet treats. Both salty and sugary foods change the composition of inner ear fluid and can produce dizziness in susceptible people, says Dr. Herdman.

Driver Fatigue

Whoever said that "getting there is half the fun" no doubt spent more time coming up with catchy slogans than going places in his car. The fact is, long stretches behind the wheel can be downright boring. And that boredom itself can be dangerous.

"People are more likely to get drowsy and fall asleep when they're in boring and monotonous situations," explains Saul Rothenberg, Ph.D., assistant director of the Sleep Disorder Service and Research Center at Rush–St. Luke's–Presbyterian Medical Center in Chicago. "And driving can be *very* boring and monotonous." No wonder experts believe snoozing behind the wheel is second only to boozing as the leading cause of traffic fatalities.

While the vast majority of long-distance travelers don't fall asleep while driving, many (commuters included) do fall victim to driver fatigue—and fatigue is almost as risky as drowsiness. Symptoms include glazed eyes or a fixed stare, slowed reaction time, forgetfulness, failure to scan the roadway or a tendency to drift toward one side. But there are ways to stay wide-eyed, so you can keep on truckin' safely.

Set Your Personal Coffee Timer

Until Detroit introduces a car with a built-in coffeemaker, you'll have to make do with periodic breaks for your caffeine pick-me-ups. What you may not know, however, is that coffee can work both for you and against you.

Yes, coffee *is* a quick pick-me-up, because the alertness-enhancing effects of caffeine start within minutes of drinking it, says Timothy Roehrs, Ph.D., director of research at the Henry Ford Hospital Sleep Disorders and Research Center in Detroit. But the effects of just one cup of coffee can last for 3 to 15 hours, which can also make it an enduring keep-me-up if you drink it too late in your journey.

So a good rule of thumb for the caffeine-sensitive is to drink your last cup about four hours before you plan to go to sleep. That way, you won't be bolt upright and wide awake just when you want to fall asleep. If coffee isn't your thing, two cola drinks or cups of tea will provide the same eye-opening punch as a cup of joe. But be forewarned that they, too, have the same lingering effect.

Watch how (and what) you eat. The only thing that will zap your energy and alertness quicker than skipping a meal is eating a big one.

"Driving on a full stomach is not a good idea because of postmeal sleepiness," says Dr. Rothenberg. "In order to maintain driver alertness, it's better to eat lightly."

Low-fat protein may be the best choice to avoid drowsiness, some experts say. Good sources of low-fat protein include lean meats, poultry, fish, yogurt and low-fat cottage cheese. Carbohydrates to avoid include potatoes, corn, bagels, muffins and *especially* snack foods like chips and crackers.

Keep your car's interior cool. "A warm car can enhance sleepiness, so try to keep your car as cool as possible," says Dr. Rothenberg. "Cold invigorates—especially when you're tired—so open a window or turn on the air-conditioning."

Snooze more the night before. Many people get driver fatigue on long-distance trips because they simply didn't get enough sleep the night before. They were too busy with packing and other predeparture hassles.

"If you know you'll be putting in long hours driving, the easiest thing to do is go to bed an hour or two earlier than normal, so you can get a better-than-usual night's sleep," says Timothy Roehrs, Ph.D., director of research at the Henry Ford Hospital Sleep Disorders and Research Center in Detroit.

Adjust your body clock—before you leave. Even more effective for long trips is to adjust your body clock so that you'll be alert during times you normally get drowsy.

For instance, if you want to do late-night driving, start going to bed one hour later each night (and rising one hour later) for three or four consecutive nights, starting about one week before departure, advises Maria Simonson, Ph.D., Sc.D., professor emeritus and director of the Health, Weight and Stress Program at Johns Hopkins Medical Institutions in Baltimore. If you want to hit the road before the rooster crows, hit the sack an hour earlier every night during the week before you leave.

If all else fails, pull over. "If you find yourself losing your edge, pull off in a safe place (such as a rest stop) and take a 20- to 30-minute nap," says Deborah Freund, a transportation specialist with the Federal Highway Administration in Washington, D.C., and project manager of a long-term study on driver fatigue. Be sure that you give yourself enough time to wake up fully before you start to drive again.

Dry Eyes

Every time you blink, a film of tears spreads over your eyes. For the wet-eyed crowd, that film can turn to an eye bath when you're watching a classic weeper like, say, *Old Yeller*. But if you suffer from dry eyes, even the tear-jerkingest flick can leave your hanky dry.

But another thing happens when you have dry eyes: They actually ache. Lacking the ability to cover or coat the cornea (the clear front surface of the eye) with a thin, protective coating of tears, your eyes start burning and stinging. At worst, it may feel as though a grain of sand is permanently embedded in your parched peepers. And because of this ongoing problem, your vision may be mildly blurred, or your eyes may become sensitive to light.

There are many causes: Medicines such as decongestants, tranquilizers and antihistamines, as well as drugs for high blood pressure, may all cause dry eyes. You can also get dry eyes if you have an allergy to contact lens products. Winter winds, air-conditioning and indoor heating are all potential culprits as well. Chronic cases often result from menopause, rheumatoid arthritis or Sjögren's syndrome, a gland condition that also causes dry mouth and vaginal dryness. Sometimes dry eyes occur for no apparent reason. But whatever the cause, here are some ways to get your peepers dewy again—and to give you a chance to shed a tear the next time you hear a sob story.

Oil your eyes with a washcloth compress. "Place a warm washcloth on your closed eyelids for five to ten minutes several times a day to help open the clogged oil glands in the eyelids," says Eric Donnenfeld, M.D., associate professor of ophthalmology at North Shore University Hospital/Cornell Medical College in Manhasset, New York.

Here's why it works. Tears are made up of three components: water, oil and mucus. Artificial tears, the kind sold in eyedropper form in drugstores, can replace the water component of your tears. But those drops don't replace the oil: Only your own eyes can do that. So the warm compress helps your eyes do the work they're supposed to, according to Dr. Donnenfeld.

Using a compress is *especially* helpful if you have "crusty" eyes when you wake up or at other times of the day, says Dr. Donnenfeld. (About 50 percent of dry-eye sufferers get this crusty condition—called blepharitis—in the morning or during the day.)

Choose the right artificial tears. Over-the-counter artificial tears are a mixture of saline and some type of film-forming substance, such as polyvinyl alcohol or synthetic cellulose. This solution can be used several times a day, because it mimics real tears and provides a soothing balm whenever your eyes feel dry.

When choosing a brand, keep in mind that thicker formulas remain in the eyes longer, so you'll need to use them less frequently. But the thicker kind can blur vision and leave a gooey residue on your eyelashes. Thinner drops, on the other hand, need to be used more frequently. "You'll need to experiment to see what drops work for your condition," says Paul Michelson, M.D., senior staff ophthalmologist at the Mericos Eye Institute in La Jolla, California.

"But only use commercially prepared, preservative-free products," warns Donald Doughman, M.D., professor of ophthalmology at the University of

Nighttime Is the Right Time for Treatment

Even when your lids are closed, eyes can dry out, which is why your doctor will probably suggest that you use either a combination tear-replacement/moisture-sealing ointment or a "moisture chamber" at night.

These over-the-counter superthick ointments, which contain petroleum and mineral oil, last longer than drops, says Paul Vinger, M.D., assistant clinical professor of ophthalmology at Harvard University in Cambridge, Massachusetts. To insert, pull the lower lid down, look up, and squeeze a dab of ointment in the trough between your lid and eye. Blink to spread the ointment around. Keep in mind that ointments can blur your vision for a while, so be sure you don't use them before driving.

Your eye doctor can supply you with ready-made moisture chamber glasses to wear during sleep, but a pair of ordinary watertight swim goggles will also do fine. In a pinch, says Mitchell H. Friedlaender, M.D., director of the Cornea Service at the Scripps Clinic and Research Foundation in La Jolla, California, you can even make your own chamber by taking a piece of plastic food wrap and securing it with petroleum jelly around your eyes. As tears evaporate, the air inside the chamber becomes slightly more humid, preventing further tear evaporation and creating a comfortable, moist atmosphere. To boost the moisture content, use ocular ointments along with your moisture chamber.

Minnesota in Minneapolis. "If it doesn't say 'nonpreserved' or 'preservative-free' on the label or box, don't buy it. Preservatives can damage your eyes."

Turn heating and cooling vents away. A blast of heat or air-conditioning may be what your body craves, but it's no good for your eyes. "When you're driving, keep air vents pointed down, away from your face," according to Dr. Donnenfeld. "And when you're home, do the same: Point heating and cooling ducts away from areas where you spend a lot of time. This is really important if your home has forced hot-air heating, because that can dry out your eyes very quickly."

Dress for the slopes. The Great Outdoors can deliver a one-two parch to dry eyes: The sun's brightness makes them supersensitive, and the wind and low humidity dry them out. That's why many experts suggest that you wear eye-protecting sunglasses or goggles for any outdoor activity. "Wraparound sunglasses are very helpful because they protect the sides of the eyes, which are vulnerable to the wind," says Dr. Donnenfeld. "But if you have *very* dry eyes, the best thing you can do is wear ski goggles when you're outside. They create a moist chamber for the eyes."

Take a blink break. Doing close work—typing at a video display terminal, driving, sewing, even watching television—can exacerbate even mild cases of eye dryness, says Dr. Michelson. "People doing tasks that require concentration tend to stare and not blink as much." And when you don't blink very often, eye moisture evaporates rapidly. So if you're doing concentrated work and notice dry eyes, look away and take a blink break whenever possible. Blinking helps restore the tear film over your eyes.

Humidify your surroundings. Moisturizing the air can keep mucous membranes from drying out during sleep, especially in the winter, doctors suggest. "When moisture is low, your eyes dry up fast," says Dr. Donnenfeld. "If you can, get a humidifier for your bedroom or other places where you spend a lot of time." And when you're using a hair dryer, don't run it any longer than necessary.

Moisten up and fly right. If you know you'll be in the arid environment of an airplane cabin, be extra vigilant in using artificial tears. And be sure the overhead air vents are pointed away from your eyes, says Dr. Donnenfeld.

Dry Hair and Split Ends

It doesn't take much hot air to turn your tresses into messes: Dry weather will do it. So will blow-drying. But don't start to think that arid attacks are the *only* way to damage your hair. Frequent shampooing and swimming in chlorinated pools do more to cripple coiffures than Delilah's scissors. Hair dyes, electric curlers and permanents also do a lion's share of damage to your mane.

Individually or in any combination, these factors can leave your hair arid, lifeless and chock-full of split ends. But here's how to offset the damage and put bounce and body on top again.

Don't hold the mayo. "Mayonnaise makes an excellent conditioner," says David Daines, owner of David Daines Salon in New York City. He advises a regular mayo bath—once a week or so. Put a dollop in the palm of your hand, then work it into your hair for *at least* five minutes before washing it out. (The preferred time for a full-blown mayo treatment is an hour, according to Daines.)

Spray on the brew. If mayo is a little too messy for your taste, you can still get help from the flip-top section of your refrigerator. "Beer is a wonderful setting lotion that gives a crisp, healthy, shiny look—even to dry hair," says Daines. Pour some of the brew into an empty pump-bottle. Then spray it onto your hair *after* you've shampooed and towel-dried but *before* you blow-dry or style. And don't worry about smelling like a lush—the odor of the beer quickly disperses.

Shampoo with care. "It's in vogue these days to shampoo every day, but shampooing washes out the hair's protective oils," explains Thomas Goodman, Jr., M.D., assistant professor of dermatology at the University of Tennessee Center for Health Sciences in Memphis.

If you must shampoo daily, use a brand that's labeled "for dry or damaged hair," suggests Michael Ramsey, M.D., clinical instructor of dermatology at Baylor College of Medicine in Houston. Among the shampoos he recommends are DHS, Neutrogena, Pert Plus, Ionil and Purpose.

Help your hair with conditioner. "Using a conditioner after shampooing can benefit dry hair," says Dr. Ramsey. When hair is dry, the outer layers—called cuticles—peel away from the shaft, resulting in notorious split ends. When you follow up with conditioner, you "glue" these cuticles back to the shaft while adding lubrication. A side benefit: Conditioner helps prevent static electricity, which creates the "frizzies."

Dry without heat. Two of the most intense sources of heat—and damage—are curling irons and electric curlers, says Joanne Harris, who operates the Joanne Harris Salon in Los Angeles and whose clients include many Hollywood stars. She suggests you rediscover the unheated plastic cylinder rollers that were used in years gone by.

For straightening, wrap slightly moist hair under and around the cold rollers, as if you were creating a pageboy hairdo. Leave them in place for about ten minutes. For curling or adding wave, try using sponge rollers overnight or sleeping with moist braids. Since blow-drying is also damaging, gently pat hair dry with a towel.

Wear a hat. One of the easiest ways to avoid dry hair is simply to wear a hat during windy weather. "Whipping winds can fray your hair like a piece of fabric," says Dr. Ramsey. Plus, a hat helps protect hair from the sun, which can also dry hair.

Snip off split ends. What to do about split ends? Snip 'em off, suggests Dr. Goodman. One round of quick snips every six weeks or so should keep those frayed ends under control.

Dry Mouth

Ever notice how drooling seems to come naturally to the very young? From the mouths of innocent babes comes enough saliva to turn a bib to a bath mat. But as we grow up, we tend to dry up. The addition of years seems to translate to a loss of saliva.

Aging alone, however, isn't the only cause of xerostomia, or dry mouth. More often we can blame it on all the 24-carat hassles that we live with in the golden age of our lives: Most cases of dry mouth can be blamed on some 400 medicines used to treat nearly everything from arthritis to ulcers. Even caffeine and over-the-counter pain relievers such as ibuprofen (Advil) can contribute to dry mouth.

Besides making your mouth feel like it's plugged with cotton, dry mouth can make swallowing, eating and even talking difficult. Worst case: Mouth tissue becomes cracked and irritated, and you begin to suffer related problems such as bad breath, lost fillings, gum infections and tooth decay. But here's how to permanently wet your whistle if you're among the one in three Americans with dry mouth.

Take a hard line against soft drinks. Drinking more is the obvious solution to dry mouth—as long as you're *not* slurping soda, orange juice or other beverages that contain either citric or phosphoric acid.

"Soft drinks are very acidic, and people with dry mouth lack the saliva necessary to neutralize these acids that can harm the teeth," says James Sciubba, D.M.D., Ph.D., chairman of the Department of Dental Medicine at Long Island Jewish Medical Center in New Hyde Park, New York, and founding chairman of the Sjögren's Syndrome Foundation.

Instead, Dr. Sciubba says carrying a flask of water and taking frequent sips is the best way to get your mouth moist again. "The key is how frequently you drink, not necessarily how much you drink," he says.

Suck on fruit pits. Pits from peaches, nectarines and cherries help increase saliva flow without adding any calories. Just be careful not to swallow them.

Eat mushy foods. Eating any food will stimulate saliva. But the best choices are soft foods and those moistened with sauces or gravies that go down the hatch easily, says Nelson Rhodus, D.M.D., associate professor of oral medicine at the University of Minnesota in Minneapolis.

Go sugarless. "Use of sugar by a patient with a dry mouth will produce tooth decay within six months," warns Dr. Sciubba. "One of the best ways to keep saliva flowing is to suck on hard candies or to chew gum, but the gum and

Brush Frequently to Beat Bad Breath

Brushing your teeth is even more important than usual when you suffer from dry mouth. Since saliva usually washes away trapped food morsels, when you're short on saliva, food hangs around longer—and that creates bad breath.

Since dry mouth almost guarantees bad breath, Nelson Rhodus, D.M.D., associate professor of oral medicine at the University of Minnesota in Minneapolis, suggests that you dip your toothbrush in baking soda moistened with water and scrub your teeth and tongue twice daily to help neutralize odor and bacteria. That's also good for your teeth, since anyone with dry mouth is at greater risk for cavities and other dental problems.

candy must be sugarless." In fact, sucking on sorbitol-containing sugarless candies, mints and gum has been found to increase saliva tenfold in some people.

Rinse your mouth with some fluoride. When saliva production is low, your risk of cavities and gum disease is high. Swishing with a fluoride mouth rinse at bedtime helps remineralize teeth and can help protect you against cavities and gum disease.

There are also artificial saliva products that help. "In our studies, we found that over-the-counter products such as MouthKote provide a nice, moist coating over mucous membranes," says Dr. Rhodus. Other products include Xero-Lube, Salivart and Evian mineral water spray.

Moisturize the air. Using a cool-air vaporizer in your home is a good way to add much-needed extra humidity to the air—especially if you're a mouth breather, says Dr. Sciubba. But make an effort to *always* breathe through your nose to prevent saliva from evaporating.

Use lemon sparingly. While full-fledged lemonade should be avoided, tasting some lemon juice diluted in water or rinsing with a bit of lemon juice and glycerin is a good way to stimulate the flow of saliva, says Dr. Rhodus. But here's the drawback: If your mucous membranes are so dry that you have developed sores, the citric acid could further irritate your mouth. (If you do have these sores, go light on lemon as well as spicy foods and anything else that can irritate your mouth.)

Dry Skin and Winter Itch

As winter approaches, our bodies turn toward flannel, our attention turns toward cheap Florida airfares, and our skin takes a turn toward something resembling Melba toast.

You can blame that toasted skin on the warm, toasty air that heats our homes, schools and offices. When it gets cold, we naturally warm up the house. The problem is, unless you add humidity to your surroundings with a humidifier or pans of water near radiators, a heated room has only about 15 percent relative humidity—as dry as Death Valley. And *that* turns our skin dry, flaky, scaly and usually itchy (and *always* bothersome).

Plus, there are other irritants to make matters worse—wind, cold, soaps, water (which dries skin when it evaporates), even added stress. Put it all together and your epidermis can dry out quicker than Aunt Gizelda's holiday fruitcake.

Dry skin and winter itch share a lot of symptoms with eczema and dermatitis, and some of the remedies for those problems can bring relief. But the key to making the winter season a merry one, itch-wise, is keeping your birthday suit well protected. Here's how.

Keep skin moisturized. Probably the most important thing you can do to prevent and treat dry skin is to moisturize *daily* with a cream-based moisturizer, advises Sheryl Clark, M.D., a dermatologist at The New York Hospital–Cornell Medical Center in New York City. "An oil-free moisturizer is recommended for those who tend to break out. Also, those with sensitive skin should choose a moisturizer without perfumes or lanolin." The brands most highly recommended by experts include Eucerin, Complex 15, Moisturel, Aquaphor and Aquaderm—all available over the counter.

But don't get soaked. You don't need expensive skin creams to keep skin moisturized. "Nothing beats plain petroleum jelly or mineral oil as a moisturizer," says Howard Donsky, M.D., associate professor of medicine at the University of Toronto and author of *Beauty Is Skin Deep.* In fact, he adds that virtually *any* vegetable oil or hyrogenated cooking oil—from Crisco oil to sunflower or peanut oil—can be used to relieve dry skin. But note: They do feel greasier than commercial moisturizers.

Don't be too hyper about your hygiene. "Bathe in cool to tepid water as briefly as possible and no more than once a day," according to Michael Ramsey, M.D., clinical instructor of dermatology at Baylor College of Medicine in Houston. "Cleansing lotions are more gentle than soaps, and they're just as effective at removing dirt," adds Leonard Swinyer, M.D., clinical professor of medicine at the University of Utah in Salt Lake City. And *don't* use a washcloth—just your fingertips. If you must use soaps, stick with mild brands such as Dove, Aveeno or Basis.

Add some oil to your bath. Make the most of your tub time by adding a bath oil rich in moisturizers—even when you apply creams *after* bathing.

Again, there's no need for the fancy stuff: Plain ol' castor oil is an excellent, low-cost choice. "It's one of the few oils that will disperse in water, and it won't leave a ring around the tub," says Varro E. Tyler, Ph.D., professor of pharmacognosy at Purdue University in West Lafayette, Indiana, and author of *The Honest Herbal.*

Make your own bath oil by mixing ½ cup of castor oil with ten drops of sandlewood-, pine-, rosemary- or mint-scented oil and storing it in a closed jar. Add one teaspoon of the mixture *each* time you bathe. For those who prefer store-bought brands, Alpha Keri body oil, Geri-Bath and Nutraderm bath oil are highly recommended. *Caution:* Be careful in the bathroom, because these oils can make tubs and floors extremely slippery.

Dry yourself damp. After bathing, pat your skin almost dry—*never* totally dry—with a towel. While the skin is still damp, apply your moisturizing lotion. "It's more effective to apply moisturizer to damp skin *immediately* after bathing than to put it on totally dry skin, because the moisturizer is what holds the water in," says Kenneth H. Neldner, M.D., professor and chairman of the Department of Dermatology at Texas Tech University Health Sciences Center in Lubbock. "A couple of pats with a towel will make you as dry as you want to be before you apply the lotion. You're trying to trap a little water in the skin, and that's the fundamental rule in fighting off dryness." If you have dry hands, he advises keeping some moisturizer near each sink in the house and using it as needed.

Be wary of wool. Clothing made of wool—or any other fuzzy or heavy material—can be particularly irritating to excessively dry skin, says Stephen M. Purcell, D.O., chairman of the Department of Dermatology at Philadelphia College of Osteopathic Medicine and assistant clinical professor at Hahnemann University School of Medicine in Philadelphia. "The last thing itchy skin needs is to have something scratchy over it. Cotton is probably the best material to wear, since polyester blends can also be irritating to some people."

Shave *before* bedtime. Shaving is tough enough on your tender skin, but meeting the cold reality of Old Man Winter right afterward makes your dry skin even worse, adds Dr. Swinyer. Unless you're hampered by severe five o'clock shadow, shave *before* bedtime, when your puss won't be subjected to such a drastic change in temperature.

And avoid eye-opening after-shaves. Their high alcohol content is too drying and zaps remaining moisture during this mean season, adds Dr. Swinyer.

Wear baggy, loose-fitting clothing. In addition to being more abrasive, tighter clothing traps perspiration, which softens the outer layer of skin, breaks down its protective barrier and worsens dry skin, says dermatologist Rodney Basler, M.D., assistant professor of internal medicine at the University of Nebraska Medical Center in Omaha. But looser-fitting clothes, particularly in "breathable" fabrics like cotton, allow perspiration to be absorbed naturally.

Dust Mite Allergies

T hey're so small that scientists have counted *thousands* of these little critters on a *single gram* of house dust. But they cause big problems for an estimated 30 million people with dust mite allergies.

These microscopic organisms, which feed off flakes of human skin and food debris (and whose feces are potent allergens), live in dust. Besides causing the familiar symptoms of hay fever—sneezing, scratchy throat, stuffy or runny nose—dust mite allergies may also contribute to stuffed-up ears, especially during winter, according to Philip Fireman, M.D., director of allergy, immunology and rheumatology at Children's Hospital in Pittsburgh. They are also the culprits causing an eczema-like skin condition, and they have triggered many an asthma attack during their long and insidious history. But even though they're minuscule and fast on their feet, dust mites *can* be robbed of their might. Here's how.

Dehumidify your surroundings. Since dust mites live in dust, the obvious solution is to keep your house hospital-clean. But it's not necessarily the dust alone that keeps them thriving. It's the humidity. While air-conditioning helps reduce humidity, if you live in a warm or moist climate, you may also want to invest in a dehumidifier.

"Dust mites really don't do well at humidities below 45 percent," says Thomas Platts-Mills, M.D., Ph.D., head of the Division of Allergy and Clinical Immunology at the University of Virginia Health Sciences Center in Charlottesville. While 45 percent humidity is fine for a home at 70°F, at higher temperatures you need lower humidity. If the temperature is closer to 80°, the humidity should be below 40 percent.

Are You Allergic to Dust Mites?

Are you among the 30 million folks who are mite-sensitive? According to Thomas Platts-Mills, M.D., Ph.D., head of the Division of Allergy and Clinical Immunology at the University of Virginia Health Sciences Center in Charlottesville, you probably are allergic to dust mites if you share these three common symptoms.

• Sneezing first thing in the morning
• Feeling the onset of allergy symptoms while making beds or doing housework
• Feeling better when you go outside

Encase your mattress in plastic. The highest concentrations of dust mites are in the bedroom, where they love to dig their eight legs into mattresses, carpeting and pillows. The answer? "Encasing in plastic is a very easy thing to do. You can buy plastic cases ready-made, or just use sheets of plastic sealed with tape to wrap the mattress like a Christmas present," suggests Richard Weber, M.D., chief of the Allergy/Immunology Division at Fitzsimmons Army Medical Center in Aurora, Colorado.

Use a bedspread. Allan Weinstein, M.D., consultant to the National Institute of Allergy and Infectious Diseases in Bethesda, Maryland, recommends you keep a bedspread on your bed during the day and remove it from your bedroom at night. "Let the bedspread collect the dust—not you," he says.

Sleep on synthetic pillows. While dust mites like synthetic pillows as much as those made from feathers or foam, pillows made from Hollofil and Dacron have one important advantage—they can be washed. Be sure to wash *all* bedding, including mattress pads, bedspreads and blankets—and do it weekly in *hot* water. It's one of the best ways to kill dust mites.

Throw down some throw rugs. Deep-pile wall-to-wall carpeting is another taboo for the mite-allergic. The best flooring is hardwood or linoleum. "Mites can't survive on a dry, polished floor," says Dr. Platts-Mills. "And that kind of floor dries in seconds." A steam-cleaned carpet takes weeks to dry.

Short-pile area rugs—throw rugs—are much more acceptable, because they can be washed at temperatures hot enough to kill dust mites. The floors underneath—courtesy of a rug's loose weave—also stay drier than they would under wall-to-wall carpeting.

Stop mites with a mask. A simple chore such as vacuuming can throw huge quantities of dust into the air, where it will hang for several minutes, says David Lang, M.D., assistant professor of medicine and director of allergy/immunology at Hahnemann University School of Medicine in Philadelphia. A small mask that covers nose and mouth, known professionally as a dust and mist respirator, can cut the allergens reaching your lungs. An inexpensive version is made by the 3M Company and can be found in most hardware stores.

Earache

If you've been spending a lot of time with a box of tissues and a bag of throat lozenges and now you're lying awake with an aching ear, you already know two things about earaches: They often accompany bad colds and sore throats, and they're always nastier at night.

A typical earache begins when a congested eustachian tube—which runs from the back of the throat to the eardrum—can't regulate pressure or fluids in the ear. Pain starts when mucus or pus builds up behind the eardrum. The more the fluid builds, the greater the pressure and pain.

While antibotic treatment can resolve the infection that's causing the pain, there are some things you can do for yourself to get temporary relief.

Warm up to relief. "The greatest pain reliever is warm, moist heat around the ear," says Stephen P. Cass, M.D., assistant professor of otolaryngology at the Eye and Ear Institute of Pittsburgh. A warm compress—such as a towel rung out in hot water and pressed against the ear—brings the most immediate relief, he says. Resoak the towel as it cools and use it as often as you need to, even while you are being treated for an underlying infection, he suggests.

Try a liquid pillow. A hot water bottle wrapped in a towel also makes a comforting pillow for an aching ear, says Dr. Cass. If you get a lot of earaches and need something more portable, you can invest in a mini hot water bottle that's made to fit directly over the ear, he says.

Press on a gel pack. Another ear-warming alternative: Use a dual-purpose first-aid gel pack that you can warm up in hot water or the microwave, suggests Anthony J. Yonkers, M.D., chairman of the Department of Otolaryngology/Head and Neck Surgery at the University of Nebraska Medical Center in Omaha. "Make sure the gel pack is not too hot, then press it right on your ear and it will make you feel better," he says.

Put your ear to the plate. Some people swear by old-time heat treatments like this: Warm up an oven-safe plate, wrap it in a towel, and rest your aching ear right on it. The plate should be warm and comforting, not hot, cautions Dr. Cass.

Find relief in your medicine cabinet. An adult with a cold or fever who develops ear pain can take aspirin, ibuprofen (Advil), acetaminophen (Tylenol) or another nonprescription painkiller, says Jerome C. Goldstein, M.D., executive vice president of the American Academy of Otolaryngology/Head and Neck Surgery in Alexandria, Virginia. Children with earaches should *never* be given aspirin, and other pain relievers should get a doctor's go-ahead. Your doctor may recommend Children's Tylenol.

Get the drop on pain. A couple of drops of warm mineral oil may soothe a sore ear, says Clough Shelton, M.D., an otolaryngologist with the House Ear Clinic in Los Angeles. Warm the oil by putting it in hot water. Test it on your wrist as you would a baby's bottle. It should feel barely warm. Use an

When to See the Doctor

If your ear hurts when you chew, it may be a tip-off that you have trouble in the jaw joint, says Clough Shelton, M.D., an otolaryngologist with the House Ear Clinic in Los Angeles. You might be a nighttime jaw clencher or have an inflamed or misaligned jaw caused by temporomandibular joint disorder (TMD)—which can be diagnosed by a doctor.

Also, sudden or severe pain in your ear without an accompanying cold or sore throat is *not* typical. See your doctor if you notice blood or pus in the ear, redness or swelling around the ear, dizziness or hearing loss. These could be signs of a severe infection that needs immediate attention.

Don't Be Bugged

Tiny insects that find their way into ears usually find their way out pretty quickly—but not always. Some get stuck inside.

What should you do if you're bugged by a bug in your ear? Using an eardropper full of alcohol, flood the ear to kill the bug, suggests Stephen P. Cass, M.D., assistant professor of otolaryngology at the Eye and Ear Institute of Pittsburgh. Then gently irrigate the ear with water from an ear syringe.

"*Do not* try to fish for it with a tweezers, pencil, fingernail or Q-Tip," he warns. You'll just push it in farther or damage your ear.

eyedropper to drip the oil in, and gently pull the outside of the ear to make sure it goes down, he says. One caution: You can't use this method if the doctor says you have a perforated eardrum.

Decongest your head. If you're really congested, Sudafed or other decongestants can shrink your eustachian tube and bring ear pain down to size, says Dr. Goldstein. Ask your doctor what might be best for you.

Stay away from wind. If wind bothers your aching ears, wear a scarf when you're outside, or put cotton in the opening of the ear, suggests Dr. Cass. But don't push the cotton down where you can't retrieve it with your fingers.

Soar above ear pain in airplanes. If your ears hurt when the pressure changes during an airplane flight, chew gum or suck on candy, especially during descent and landing, which is the most troublesome time of changing pressure. The chewing or sucking will activate the muscles that send air to your inner ears, says Dr. Shelton. When you hear your ears "pop," you'll feel better, because pressure in the ear is balanced.

If chewing doesn't work, close your mouth, relax your cheek muscles, hold your nose, and blow *gently* until you feel relief, Dr. Shelton says.

Take a dose *before* and *after.* Experienced flyers who expect painful flights can take Sudafed or use a nasal decongestant at the recommended dose for a day *before* they fly, says Dr. Yonkers. And if the pain is unresolved after you land, use decongestants for a day *after* your flight, too, adds Dr. Shelton.

Earlobe Pain

Your new silver earrings with copper inlays were *perfect* with that outfit. And even though they made your earlobes itch after a couple of hours, you kept on wearing them for a couple of more. So today you're gingerly fingering two tender, red, weeping earlobes.

Blame your angry earlobes on nickel, which is in virtually *all* jewelry. One in ten women is allergic or sensitive to this common metal, according to William Epstein, M.D., professor of dermatology at the University of California, San Francisco, School of Medicine. But if you notice the reaction—known as dermatitis—and treat it before mere inflammation becomes real infection, you can easily do a favor for your inflamed earlobes.

Remove your earrings. You won't "build up resistance" to the nickel that's causing your skin to rebel—so once you've taken off the offending earrings, keep them off. "Once you're allergic to something, assume you're always going to be allergic to it," says Hillard H. Pearlstein, M.D., assistant clinical professor of dermatology at Mount Sinai School of Medicine in New York City.

Try a lobe bath. Clean your lobes with hydrogen peroxide, says Nancy Sculerati, M.D., assistant professor of otolaryngology and director of pediatric otolaryngology at New York University Medical Center in New York City. Mix equal parts peroxide and water. (Rubbing alcohol also works, but it tends to sting, she says.) Pour the solution over the earlobe, or apply it with gauze, and let the runoff drip into a sink. Don't apply the liquid with cotton balls if the ear is weepy, says Dr. Sculerati, because the cotton will stick to the earlobe.

Stop the itch. To soothe itchy rashes that are oozing or weeping, use Domeboro powder, which you can get in a drugstore, according to D'Anne Kleinsmith, M.D., a cosmetic dermatologist with William Beaumont Hospital near Detroit. Mix the powder with water at *half* the recommended strength, says Dr. Kleinsmith.

When to See the Doctor

Ears are prone to sunburn because they stick out like wings on a plane," says Hillard H. Pearlstein, M.D., assistant clinical professor of dermatology at the Mount Sinai School of Medicine in New York City. "That's why they're extremely susceptible to cancerous change." Any change in the texture or color of the skin on the ears warrants a trip to a dermatologist.

Also, small, hard lumps in the earlobes—called fibromas—are common, says William Epstein, M.D., professor of dermatology at the University of California, San Francisco, School of Medicine. A fibroma usually is not serious, but only a doctor can tell. "If one comes up where it hadn't been before, or if one grows, a doctor should look at it," he says.

Dip a washcloth or gauze pad in the solution and hold it on the ear for a minute or so. Let the ear dry, then repeat once. This will have a "drawing" effect on the earlobe and will help dry up the dermatitis, says Dr. Kleinsmith.

Recommended frequency: Use the compresses three times a day at first, then taper off treatment during the next three or four days. As soon as the oozing or crusting stops, stop using the compresses, Dr. Kleinsmith says, or you'll dry your skin too much.

Fight the itch with cream. Mild dermatitis might meet its match if you fight it with 1 percent hydrocortisone cream, available without prescription at most drugstores. Dr. Epstein suggests applying some cream directly to the earlobes, following the package directions. If this doesn't help, he says you may need a prescription for a stronger steroid treatment.

Keep both hands on the table. "Pay attention to your hands," says Dr. Epstein. If you pick or pull at your irritated earlobes, the dermatitis could worsen into a low-grade infection, he says. You'll know it's on its way when the earlobe thickens or becomes sore.

Apply antibiotics. For mild, superficial infections, limited to a tiny earlobe area, you can buy Neosporin or Polysporin antibiotic ointment, says Kenneth H. Neldner, M.D., professor and chairman of the Department of Dermatology at Texas Tech University Health Sciences Center in Lubbock. Keep the earlobe clean with antibacterial soap, and use an antibiotic ointment two or three times a day, he says. The infection should go away in a few days. If it doesn't, see a dermatologist.

Keep those openings unclogged. If your earring holes become clogged with dry skin or oil, douse them once a day with a mild astringent such as Sea Breeze, witch hazel or alcohol, suggests Dr. Pearlstein. This will help prevent waxy, dried body oil (sebum) from coagulating in the holes.

Go for the gold. When your dermatitis has cleared up and you're ready to try on earrings again, buy high-grade gold or pure silver, suggests Dr. Neldner. One warning before you empty your bank account, however: There's no guarantee this will solve your problem, because even 18-karat gold contains nickel, says Dr. Pearlstein.

"You may be able to wear pearl, ceramic, glass or plastic earrings with gold posts or surgical steel posts and be just fine, though," says Dr. Kleinsmith.

Coat them with polish. "You can try painting the backs of bothersome earrings with clear nail polish," suggests Dr. Kleinsmith. The lacquer creates a barrier between the metal and your skin. Use Almay or Clinique nail polish, which contain no formaldehyde, to reduce your chances of having a reaction to *that* common allergen, she says.

Earwax

E arwax is a recycling center. Most of the time, your ears produce just enough protective wax to trap dust in your ear canal and move it to the ear opening. Then the wax and dust are bathed away whenever you wash around your ears.

But sometimes the wax gets all jammed up—which is uncomfortable, annoying and sometimes downright itchy. Not only that, wax-plugged ears are more susceptible to infection. So if you find yourself with too much wax, here's how to deal with it.

Irrigate earwax. "Gently irrigate your ear with body-temperature water," suggests Stephen P. Cass, M.D., assistant professor of otolaryngology at the Eye and Ear Institute of Pittsburgh.

To do it right, you'll need a rubber ear syringe (available at most pharmacies) and a sinkful of water. (If it's the correct temperature, it will feel neither warm nor cold when you dip your hand in.) Hold your head over the sink while you very gently squirt the water into your ear, letting water and wax run out into the sink. Be sure to dry the ear canal after washing. To do this, fill an eyedropper with rubbing alcohol and squeeze the alcohol into the ear. It will absorb moisture and dry the ear.

If you're prone to excess buildup of wax, use the syringe to irrigate your ears once or twice a month as a precaution, suggests Jerome C. Goldstein, M.D., executive vice president of the American Academy of Otolaryngology/Head and Neck Surgery in Alexandria, Virginia. (But you shouldn't squirt anything in your ear if you have any kind of eardrum damage—so check with your doctor first, and again if you feel any pain.)

Baby your ears. If the wax refuses to budge, you may need to soften it up before you irrigate. One way is to use baby oil, according to Anthony J. Yonkers, M.D., chairman of the Department of Otolaryngology/Head and Neck Surgery at the University of Nebraska Medical Center in Omaha. "Warm

Do You Have Too Little of a Good Thing?

Yes, it is possible to have too *little* earwax. People who have skin conditions like eczema and psoriasis sometimes have an earwax deficit.

The cure?

"People can replenish earwax by putting a coat of Vaseline in the ear canal," says Anthony J. Yonkers, M.D., chairman of the Department of Otolaryngology/Head and Neck Surgery at the University of Nebraska Medical Center in Omaha. Use your finger to apply the coating to the outer edges of the ear opening only.

And if your wax shortage causes itching, augment this treatment with an over-the-counter itch reliever such as hydrocortisone cream, suggests Stephen P. Cass, M.D., assistant professor of otolaryngology at the Eye and Ear Institute of Pittsburgh. Apply the cream to the outer ear and the itching should ease in a few days.

189

up the oil to body temperature, then place a few drops into the ear twice a day. It will melt or soften the wax, and you can irrigate it out," Dr. Yonkers says.

Try peroxide. Another softening-up method: "Fill the ear with a dropper-ful of peroxide, and let it bubble and work for five minutes or so," suggests Dr. Goldstein. If you need to, put a piece of cotton in the opening of the ear canal, so you can sit up while the peroxide goes to work. Then flush it away with water.

Clear your canals with nonprescription treatments. Many over-the-counter earwax treatments, such as Murine and Debrox, are actually lubricant-based peroxide solutions. "They work, too," says Frank Marlowe, M.D., an otolaryn-gologist for the Medical College of Pennsylvania in Philadelphia. Plus you get a side benefit from the lubricant: It relieves dry skin in the ear canal. (That dry skin can become enmeshed with wax, causing formation of a wax ball that blocks the ear canal.)

A stool softener might sit well with you. If you have impacted wax, try using Colace, a stool softener found in most drugstores, suggests Dr. Cass. Using an eyedropper, put a couple of drops of liquid Colace in each ear. You can leave it there from a few minutes to an hour or two (depending on how stubborn the wax is), then irrigate your ears with water.

Don't use a Pik or a poke. No matter how much earwax accumulates in your ears, don't be tempted to probe for it with paper clips, tweezers or any small object—*including cotton-tipped swabs*—warns Dr. Cass. You'll push wax farther into your ear, and you might scratch or damage an eardrum. And don't use a Water Pik–type device—that's for teeth only. If you're going to irrigate your ears, use *only* an ear syringe.

Eczema and Dermatitis

S ome people know it as eczema. Others know it as dermatitis, the newer classification for any of several different types of skin inflammation. But anyone who's ever had these bothersome skin rashes—characterized by red, oozing, scaly and itchy patches—has probably referred to them by names that would make a sailor blush.

That's a lot of @$®&#®! and even more scratching, since untold tens of millions suffer some form of eczema/dermatitis each year. There are *at least* five different "groupings" of these skin irritations. The symptoms for each group are a little different, but all have one thing in common—misery.

Get clean—without soaps. "The smartest thing you can do is to use the most gentle cleanser you can find—definitely *not* regular toilet soaps," advises Nelson Lee Novick, M.D., associate clinical professor of dermatology at Mount Sinai School of Medicine in New York City. "They clean just as well and are much less irritating to the skin. You'll find them in your drugstore labeled as cleansing 'bars' or 'cakes,' or you can go with a liquid cleanser that's labeled as 'nonirritating,' such as Moisturel sensitive skin cleanser."

The same goes for shampoos: "Use baby shampoo or other mild types," suggests Dr. Novick.

Heal with oatmeal. "Oatmeal baths made from powders such as Aveeno provide effective but temporary relief from the itching of eczema and dermatitis," says Stephen M. Purcell, D.O., chairman of the Department of Dermatology at Philadelphia College of Osteopathic Medicine and assistant clinical professor at Hahnemann University School of Medicine in Philadelphia.

Relieve the itch with ice. "An ice pack made by putting ice cubes in a plastic bag and placing it on the itchy area makes an inexpensive and effective itch fighter," adds Michael Ramsey, M.D., clinical instructor of dermatology at Baylor College of Medicine in Houston. Make sure that the ice pack is wrapped in a towel.

For Controlling Eczema . . .

Here are some other things that you should avoid if you're prone to eczema.

- Baby lotions: The added fragrances and lanolins are common causes of skin allergies, says John F. Romano, M.D., a dermatologist and clinical assistant professor of medicine at The New York Hospital–Cornell Medical Center in New York City.
- Colored toilet paper and tissues: Their dyes are irritating to many, so when it's time to wipe, stick with white, advises Howard Donsky, M.D., associate professor of medicine at the University of Toronto.
- Stuffed animals: Fuzzy and furry toys and pillows can bother those with sensitive skin, says Jerome Z. Litt, M.D., assistant clinical professor of dermatology at Case Western Reserve University School of Medicine in Cleveland.
- Real animals: Sorry, but man's best friend—particularly long-haired breeds—is anything but friendly to those with eczema, adds Dr. Litt. He advises keeping dogs and cats outdoors—at least until your skin improves.
- Fake fingernails: They cause very real dermatitis in some people. Dr. Donsky blames the problem on acrylics in some artificial and sculptured fingernail products.
- Live Christmas trees: Metal trees may not be as appealing, but Dr. Litt says that they're less allergenic to eczema sufferers than the real thing.
- Quick changes in air temperature: Quickly going from a nice, warm room into the cold outdoors, or vice versa, plays havoc with your skin, says Dr. Donsky. Spending some "in-between" time in a mudroom or wearing layers of cotton clothing—and peeling them off slowly—can help.
- Metallic jewelry: If you're prone to nickel allergies—the most common form of contact dermatitis—then avoid watchbands, earrings and jewelry that cause a skin reaction. Buying earrings? Look for earring posts that are stainless steel.

And milk is "udderly" effective. For weeping eczema, which "oozes," a compress of cold milk is another way to soothe itchy skin, suggests John F.

Romano, M.D., a dermatologist and clinical assistant professor of medicine at The New York Hospital–Cornell Medical Center in New York City. Pour some cold milk onto a gauze pad or thin piece of cotton and apply it to the skin for about three minutes. Resoak the cloth and reapply at least two more times for three-minute soaks. Repeat several times a day, but make sure to rinse your skin in cool water after each application, because the milk will smell.

Avoid *most* antiperspirants. The active "drying" ingredients found in most antiperspirants—aluminum chloride, aluminum sulfate and zirconium chloro-hydrates—are too irritating to those with dry, sensitive skin, cautions Howard Donsky, M.D., associate professor of medicine at the University of Toronto and author of *Beauty Is Skin Deep*. "I recommend that people use an antiseptic soap such as Dial or Zest. Also, Tom's of Maine natural deodorant is a very gentle product."

But stay dry and odor-free. Baking soda is an excellent alternative to commercially sold antiperspirants, adds Dr. Novick. Besides being less expensive, it absorbs excess moisture without irritating dry or sensitive skin.

Keep nails short and clean. Short nails are less effective at scratching—and you don't want to scratch. "Not only will scratching aggravate your skin, but it can break and damage it, contributing to secondary bacterial infections," says Jerome Z. Litt, M.D., assistant clinical professor of dermatology at Case Western Reserve University School of Medicine in Cleveland. Clean, short nails are less likely to irritate or cause infection in case you do scratch.

Sit on your hands. In Sweden, where the cold winter air makes skin incredibly dry, researchers have been very successful in teaching eczema patients "antiscratching therapy." In the first of two sessions, patients were taught to press firmly on the itchy area for one minute whenever they had an urge to scratch—and then immediately move their hands to their thighs or to an object. In the second session, patients avoided the itchy area entirely—instead moving their hands *directly* to their thighs or an object. After four weeks, patients given this therapy and a hydrocortisone cream had *twice* the improvement, compared with those given only the cream.

Humidify your surroundings. As with winter itch or any form of dry skin, "anything you can do to add moisture to the air is going to help," explains Dr. Novick. "I recommend either buying a cold-air humidifier or placing shallow pans of water near radiators and on wood stoves to add humidity."

Keep showers extra short. "Your showers should last about three minutes—and *no longer* than five minutes," adds Dr. Novick. "The only baths you should take are oatmeal baths, because baths encourage you to stay in the tub longer—and water *adds* to your dryness. Hot water is especially drying, so keep the water as cool as possible."

And use only your fingertips to wash—*not* washcloths or sponges—and then pat yourself dry.

Don't forget your emollients. Those containing urea or lactic acid are best for relieving itching, says Hillard H. Pearlstein, M.D., assistant clinical professor of dermatology at Mount Sinai School of Medicine. Carmol 10, Carmol 20 and Ultra Mide 25 contain urea, and Lac-Hydrin Five contains lactic acid.

Wash once, rinse twice. Laundry detergents are another no-no, because these powerful soaps are especially irritating, adds Dr. Purcell. "It's wise to double-rinse your laundry to make sure the detergent rinses out and won't come in contact with your skin."

Don't use dryer sheets. "Some of the chemicals in fabric-softening dryer sheets remain on the skin and can be irritating to people with eczema," says Rodney Basler, M.D., a dermatologist and assistant professor of internal medicine at the University of Nebraska Medical Center in Omaha. "However, fabric softeners you add to the washing machine don't seem to irritate."

Don't be a fool if you use a pool. "If you do a lot of swimming in chlorine-filled pools, you have to take even more precautions," according to Dr. Novick. "*Immediately* after leaving the pool, rinse off your body in cool water and apply a moisturizer."

Buy American when it comes to cosmetics. The general rule is, avoid cosmetics if you're bothered by eczema or dermatitis. But if you must wear them, buy American. That's because some cosmetics made in Japan, Italy, France and other foreign countries contain formaldehyde, which can cause allergic dermatitis in many people, says Mary Ellen Brademas, M.D., chief of dermatology at St. Vincent's Hospital and assistant clinical professor of dermatology at New York University Medical Center, both in New York City.

Relax. "Stress is a definite contributing factor in eczema as well as other skin conditions," says Dr. Basler. "If you are feeling stressed out or are particularly worried about something, it will only aggravate your condition."

Emphysema

A typical set of lungs contains about 300 million tiny, elastic air sacs that, with every breath, add oxygen to the blood and remove carbon dioxide. Emphysema occurs when the elasticity in these sacs changes and they enlarge and rupture—making it impossible to fully exhale.

Father Time can take some of the blame, since most people experience a change in lung elasticity as they age (though usually not enough to cause serious problems). And maybe you can cast some blame on genes, too, as a small percentage of folks *inherit* a protein deficiency that causes emphysema. But if you want to point the finger at culprit number one, it's demon weed: Most emphysema strikes long-term smokers and is a direct result of smoking.

Emphysema is serious business. It can make breathing difficult and simple chores nearly impossible. It also increases the risk of heart disease by interfering with the passage of blood through the lungs. For many people, even eating becomes difficult. But even though it's usually irreversible, here's what you can do to deemphasize emphysema and breathe easier.

Munch a bunch. Since people with emphysema cannot fully exhale, the lungs enlarge with trapped air. The enlarged lungs push down into the

When to See the Doctor

Emphysema is a serious condition that requires medical supervision. And other respiratory conditions, such as a cold or flu, can make it a lot worse. So besides paying special attention to preventing these ailments, call your doctor for immediate advice at the first indication that you've caught a "bug"—such as fever, chills or severe coughing.

abdomen, leaving less room for the stomach to expand—making eating uncomfortable.

"Many people with emphysema find it's much better to eat many smaller meals instead of three large ones," says Barry Make, M.D., director of pulmonary rehabilitation at the National Jewish Center for Immunology and Respiratory Medicine in Denver. "When you eat a large meal, it puts more pressure on the stomach and pushes up the diaphragm, which makes it more difficult to breathe. Besides eating a lot of little meals, it's also important to take small bites, to eat slowly and to chew your food well, which will make it easier on your breathing."

"A lot of people with emphysema lose weight or have trouble keeping weight on because eating can become so difficult," adds Mark J. Rosen, M.D., chief of the Division of Pulmonary and Critical Care Medicine at Beth Israel Medical Center in New York City. "You want to avoid weight loss, so be sure to eat enough."

Profit from produce. Some of the most advantageous eats you can have are fresh fruits and vegetables high in vitamin C and beta-carotene. "Some evidence suggests that vitamin C and beta-carotene may help protect against a decline in lung function," says Joel Schwartz, Ph.D., an epidemiologist and senior scientist at the Environmental Protection Agency in Washington, D.C. "It may be a very minimal effect in those with emphysema, but eating foods rich in these nutrients certainly won't hurt and may help."

Good sources of vitamin C include citrus fruits, strawberries and other fruits, as well as peppers and broccoli. Beta-carotene is abundant in sweet potatoes, squash, carrots and other fruits and vegetables with a yellowish orange color.

Stop smoking *now!* "When you stop smoking, you slow the deterioration of your lungs, and that's probably the best thing you can do once you've been diagnosed with emphysema," says Dr. Rosen. "Besides that, you will boost your feeling of well-being. And you'll be able to exercise longer, which will improve your comfort in breathing."

Failing to quit, on the other hand, speeds the deterioration of your lungs. It's also wise to avoid any exposure to secondhand smoke as well as any substances that may trigger allergies.

Get your heart pumping. "Aerobic exercise is very important for people with emphysema because it strengthens the heart and can help improve your breathing," says Dr. Rosen. "Walking is probably the best thing you can do, and you should try to do it every day."

Breathe Easier with These Techniques

Besides following a regular exercise program, you can strengthen your breathing muscles—and make yourself more comfortable—if you practice special breathing techniques.

One of the most effective is also the simplest: Just blow out. Here's how: To practice, exhale twice as long as you inhale, suggests Henry Gong, M.D., professor of medicine at the University of California, Los Angeles (UCLA), and associate chief of the Pulmonary Division of the UCLA Medical Center. For 30 minutes a day, concentrate on blowing out slowly through pursed lips to help keep the airways open.

Learning to breathe from your diaphragm is also helpful, since it's the most efficient way to breathe. To make sure you're breathing from your diaphragm—and *not* your chest—try this exercise.

Lie down with a book on your stomach, then watch what happens to the book when you breathe. If it moves up and down, you're breathing from your diaphragm; if not, you're chest breathing. Practice belly breathing (that is, using your diaphragm rather than your chest and shoulders) until you're doing it naturally every day.

Although you'll probably tire quickly, try to slowly build your endurance so that you can walk for about 20 minutes at least three days a week. Riding a stationary bicycle, swimming and participating in low-impact aerobics classes are also good, adds Dr. Make.

Build your body, too. What good are bulging biceps when you have trouble breathing? "The muscles in your shoulders, arms and upper chest comprise one of the two muscle groups that participate in breathing," says Dr. Make. (The other is the diaphragm.) Whether it's doing some simple exercises while holding wrist or hand weights or starting a full-fledged weight-training program, anything you can do to build your upper body strength will help your breathing. But make sure you breathe correctly while pumping iron: Exhale through pursed lips as you lift, and inhale as you relax.

Dress in the baggy look. Wearing clothing that fits loosely around your chest and abdomen allows plenty of room for them to expand freely, keeping breathing more comfortable. You might want to try suspenders instead of a belt, a camisole instead of a bra and going without a girdle.

Endometriosis

As if those monthly cramps weren't enough, now your period has been punctuated with new pain: Maybe your lower back aches more than an overaggressive bellboy's or you feel pain during bowel movements or sex.

Your doctor may tell you it's endometriosis, a condition that occurs when the tissue that lines the uterus becomes implanted on other pelvic organs—usually on the ovaries, the fallopian tubes or the ligaments that support your uterus. It may affect the bowel, bladder or ureters as well. This misguided tissue imitates the menstrual cycle, leaving a discharge that can't exit the body and causing inflammation and scarring. It can also cause infertility in a small percentage of women.

Pregnancy and breastfeeding can end symptoms of endometriosis, but here are some easier and faster ways to get relief.

Get into workouts. While a rigorous workout may be the last thing on your mind when pain strikes, plenty of exercise is often recommended. Research shows that women who exercise regularly have less endometriosis pain and easier periods in general.

"Exercise decreases estrogen production—and estrogen makes the disease worse," explains Owen Montgomery, M.D., an obstetrics/gynecology specialist at Thomas Jefferson University Hospital and Jefferson Medical College of Thomas Jefferson University, both in Philadelphia. His recommendation: a *vigorous* workout three to six times a week for at least 30 minutes each time.

Eat for a stronger immune system. Just as diet influences the severity of other diseases, it may have a role in causing endometriosis pain. "There are data suggesting an association of autoimmune disease with both the risk of developing endometriosis and the extent or severity of endometriosis," says Dan Martin, M.D., clinical associate professor of obstetrics/gynecology at the University of Tennessee and a reproductive surgeon at Baptist Memorial Hospital, both in Memphis. To build a stronger immune system, eat plenty of fresh fruits and vegetables that are rich in vitamins. Vitamin C is especially important, so fill up your plate with vegetables and fruits such as broccoli, red bell peppers, oranges, strawberries and cantaloupe—all high in viatmin C.

Don't forget fish. Rich in omega-3 fatty acids, fish such as mackerel, herring and sardines are also helpful, because they suppress prostaglandin production, suggests gynecology and fertility specialist Camran Nezhat, M.D., director of the Fertility and Endoscopy Center and Center for Special Pelvic Surgery in Atlanta. Prostaglandin is a hormone in the uterine lining that causes cramping.

Try hands-on healing. Acupressure relieves pain in some women, says Susan Anderson, an endometriosis sufferer who is a member of the national board of the Endometriosis Association, a self-help group based in Milwaukee. When pain begins, press the area on the inside of your leg about two inches above your ankle bone. To locate that spot, press with your thumb until you locate an area that feels tender. Another spot where pressure can ease pain is the web of your hand, at the base where the bones of your thumb and index finger meet. "If it doesn't hurt when you press, then it's not the right spot. Know that it will hurt, but you need to keep pressing, and you should feel relief in the pelvic area," says Anderson.

Keep a calendar of symptoms. If you know when endometriosis pain is likely to occur each month, you can plan around it. Dr. Montgomery recom-

When to See the Doctor

Endometriosis has been called "the great imitator" because its symptoms often mimic those of other ailments, such as irritable bowel syndrome, urinary tract infections, even tubal pregnancies. Because a doctor's diagnosis is needed to determine the cause of pain, be sure to consult your doctor before you try any kind of self-treatment, says Owen Montgomery, M.D., an obstetrics/gynecology specialist at Thomas Jefferson University Hospital and Jefferson Medical College of Thomas Jefferson University, both in Philadelphia. Dr. Montgomery recommends keeping a calendar of symptoms to help the doctor determine whether you have endometriosis or a different ailment.

mends keeping a chart of your symptoms for a few months until you see a pattern.

"Charting helps you get control of your disease, so you can plan your life better," he says. "For instance, if you know that you always have severe pain on the 22nd day of your cycle, you can avoid planning important events for that day. You can also plan your pain relief medications prior to that day, so you won't wake up on the 22nd day with severe pain."

Switch off caffeine and nicotine. Caffeine found in coffee, tea, chocolate and cola has been found to aggravate symptoms, says Dr. Nezhat. And while there's no scientific proof, most experts suspect that smoking aggravates endometriosis symptoms and pain. If you smoke and drink coffee or tea, consider giving them up—at least during your period.

Heat yourself up. Taking ibuprofen (Advil) is probably the easiest thing to do, but many women find a heating pad and warm beverages bring relief from abdominal pain and cramping, says Mary Sinn, R.N., nurse manager of the Medical Surgical Department and former coordinator of the WomanCare Unit at Gnaden Huetten Hospital in Lehighton, Pennsylvania.

Or cool yourself down. If heat doesn't help you beat endometriosis, you may be among those women who get more relief from an ice pack wrapped in a towel and placed on your lower abdominal area, adds Sinn.

Eyestrain

Eyestrain can happen to anyone. In fact, it usually happens to *everyone*, especially if you're over age 40. You're likely to have eyestrain at least occasionally if you use a computer, watch TV, drive a car or live in a smoggy city.

You know you've got eyestrain when normally clear images (such as words on the computer screen or print on the page) begin to appear blurry. Your eyes start to ache so much that you just want to close them for a while. Well, that's *one* thing you can do. But here are some other ways you can put a lid on eyestrain.

Try time-outs from close work. "When you're using a computer or doing any other type of close work that strains your eyes, stop every hour for about two minutes and give your eyes a rest," suggests Eric Donnenfeld, M.D., associate professor of ophthalmology at North Shore University Hospital/Cornell Medical College in Manhasset, New York. "Just close your eyes and do nothing for a couple of minutes."

Stop reading—and refocus. "When you're reading, stop every 30 minutes or so and focus on something far away for a few seconds," adds Merrill M. Knopf, M.D., an opthalmologist in Long Beach, California, and an officer of the California Association of Ophthalmology. There's a muscle in your eye that contracts when you're doing close-up work, Dr. Knopf explains. By refocusing,

Fine-Tune Your Workstation

If you're a frequent computer user, you have probably discovered how important it is to reduce the glare on your computer screen in order to minimize eyestrain. "It's not so much the intensity of the surrounding light that's important; rather, it's the positioning," says Merrill M. Knopf, M.D., an opthalmologist in Long Beach, California, and officer of the California Association of Ophthalmology. "The light source should be positioned close enough to you that it's comfortable but far enough away that it doesn't shine on your screen or into your eyes." Of course, placing a special antiglare shield on the screen also helps.

But here are some lesser-known tips to help prevent video-screen eyestrain from R. Anthony Hutchinson, O.D., an optometrist in Encinitas, California, and author of *Computer Eye Stress: How to Avoid It, How to Alleviate It.*

- Adjust your computer monitor so that the letters on the screen are at least five times brighter than the background.
- When buying a monitor, choose one with amber or green letters, because they're easiest on your eyes. Screen size isn't significant, but letter size is: Capital letters should be at least ⅛ inch high.
- Avoid overhead fluorescent lighting when using your computer, because its flickering can interact with the flicker on your screen, causing eyestrain. (Even though you can't see the fluctuation in light, a fluorescent tube actually flickers about 60 times a second).

you relieve the spasms in that eye muscle. If you want something to look at, hang a sheet of newspaper on a far wall and try to read the larger print.

Take a tea break. Warm eyebright tea is a gentle balm for eyes that are strained. "Take a towel and soak it in brewed eyebright tea," says Meir Schneider, director of the Center for Self Healing in San Francisco and author of *Self Healing: My Life and Vision.* "Lie down, place the warm towel over your closed eyes, and leave it there for 10 to 15 minutes. It will make your eyestrain go away."

Be very careful not to let the towel drip tea into your eyes, though—and be sure the tea has cooled down enough before you soak the towel in it. Note: Eyebright tea is not a real tea but a mixture of herbal ingredients, sold in loose tea form at most health food stores, specifically for eyestrain.

Put your eyes "on the blink." Your eyes have their own personal masseuse—the eyelids. "Make it a point to consciously blink your eyes frequently and not squint," says Schneider. "Each blink cleanses your eyes and gives them a tiny little massage."

Get glasses. Most eyestrain is the result of vanity, says Dr. Donnenfeld. "Obviously, you're going to strain your eyes if your vision is off, so get a pair of glasses if you need them." If you have good distance vision and just have trouble seeing up close, reading glasses, sold in most drugstores, are sometimes enough to cure eyestrain.

Exercise your eyes. Standing about five feet from a blank wall, have someone toss a tennis ball at the wall while you try to catch it each time it bounces off. Or hold your thumb out at arm's length. Move it in circles and Xs, bringing the thumb closer, then farther away, as you follow it with your eyes. Both exercises help offset damage caused by eyestrain and improve the brain-to-nerve-to-muscle connection of your vision, says Don Teig, O.D., an optometrist and sports vision specialist in Ridgefield, Connecticut.

Fallen Arches

The belly isn't the only part of your body subject to middle-age spread. As we get older, the years of walking and standing can cause feet to spread and flatten out as ligaments that support the arch lose their holding power. The result: the condition known as fallen arches, or flat feet.

"Keep in mind that we're talking about 26 bones in the foot that are supported by a series of ligaments, muscle tendons and other connective tissue," says Glenn Gastwirth, D.P.M., deputy executive director of the American Podiatric Medicine Association in Bethesda, Maryland. "Over a period of time, the ligaments stretch out or 'give' under the pressure of your weight—especially if you're overweight. So what usually happens is you go shopping for new shoes one day and suddenly realize that you now need a size 8 when you've always worn a size 6. You may think your foot has grown, but what really happens is that the foot has spread out, both in width and length."

Here's how to delay or even prevent fallen arches or reduce arch pain if it's already happened.

Tie 'em on. One reason fallen arches are most prevalent in women is that pumps and other shoes with "flimsy uppers" don't give the same support as the

When to See the Doctor

If you have sudden pain or swelling in your foot, either out of the blue or as the result of an injury, you should pay a visit to a foot specialist, according to Philip Sanfilippo, D.P.M., a podiatrist in San Francisco.

"Sudden pain can be a sign of a ruptured tendon, especially among older people," says Dr. Sanfilippo. This is a serious foot condition that requires a doctor's attention as soon as possible.

lace-up shoes more typically worn by men, says Philip Sanfilippo, D.P.M., a podiatrist in San Francisco. "You're less likely to get fallen arches if you wear lace-ups or other styles that provide more support in the upper (the top of the shoe)." He points out that loafers, pumps and slip-ons don't give sufficient support to feet that are prone to developing fallen arches.

Get shoes made for walking or running. One way to support your arch is to wear good-quality running or walking shoes, says Dr. Gastwirth. "These shoes generally provide good support to the foot."

Add support. The top-of-the-line arch support is an orthotic insole, which may cost $900 or more and must be custom-made. "But many people with sore arches will get relief with over-the-counter arch supports for about $10," suggests Judith Smith, M.D., assistant professor of orthopedic surgery at Emory University School of Medicine in Atlanta. "The thing to remember about arch supports is that your shoe must have enough depth to accommodate them. Otherwise, you'll get a lot of rubbing on the top of your foot, or your heel will come out of the shoe." Most men's shoes are deep enough to accommodate the insoles; women should take their shoes with them to the drugstore when buying the insoles to ensure a good fit.

If your heels are high, keep them wide. High heels may be your Achilles' heel—especially if you wear them constantly. "Flatter shoes are no doubt

If the Shoe Fits These Criteria . . .

Wearing good-quality running or walking shoes is one of the best ways to prevent or treat fallen arches. But "good quality" doesn't necessarily mean high price tag.

"A lot of moderately priced shoes also have what you should be looking for," says Philip Sanfilippo, D.P.M., a podiatrist in San Francisco. "You want a shoe with a stiff heel counter, meaning that your heel doesn't slide around when you're wearing the shoe. Look for models that have extra reinforcement on the *inside* of the heel. Also, the shoe should bend where the foot bends—across the ball of the foot. And it's essential to find a shoe that *fits* well, so it completely supports your foot." A shoe that fits poorly will not be helpful, even if it has the correct shape and design.

better," says Dr. Sanfilippo. Flat heels help prevent fallen arches and are kinder to your feet if fallen arches have already occurred. "If you *must* wear high heels, choose styles with a wide heel. Stay away from stiletto heels."

Roll away pain. "If you're feeling pain in the arch area, you can get some relief by massaging the bottom of your foot," says Dr. Gastwirth. "A regular massage while you're watching TV can do wonders."

Stretch out. Doing the same type of stretching exercises that runners do in their warm-up can help reduce arch pain caused by a tight heel cord. One of the best exercises is to stand about three feet from a wall and place your hands on the wall. Leaning toward the wall, bring one foot forward and bend the knee so that the calf muscles of the other leg stretch. Then switch legs. "Stretching is particularly important for women who spend all week in heels and then wear exercise shoes or sneakers on weekends," says Dr. Gastwirth.

Get measured *each* time you buy new shoes. "Don't assume that since you always wore a particular size, you always will," says Dr. Sanfilippo. "Too many people try to squeeze into their 'regular' shoe size and wind up with serious foot problems or sores on their feet. When your arch is falling, your feet may get longer or wider and you may or may not feel pain, so getting your foot measured *each* time you buy shoes is a good indicator of your arch's degeneration."

Examine your shoes. "If the heel is worn down, replace it. But if the back portion of the shoe is distorted or bent to one side, get yourself into a new pair of supportive shoes like those made specifically for walking," according to Dr. Gastwirth. That's because flat feet can affect your walking stride, and failing to replace "worn" shoes may lead to knee or hip pain.

Fatigue

Everyone suffers from fatigue now and then—usually as the result of being under too much physical or mental strain. The usual Rx is some R and R. But if you're all caught up on your rest and relaxation and you *still* feel pooped, it's time to wonder why.

Of course, anyone who feels totally drained most of the time should pay a visit to the doctor. But for the usual, run-of-the-mill worn-out feeling, here are some ways to perk up your get-up-and-go.

Add some stress to your life. It's no surprise that too much stress can knock you out. But if there's not *enough* stress in your life, you can feel fatigued because of boredom and lack of motivation. "It's sort of like the tension or stress on a violin string," says Paul J. Rosch, M.D., clinical professor of medicine and psychiatry at New York Medical College in Vallhalla and president of the American Institute of Stress in Yonkers. "If you have too much, the string will snap. If you have too little, you'll get a dull, raspy sound. But just the right amount creates a beautiful tone. Similarly, we need to find the right amount of stress that allows us to make beautiful music in our lives."

The key is to add the kind of stress that will make you feel challenged, not beaten. "I suggest becoming a volunteer," says consumer health expert John Renner, M.D., clinical professor of family medicine at the University of Missouri at Kansas City. The only additional stress is your commitment to show up on time and do the job, but you have the challenge of working with people and producing results.

But avoid stress carriers. "Some people are Typhoid Marys of stress, and just being around them can fatigue you," says Maria Simonson, Ph.D., Sc.D., professor emeritus and director of the Health, Weight and Stress Program at Johns Hopkins Medical Institutions in Baltimore. "They tend to be the people who are insensitive, complainers and blamers. The best thing you can do is try to stay clear of them."

Close your mouth for better breathing. One often-overlooked cause of fatigue is poor breathing. People who breathe shallowly and rapidly get fatigued easily because the body gets less oxygen. The problem is often due to mouth breathing, says Robert Fried, Ph.D., director of the Biofeedback Clinic at the Institute for Rational Emotive Therapy in New York City and author of *The Psychology and Physiology of Breathing in Behavioral Medicine.*

Remedy the situation by breathing slowly and steadily through your nose. Expand your abdomen *and* keep your chest down with each breath; that way, you use your whole diaphragm.

Give (inner) peace a chance. Meditation is a great way to offset fatigue, and anyone can do it. Start by turning on some soft music, lying back on the sofa and telling yourself that you're feeling relaxed, says Dr. Simonson. "Concen-

When to See the Doctor

When that tired, worn-out, run-down feeling won't go away no matter what you do, it's a good idea to see the doctor.

Fatigue can be a warning sign of serious illness, including diabetes, lung disease and anemia, according to Rick Ricer, M.D., associate professor of clinical medicine at Ohio State University College of Medicine in Columbus.

In some cases, fatigue can be a symptom of hepatitis, mononucleosis, thyroid disease or cancer, according to doctors. And a pattern of extreme fatigue could be one sign of chronic fatigue syndrome, which is more debilitating than normal fatigue and requires a doctor's diagnosis and treatment.

So be sure to see a doctor if you can't shake off that pooped-out feeling.

trate on the softness of the music and breathe deeply. With each exhalation, repeat a word, phrase or prayer that brings feelings of peace. (Many people say the word *peace*.) While doing this, imagine yourself on a beach . . . imagine the breeze, the waves and the seagulls." If your doctor has found no reasonable cause for fatigue, Dr. Simonson recommends meditation twice a day for 20 minutes each time.

Color your world. "If you live in a dark, dark house, you're going to feel fatigued," says Rick Ricer, M.D., associate professor of clinical medicine at Ohio State University College of Medicine in Columbus. Add some color and more light to your life, he suggests. Studies show that wearing red or being in red surroundings energizes. The color green has been found to evoke peacefulness and serenity, while brown helps induce feelings of warmness and camaraderie.

Use your head to exercise your body. Studies show that as you exercise, no matter what kind of daily exercise you choose to do, your body becomes better at handling the everyday emotional and physical stressors, says Ralph Wharton, M.D., clinical professor of psychiatry at Columbia University in New York City. "Just be sure you exercise with regularity and a minimum of three times a week for 30 minutes each time."

If exercise causes pain, of course, you should see your doctor first. And whatever you do—walking, running, aerobics—ease into it slowly. If you are a regular exerciser, stick with lighter-than-usual workouts until you begin to feel more energetic.

Don't be a sundown sprinter. Beware of late-night activity, whether it's a light workout or intense training. Most experts agree that exercising after 7:00 P.M. can cause a disruption of regular sleeping habits, which can translate into fatigue the following morning.

Stomp out cigarettes. Smoking is an oxygen robber that can cause fatigue. But doctors say you shouldn't expect an immediate energy boost upon quitting. Nicotine is a stimulant, and withdrawal from smoking can cause temporary tiredness.

Lose weight . . . but not too quickly. It's true, lugging around extra weight can tire you out faster, but don't try to lose too much too soon. Crash diets can send your energy into a nosedive. (Because ultra-low-calorie diets concentrate on one type of food, such as grapefruit, they don't give you all the nutrients you need for sufficient energy.)

When your calorie intake is restricted too much, it's very stressful for the body, according to Manfred Kroger, Ph.D., professor of food science at Pennsylvania State University in University Park. "And one of the many symptoms of this type of stress is fatigue."

For responsible dieting, men should consume at least 1,500 calories a day, and women should have 1,200 calories or more.

Turn off the tube. Sure, television helps you unwind after a hard day of hassles—but maybe you're unwinding too much. TV is notorious for lulling folks into a state of lethargy. Instead of watching the tube, try something a little more mentally stimulating, like reading, says Dr. Ricer. "That will be more energizing."

Fever

W hen your forehead feels hot enough to fry an egg, your body is shaking like Jell-O and your teeth are chattering, it's hard to believe that fever is your friend.

But it is.

A fever isn't a disease. It's a *symptom* of an infection, typically caused by a cold or the flu. When you have a cold, for instance, your immune system signals to

---

When to See the Doctor

I t's a myth that high temperatures can 'boil your brain,'" says Thomas Rosenthal, M.D., associate professor of family medicine at the State University of New York at Buffalo. "Most adults can tolerate five points above the normal body temperature." Brain damage doesn't happen until your temperature reaches 107°F, which rarely happens, he says. Adults over age 60, however, are less likely to mount an immune defense. For them, fever may be more taxing on the heart and thus more risky. With that in mind, contact the doctor immediately for:

- Fever above 103° in an adult.
- Fever of 101° if you're over age 60.
- Fever above 102° in a child (or if the child is vomiting or convulsing or has a headache).
- Any fever in a baby under three months old.
- Any fever if you have a chronic illness such as diabetes, heart disease or lung disease.
- Fever that lingers more than three days.
- Fever accompanied by a rash, severe headache, stiff neck, confusion, back pain or painful urination.

---

your brain that it needs more body heat in order to attack infectious cells, and your body temperature rises.

There are some tried-and-true procedures that can help bring down the fever and make you more comfortable. Here's what doctors recommend.

If it's mild, hands off. Some doctors believe a mild fever (under 100°F in adults) should not be treated.

"Taking antipyretics such as aspirin or acetaminophen (Tylenol) brings down the fever, but there's also some evidence that immune activity is suppressed," says Donna McCarthy, Ph.D., assistant professor of nursing at the University of Wisconsin–Madison.

Don't be stoic—pop a pill. On the other hand, there's no good proof that *not* treating fever helps your recovery, says Thomas Rosenthal, M.D., associate

Tools for Temperature Taking

Like trying to invent better mousetraps, inventing a better thermometer poses a real challenge. But there are definitely some interesting variations. Here's a rundown of the old and the new.

- Just for kids: Rectal thermometers with a bulb at one end are used until a child is old enough to hold a thermometer in his mouth. With the child lying facedown on your lap, hold the buttocks and insert the lubricated bulb one inch into the rectum. Hold it in a minute or two. Rectal temperatures register one degree higher than body temperature. After use, wash the thermometer thoroughly in cold, soapy water.
- Recommended for adults: The "standard" glass thermometer filled with silver mercury or red alcohol is still recommended for temperature taking, says Donna McCarthy, Ph.D., assistant professor of nursing at the University of Wisconsin–Madison. "Place the thermometer in the deep pocket alongside the tongue, not under the tongue," says Dr. McCarthy. "The pocket ensures an accurate reading, because it's closer to the artery where the heat originates." For the record, the proper way to use one is to shake it until the mercury is below 96°F, place it in the mouth and leave it for three minutes.

professor of family medicine at the State University of New York at Buffalo. "Let your comfort be your guide," says Dr. Rosenthal. "If you have headache or muscle aches, by all means take an aspirin or acetaminophen. Both are equally effective, and you should feel effects in a half-hour." (Children should be given only child-size doses of acetaminophen: Aspirin is not advised by pediatricians because of its link to Reye's syndrome, a potentially fatal neurological disease.)

Have a massage. If you go the nondrug route, having a massage and listening to soothing music helps boost comfort, says Dr. McCarthy.

A warm bath is best. "The old-fashioned advice to immerse a fevered person in cold water is outdated," says Dr. Rosenthal. "A cold bath makes the body temperature drop too quickly. You'll shiver—which raises your temperature

- Temperature "strips": These strips turn colors as your temperature rises, so it's no wonder kids like to use them in front of a mirror. While forehead strips are not supersensitive, you can distinguish between a temperature of 100° and 102°F by looking at the colors, says Herbert Patrick, M.D., assistant professor of medicine and medical director of the Respiratory Care Department at Jefferson Medical College of Thomas Jefferson University in Philadelphia. The mouth strips are more reliable but must remain in the mouth a full two minutes.
- Electronic thermometers: Primarily for use in doctors' offices, an electronic thermometer consists of a steel probe covered with a disposable sheath. It's attached to a cord hooked to a monitor that flashes a digital readout in a mere 15 seconds. Even faster are models that can be inserted in the ear. The drawback? They cost more than $100.
- Digital thermometers: These affordable, plastic, paddle-shaped probes contain a tiny computer chip that receives an electric signal. Within a minute, the beep alerts you to the temperature displayed in the window. You don't have to shake them, but you must wash the tip and keep a battery on hand. They are available at most pharmacies.

even more, because the rapid muscle movement generates body heat." For the same reason, he adds, you should avoid alcohol rubs, which also cool the skin too quickly.

Fill 'er up. With fever, your system is pumped up, and you lose double or triple your normal water loss without even knowing it, says Dr. Rosenthal. Drinking lots of liquid makes it easier to sweat and get rid of the heat.

Back off from heavy exercise. Both fever and exercise boost your body's heat production, making your heart work harder. Also, if you can't lose the extra heat fast enough, heat exhaustion could result. "The 'work' of fever is enough of a workout to skip exercise for a day," says Herbert Keating, M.D., chief of medicine at the Veterans Administration Medical Center in Des Moines, Iowa.

Flatulence

Theoretically, flatulence should leave us unruffled. It's just excessive intestinal gas in the stomach or intestine. Flatulence's famous sidekick, of course, is the aroma you might like to blame on somebody else. The trouble is, look around for someone to blame, and whoops, they've all *disappeared.*

The odor of flatus actually comes from trace gases that make up less than 1 percent of intestinal gas. Unfortunately, humans turn positively bloodhound when it comes to perceiving intestinal gas. We can detect this odor in amounts as low as 1 part per 100 million.

Flatulence can be painfully embarrassing as well as plain old painful, and it happens a lot. Eight to 20 gas elimination episodes a day is normal, and there are times when you may have even more. If you are sedentary, have premenstrual bloating, have difficulty digesting carbohydrates or have just gone on a brand-new high-fiber diet, an ill wind may be blowing your way. Problems digesting milk and dairy products can also create a problem with gas. (See page 332 for more information about lactose intolerance.)

Here's some degassing advice from the experts.

Befriend These Offenders . . . Gradually

Do you love beans? Crave broccoli? Champ at the bit for the first fresh ears of corn every summer? All these high-fiber foods can cause gas problems—but so can a lot of less fibrous, fattening foods such as cream, ice cream and pastries. If you happen to be a gassy gourmet, monitor your reaction to these foods known to be the biggest offenders.

Apples	Lima beans
Apricots	Milk
Baked beans	Oats
Bananas	Onions
Bran cereals and muffins	Pastries
Broccoli	Peaches
Brussels sprouts	Pears
Cabbage	Potatoes
Cauliflower	Pretzels
Citrus fruits	Prunes and prune juice
Corn	Radishes
Cream	Raisins
Cucumbers	Rutabagas
Dried beans	Sauerkraut
Dried peas	Sorbitol and mannitol (artificial
Eggplant	sweeteners)
Ice cream	Tomatoes
Ice milk	Wheat bread
Kohlrabi	Wheat germ
Lentils	

Rock in the breeze. Try rocking in a rocking chair! It's been found to relieve painful gas buildup in women who've just had a cesarean section delivery, reports Helen Ptak, Ph.D., director for research at the University of Southern Mississippi's College of Health and Human Sciences in Hattiesburg. "And it works for other people as well," she adds. The rocking stimulates the nervous system and may exert a little pressure on the abdomen, which makes it easier to pass gas. "But you can't just rock. You need to put your feet on the floor and put some 'wham' in it," says Dr. Ptak.

Take time for tea. Peppermint, spearmint, anise and caraway contain oils that settle the stomach, according to William J. Keller, Ph.D., professor and head of the Division of Medicinal Chemistry and Pharmaceutics at Northeast Louisiana University School of Pharmacy in Monroe and secretary of the American Society of Pharmacognosy. "Herbal tea is a good form to take them in," he says. And they taste good. Spearmint and peppermint teas are readily available in the tea section of your supermarket; anise and caraway may require a stop at the health food store.

Zero in on the culprit. "One vegetable in the salad might be responsible for a disproportionate portion of discomfort," says Bruce Yaffe, M.D., a gastro-enterologist affiliated with Lenox Hill Hospital in New York City. We all want to get more fiber in our diet, but some of those high-fiber foods are real gas

Bean Busters You Can Bank On

After all the fuss (and fumes), why do you want to bother with beans anyway? Because they're high in fiber, low in fat, extremely versatile in recipes and absolutely delicious!

There are a number of ways to minimize gas problems and still eat beans. Bruce Yaffe, M.D., a gastroenterologist affiliated with Lenox Hill Hospital in New York City, recommends that you eat only small portions of beans at any one sitting. And don't mix them with other gassy foods in the same meal or recipe. Here are some other ways to lower the bean impact.

- Try gentler beans, such as split peas, limas and lentils, before gradually introducing yourself to others. Among the mildest are Anasazi beans, which are sweet, mealy and excellent for baking. You can find them in most health food stores.
- Beans are less likely to cause a problem if you soak them for four to five hours or overnight, then drain, rinse, and cook in fresh water. Be sure to cook them thoroughly.
- Try canned beans in your recipes (they're usually well cooked).
- The oh-so-healthy soybean can pack a powerful intestinal punch. So enjoy the benefits of soybean products such as tofu or soybean curd instead of gas generators. Most of the hard-to-digest sugars are washed out of the way with the whey in processing.

promoters. To find out which ones balloon into problems, "start with a simple lettuce and tomato salad," Dr. Yaffe suggests. Then over a period of time, meal by meal, add the new vegetable ingredients one at a time. That way, you can find out which of the veggies is the troublemaker.

"Some people are particularly bothered by onions, or garlic, or peppers, but not beans," points out W. Steven Pray, Ph.D., R.Ph., professor in the Southwestern Oklahoma State University School of Pharmacy in Weatherford. "We're all different."

Remember the two Ps. Think posture and position. If you have a problem with gas, you should probably be eating your meals when you're sitting at the table, not when you're lounging or lying down. "When you drink or eat lying down," Dr. Pray says, "the gas in your stomach cannot escape." Slouching can cause problems, too, so watch that posture.

Breathe air, don't swallow it. "Eat slowly, chew thoroughly, and don't gulp," says Dr. Yaffe. The reason? "When you gulp, you swallow air, and swallowing air will only make things worse." Chewing gum, ill-fitting dentures and sucking on hard candy can also cause you to swallow a lot of excess air, he says. To avoid those gulps that go to gas, steer clear of carbonated beverages and beer. And it's another reason not to smoke.

Dry up that drip. "The most important thing I've discovered in my medical career," says Dr. Yaffe, "is that postnasal drip often leads to air swallowing and increased gas production. People who have mucus in the backs of their throats are always swallowing." (For tips on postnasal drip, see page 409.)

Give bravos for Beano. Beano, a product introduced in 1990, lets people with gas problems befriend the bean again. The food enzyme in Beano breaks down indigestible sugars found in gas-producing vegetables and legumes. "I've had people come to me with tears in their eyes after trying Beano," says Dr. Pray. "They can eat foods they haven't eaten in 20 years." Take three to eight drops of Beano with the first bite of food (beans especially) and you may feel a lot more comfortable afterward.

Reach for simethicone for a sigh of relief. For persistent discomfort or fathom-less flatulence, there are a variety of over-the-counter medications containing simethicone, such as Gas-X, Mylicon Gas and Phazyme-95. A defoaming agent, simethicone "relieves symptoms of bloating, pressure and fullness due to gas," says Dr. Pray.

Fleabites

When it comes to motherhood, few are more prolific than the lowly flea. In just a few months, a single pair of fleas can produce up to 2,000 eggs. Nearly all the eggs are laid on your pet and then fall off to hatch in your carpet, furniture, bed sheets or elsewhere around your home or in the yard. Then each new female can hatch thousands of its own offspring.

This population explosion translates to a heck of a lot of fleabites. While Fido or Kittypuss is their main choice of entrée, your ankle or foot also makes a tasty treat when pets aren't around.

Fleabites leave you with redness or a rash as well as severe itching. But here's how to turn the tables on fleas and take the itch out of their annoying nips.

Cool the itch with cold. If you've had fleas noshing on your ankles and legs, you probably headed for a hot shower to wash them off and stop the itching. It's the wrong approach. "*Cold* is one of the best ways to stop any itch," says Charles H. Banov, M.D., clinical professor of medicine and microbiology/immunology at the Medical University of South Carolina in Charleston and past president of the American College of Allergy and Immunology. "When people go right into a hot shower, that only brings blood to the area and aggravates the itching. In fact, I wouldn't even recommend a shower, because the pressure of the water might trigger itching. I'd advise a cool bath or applying a cold towel to the area."

Use lotion to kill their motion. Calamine lotion is the old standby for itch relief from fleas, but another household regular may be good at keeping them away. Avon's Skin-So-Soft, a bath oil, has long been known as a mosquito repellent. Now researchers at the University of Florida in Gainesville have found that it works just as well on fleas. In tests, flea counts dropped 40 percent in just one day after dogs were soaked with a solution of 1½ ounces of Skin-

A Flea-Free Pet Is Your Best Insurance

The easiest way to prevent being bothered by fleabites is to make sure your pet isn't bothered by fleas. For a flea-free dog or cat, try these tried-and-true treatments.

Give pets a dip. "A flea shampoo kills only the fleas that are on your pet at that time. But as soon as your dog or cat goes outside, it picks up a new bunch of fleas. So flea shampoos aren't enough—you also have to give your pet a flea dip," says Paul Donovan, V.M.D., a veterinarian and director of the Alburtis Animal Hospital in Alburtis, Pennsylvania. Dips last anywhere from 10 to 30 days (depending on the product). "The idea is to pour the dip while the animal is still in the tub. Let the animal drip-dry for a couple of minutes, then turn it loose, so the product dries on the coat."

Add garlic to their Gravy Train. While there's no scientific proof, many pet owners swear that adding garlic or brewer's yeast to a pet's daily diet—or even rubbing it directly on the animal's coat—is a surefire flea zapper. Fleas don't go for the flavor, it's said, and they'll go elsewhere for their meals.

Don't rely on flea collars. They are one of the least effective methods of flea control because they usually don't deliver what they promise.

"They have little or no repellency, so they work too slowly to do any good," says David Thompson, D.V.M., a veterinarian and director of the Animal Hospital of Asheville in Asheville, North Carolina. "Authorities in the field suspect the fleas are killed so slowly that they can grow to reproductive age, lay their eggs and keep on infesting your pet and home even in the presence of the collar."

Take extra care with kitty. Because most cats dislike water and are not fond of hissing sounds, you can guess that cats don't like flea-control sprays, says Marvin Samuelson, D.V.M., director of the Animal Dermatology and Allergy Clinic in Topeka, Kansas.

Dips are generally effective if your cat will tolerate a soaking. You might try using a flea-killing foam made especially for cats. (A dog preparation may be too potent.)

So-Soft in a gallon of water. The researchers believe that fleas, which have a keen sense of smell, don't like the product's woodland fragrance. Advice: Smear Skin-So-Soft on flea-bitten areas of your body to prevent repeat bites.

Sock it to 'em. To determine if your pets have brought fleas into your home, walk across the floors (particularly carpeted areas) wearing white socks. The fleas will go for the socks, since they are attracted to vibrations and warmth, says Jeffrey Hahn, assistant extension entomologist for the University of Minnesota Extension Service and University of Minnesota Department of Entomology in St. Paul. You'll be able to spot them easily before they get to your skin. If your socks are dotted, you've got fleas. So give rugs a good regular vacuuming, then apply a flea-control product made especially for rugs. Various brands are sold in pet shops.

Debug with some earth. Spread a little diatomaceous earth in the nooks and crannies and under furniture where you can't reach by vacuuming, suggests Richard Pitcairn, D.V.M., Ph.D., a veterinarian at the Animal Natural Health Center in Eugene, Oregon, and coauthor with Susan Hubble Pitcairn of *Dr. Pitcairn's Complete Guide to Natural Health for Dogs and Cats.* Diatomaceous earth is a natural earthlike substance, the residue of microscopic animals that once lived in the sea. Its crystalline structure cuts through the waxy coating on fleas, causing them to dry out and die. Don't use the type used in pool filters, however. It is ground too fine and may be dangerous if inhaled. A natural, unprocessed form—Diatom Dust—is available from Eco-Safe Products, 7000 U.S. Route 1 North, St. Augustine, FL 32095. Be sure to wear a dust mask when you spread it.

Wash *all* bedding—yours *and* your pet's—in hot water. If you have indoor pets, it's just a hop, skip and flea-jump from your pet's hide to your snowy sheets. And once a flea or two are in bed, you'll get bitten while you sleep. So once a week, carefully roll up your bedding (to avoid dropping fleas or their eggs on the floor) and wash it in a hot, soapy cycle in your washer. Then dry it in a hot cycle of your dryer, say Dr. Pitcairn. This is especially important in the summer, when flea activity is highest.

Flu

Do you feel the onset of a brain-mashing headache—along with major muscle aches, bone-tiring fatigue, vomiting and a fever that makes you sweat and shiver? These are all clues that the flu has its hold on you. Anyone who's had the flu before will probably be tempted to get a flu shot before the season begins—and a shot can prevent the flu or lessen its severity. But if it strikes, most of the recovery action is on the home front. Here are some things you can do to make your flu flee.

By all means, feed your flu. You need vitamins and minerals to mount an effective defense against the flu bug, says Herbert Patrick, M.D., assistant professor of medicine and medical director of the Respiratory Care Department at Jefferson Medical College of Thomas Jefferson University in Philadelphia. Aim for well-balanced meals, or at least try some bland fruit such as mashed bananas or applesauce.

Sip your nutrition. "Drinking your nutrients is a good idea when you have the flu, especially if you're not up for eating solid foods," says Frederick Ruben, M.D., professor of medicine at the University of Pittsburgh and spokesperson for the American Lung Association. Wash down your meals with a vitamin-rich juice such as vegetable juice, or have a bowl or two of soup. The more fluid you drink, says Dr. Ruben, the more your tissues are hydrated, and the more mucus flows.

Beware of fluid flu remedies. Combination cold/flu liquid remedies can contain as much as 80-proof alcohol. "That's equal to the amount in a shot of liquor," says Dr. Ruben. Alcohol can depress your immune system and also dry out your mucous membranes, so you should avoid it when you have the flu, he says.

Toss your old toothbrush. The virus continues to linger on wet toothbrush bristles, and you can reinfect yourself day after day, says Dr. Patrick. To prevent

When to See the Doctor

If you are over age 65 or have certain chronic conditions such as heart disease or lung disease, doctors recommend getting a flu shot *before* flu season begins. Residents of nursing homes and most medical personnel are also advised to have flu shots, which can usually prevent the flu entirely or lessen its severity.

If you do get the flu, you should see a doctor immediately if you have any of the following symptoms.

• Hoarseness
• Pains in the chest
• Difficulty breathing

Also, be sure to consult a doctor if you have vomiting that continues for more than a day or severe abdominal pain. Prolonged vomiting can leave you dehydrated, which is especially risky for young children and elderly people. And abdominal pain can be a sign of another problem, such as appendicitis.

this, throw away your toothbrush three days after the onset of the flu and use a new one.

Steer clear of crowds. There *is* a season when you're more likely to be hit by this viral bully, according to Dr. Patrick. "Spending time in offices, malls, theaters or other crowded environments between December and February increases your chances of ending up flat on your back with the flu, especially if your resistance is low," he says.

Consider postponing that flight. More than a decade ago, researchers from the Alaskan division of the Centers for Disease Control and Prevention (CDC) in Atlanta traced an outbreak of flu to a single infected passenger in an airplane. Due to a faulty ventilation system, the air inside the cabin recirculated the flu virus as the plane sat waiting for takeoff. Later, 38 of the 54 people on the flight came down with the flu. There have not been follow-up studies, "but an airplane has cramped quarters and air blowing all around, which may create a high-risk situation for exposure to airborne infectious diseases," says Nancy Arden, chief of the Influenza Epidemiology Division of the CDC. If you have any kind of chronic condition (such as diabetes or heart or lung disease), a bout with the flu could be serious. You may want to reduce risk of exposure by avoiding long trips in peak flu season, from December through February.

Develop the hand-washing habit. "Ordinary soap kills the flu virus, but in order to reduce your chance of infection, you've got to remember to wash your hands throughout the day, not just before meals or after going to the bathroom," says Carole Heilman, Ph.D., chief of the Respiratory Diseases Branch at the National Institute of Allergy and Infectious Diseases in Bethesda, Maryland. When a family member is sick, you can use a disinfectant spray on the sink and countertops. Use hot, soapy water to wash towels, telephones and dishes.

Go for the tiny droplets. Humidifying a room can help lick the flu, according to Dr. Patrick. The vapor emitted by a room humidifier moistens the mucous membranes in your nose and throat, so germs are more easily trapped and expelled.

If you use an ultrasonic room humidifier, be sure to rinse it out daily to prevent mold and fungus growth in the water reservoir, says Dr. Patrick. (And you should run a hot-water-and-bleach mixture through the machine at least once a week, following directions on the humidifier.) Better yet, use a hot steam humidifier that moisturizes *and* kills any microbial growth in the water.

Breathe deeply . . . and meditate. Relaxation techniques may protect you from influenza and other infections, according to the results of a study at the University of Pittsburgh School of Medicine that involved the use of self-hypnosis for relaxation. But you don't have to do self-hypnosis to get the benefits of relaxation therapy. Other ways to relax include deep breathing and stretching, meditation and yoga.

Don't exercise. Once you have been hit by the flu, get in bed and cancel your daily run. "There is some evidence that pushing yourself when you have the flu can depress your immune system and slow your recovery," says David Nieman, Ph.D., a health researcher at Appalachian State University in Boone, North Carolina.

After your symptoms clear—which usually takes about a week—wait another two weeks before returning to your regular exercise schedule.

Flushing

I t can be plenty embarrassing to look embarrassed—especially when your only faux pas is having a face full of hypersensitive blood vessels.

For unknown reasons, the tiny blood vessels in some people's faces make them frequent flushers. Vessels in the nose, cheeks and other facial areas react to the slightest provocation—a glass of wine, a blast of cold air or a cloud of steam. And when an embarrassing moment comes along, a blush for these flushers can last for hours.

It doesn't need to spoil your day. In fact, some people won't even notice if your face is turning red now and then. But if you're bothered by it, here are a number of ways to take some of the excess color out of your cheeks.

Avoid the triggers. The easiest way to foil flushing is to avoid the food and drink that often cause it, say experts. Alcoholic beverages, for example, can cause blood vessels to dilate, according to Jonathan Wilkin, M.D., professor of medicine and pharmacology and director of the Dermatology Division at Ohio State University in Columbus. So if you find that a glass of burgundy gives you crimson cheeks, switch to another beverage. And you may have to forget about ordering enchiladas with jalapeño peppers or other spicy foods. These foods contain ingredients that tend to dilate blood vessels, according to Dr. Wilkin.

Let your soup cool down. Food shouldn't be piping hot, says Dr. Wilkin. Consuming hot foods and beverages heats the blood that eventually makes its way to the hypothalamus, your body's thermostat. When your body gets the signal that something hot is on the loose, it responds by dilating the blood vessels near the skin's surface, causing a flush.

Suck on ice chips. "Some people can temporarily stop flushing by sucking on ice chips," says Dr. Wilkin. Holding ice chips in the mouth provokes a heat-opposing response.

When to See the Doctor

Some prescription drugs, such as high blood pressure medications, may cause persistent flushing, according to Jonathan Wilkin, M.D., professor of medicine and pharmacology and director of the Dermatology Division at Ohio State University in Columbus. If you suspect that this may be the problem, be sure to check with your doctor.

If you flush so often that your face seems to be getting more intensely red—or if the flushing lasts longer than ever—ask your doctor about it. In some cases, flushing can be a sign of rosacea, the disfiguring condition that can result in a reddened, bulbous nose. (W. C. Fields had rosacea.) Under a doctor's care, however, problems related to dilated blood vessels can be corrected with medicine or surgery.

Don't quit caffeine cold turkey. The caffeine in cola, tea and coffee is a blood vessel constrictor. If you give up caffeine, blood vessels may overly dilate and bring on flushing. "If you want to wean yourself from caffeine, it's better to taper off a cup at a time," says Dr. Wilkin.

Wear a petroleum jelly face mask. "On wintry days, a thin shield of Vaseline on your face helps prevent the flushing that occurs when blood vessels dilate in response to the cold," according to dermatologist Joseph Bark, M.D., past chairman of the Department of Dermatology at St. Joseph's Hospital in Lexington, Kentucky. On warm days, he adds, a layer of sunscreen can block the warmth that triggers flushing. Also, limit your time outdoors on really hot or cold days, and don't overdress or underdress.

Treat your cheeks like fine silk. Avoid any products that cause redness or stinging, such as harsh soaps and hair sprays, says Jan Garver, R.N., nurse manager in the Dermatology Clinic at Ohio State University in Columbus.

Take a pill before showering. For some people, hot or cold water on the skin can turn it a rosy red that does not easily fade, according to Paul Lazar, M.D., professor of clinical dermatology at Northwestern University Medical School in Chicago. If you want to avoid being red-faced in the morning, take an antihistamine 30 minutes before bathing and you'll keep water-triggered blushing at bay. Because antihistamines have been known to cause drowsiness, you may want to plan your day accordingly.

Just say no to niacin. Flushing is a common side effect of certain over-the-counter supplements, according to Dr. Wilkin. Niacin supplements, for example, "can make you flush horrendously," he says.

Use greenish makeup. If you have persistent blushing, neutralize a red face with sheer, green-tinted, cover-up makeup, specially formulated for red-faced people, says Dr. Wilkin.

Food Poisoning

E at some potato salad left unrefrigerated, or have some luncheon meat handled by someone with unwashed hands, and you may find out what stomach rebellion is all about.

Food poisoning may be the result of eating food or drinking water that's been contaminated with infectious bacteria. Some bacteria work by secreting toxins that affect the whole body, including the digestive tract. Others work by directly attacking the lining of the intestines. Typically you'll experience abdominal cramps, diarrhea or vomiting within 24 to 48 hours after dining; you may also experience sweating, itching or even a slight fever. These symptoms usually end after a day or two.

Food poisoning can strike anyone. "How you feel can range widely, depending on the type of bacteria you are infected with and your own state of health," says William B. Ruderman, M.D., chairman of the Department of Gestroenterology at the Cleveland Clinic–Florida in Fort Lauderdale. It usually hits hardest when your immune system is already weak from previous illness or immunity-weakening drugs.

When you find yourself infected with bacteria or a virus that causes food poisoning, you may simply have to be miserable for a short time, until your immune system responds and fights off the infection, says Dr. Ruderman. But as bad as that spell may be, there are some things that you can do to coddle your innards while you wait for the misery to pass.

Drink water. "You are losing liquids very quickly when you have food poisoning. Therefore, it is extremely important to replenish your system," says Joseph Madden, Ph.D., director of the Division of Microbiology at the Center for Food Safety and Applied Nutrition, a branch of the Food and Drug Administration in Washington, D.C.

"Start with a few sips of water," says Dr. Ruderman. "Once you can keep water down, it is better to take in fluids containing sugar, because they are better absorbed by the body." Try clear fruit juices. If vomiting is a problem, though, wait several hours before taking in liquids.

Slurp on a sports drink. Drinks like Gatorade contain electrolytes, which are essential elements such as potassium and sodium that influence the way water is distributed throughout your body. "When you're vomiting or having diarrhea, these elements get lost along with liquid during dehydration," says Dr. Madden. "The sports drinks like Gatorade help replenish these necessary elements as well as rehydrate your body with water." Rehydration is more important than replacement of electrolytes, so sports drinks can be diluted 50-50 with water.

When to See the Doctor

Most cases of food poisoning don't require medical attention. Doctors say that in a day or two, your vomiting, diarrhea, cramps and other below-the-belt discomfort should ease, and you'll be back to normal.

However, if you have any of the following warning signs, which could signal a more significant problem, it's wise to see your doctor.
- Prolonged inability to hold down fluids
- High fever
- Abdominal cramps that are worsening
- Bloody diarrhea
- Prolonged symptoms that don't improve after 24 to 48 hours

Be a Bacteria-Banishing Cook

With a little care in the kitchen, you may never experience food poisoning. Food needs to be cooled, cooked and reheated properly to prevent microbe contamination. Here are some kitchen-wise tips from the experts.

- Keep your refrigerator at 40°F or below and your freezer at 0° to stop bacteria from multiplying.
- It's best to throw out fish, meat or poultry that has been in the refrigerator for more than four days. For longer storage, you should use the freezer. Be sure to read labels on processed foods to find the correct storage times.
- To keep juices from dripping on other foods stored in the refrigerator, put a plate under raw meat, poultry and fish.
- When storing leftovers, divide them into small, shallow containers for quick cooling.
- Make sure leftovers are thoroughly reheated. "Leftovers need to be heated to a temperature as hot as or even hotter than they were originally cooked at," says Joseph Madden, Ph.D., director of the Division of Microbiology at the Center for Food Safety and Applied Nutrition, a branch of the Food and Drug Administration in Washington, D.C. "This is the best way to kill the bacteria that may have multiplied since the original cooking of the food."
- Any food being prepared in the microwave should be rotated for

Relax. "Most of the time, food poisoning problems tend to resolve themselves without needing intervention," says Dr. Ruderman. Once your body's immune system takes over, relief is on the way, and you'll be feeling better soon. Just rest and drink fluids, and when you feel a little better, start to establish a diet.

Leave the over-the-counter drugs on the counter. If you feel the urge to reach for an antacid, stop yourself. "They don't really help," says Dr. Ruderman. If you're suffering from traveler's diarrhea, however, Pepto-Bismol is beneficial for relieving the symptoms until you feel better.

even cooking. Microwaves can sometimes leave cold spots in food, which harbor bacteria.

- Frozen food should be thawed in the refrigerator, the microwave or a wrapped package under cold water—not by leaving it on the counter. Bacteria grow very quickly when food is thawed on a countertop.
- Scrub counters with warm, soapy water and bleach to combat countertop bacteria.
- Use a plastic cutting board instead of a wooden one. Be sure to thoroughly clean the cutting board after you've finished using it. Better yet: Use *two* cutting boards—one for meat and one for vegetables.
- Kitchen towels, sponges and cloths are full of bacteria. Wash or replace them often to keep the bacteria out of the kitchen.
- Scrub vegetables before you use them. Harmful bacteria are sometimes found in the soil where root vegetables have grown, but thorough cleaning will make the vegetables safe to eat.
- And if you've been feeling sick and you suspect that you may have food poisoning, you should avoid kitchen duty completely. "Even if a person has a mild case of food poisoning, doing food preparation can cause contamination for an entire household," explains Judith Alsop, Pharm.D., coordinator for the Poison Control Center in Sacramento, California.

Ease into a bland diet. When you feel ready to begin eating, a bland diet is recommended. This means eating easily digestible foods such as cereal, pudding or chicken soup. Be sure to avoid foods that are fried, smoked or salty as well as raw vegetables, pastries, preserves, candies, alcohol and spices and condiments.

Get a lift from a sugary drink. If you're feeling weak, sip on a flat soft drink. "The advantage of soda is that it has sugar in it," says Dr. Ruderman. "This will give you some energy."

Foot and Heel Pain

If your feet burn, swell, ache or otherwise bring you pain, your misery is in good company. "Nearly nine of every ten people have some kind of general foot pain," says Terry Spilken, D.P.M., a podiatrist and adjunct faculty member at the New York College of Podiatric Medicine in New York City.

But here's how to stay one step ahead of general foot and heel pain not related to any specific ailment.

"Massage" with water. "The best treatment for general foot and heel pain is nightly soaks alternating between cold and hot water," says Dr. Spilken. "That means you should soak your feet in cold water for five minutes, then soak them in hot water for five minutes and repeat. This has a 'massaging' effect that invigorates feet by opening and closing blood vessels."

Another invigorator: Rub moisturizing lotion into your feet before going to sleep each night. "The lotion will actually make it easier to give your feet a good massage," says Dr. Spilken.

Get some heat on your feet. Ask your doctor about ointments made with capsaicin, the active natural ingredient in hot peppers. Strange as it seems, these products relieve the blaze caused by burning feet—particularly among those with diabetes. Applying the lotion will cause a burning sensation in a significant number of people, according to George Dailey, M.D., head of the Division of Diabetes and Endocrinology at the Scripps Clinic and Research Foundation in La Jolla, California. This feeling is lessened, however, the more you use the ointment. In various studies, diabetics who treated their burning feet with capsaicin got greater improvement and were able to walk more easily than those not using the cream. "Since it's applied topically, patients can avoid a lot of the side effects they might get from an oral drug," says Dr. Dailey.

A "hot pepper" ointment called Zostrix is available over the counter but is sometimes hard to find. Ask your pharmacist to order it for you if necessary. But check with your doctor first, since this therapy isn't for everyone.

Lower your mileage with new shoes. Recreational walkers and runners need to temporarily lower their mileage when they get new athletic shoes to avoid much of the "break-in" pain. "Because of the advances in shoe development, modern athletic footwear usually doesn't lead to injury in normal use—but changing from one pair to another can," warns Angus McBryde, M.D., professor of orthopedics at the University of South Alabama in Mobile.

Stretch out your calf. Stretching your heel cord or Achilles tendon at the back of your foot can reduce or relieve heel pain, says Gilbert Wright, M.D., an orthopedic surgeon in Sacramento, California, and spokesman for the American Orthopedic Foot and Ankle Society. To stretch, stand three feet from a wall and place your hands on the wall. Lean toward the wall, bringing one leg forward and bending at the elbows. Your back leg should remain straight, with the heel on the floor, and you should feel a gentle stretch in the calf muscle. Then switch legs.

Buy shoes in the right *shape*. "Although we're brought up to think that shoe *size* is the most important aspect of a good fit, just as important—or even more so—is buying shoes with the right *shape*," says Houston podiatrist William Van Pelt, D.P.M., former president of the American Academy of Podiatric Sports Medicine. When you buy running or walking shoes, you can select a shape that fits the curve of the arch on the inner side of your foot. "Feet come in three basic shapes: curved, slightly curved and straight," says Dr. Van Pelt. Although there can be variations to the rule, generally those with high arches need a curved shoe, those with flat feet need a straight shoe, and those in between need a slight curve.

Foot Odor

What gives? You already wash your feet regularly (with warm soapy water). You change your socks at least once a day. And your shoes are clean enough to prevent high school biology classes from making field trips in your closet to collect mold spore samples.

Still, those dogs of yours smell bad enough to make those around want to howl at the moon in agony. So the next time you remove your shoes (that is, *after* you and the rest of your ZIP code come back to consciousness), try these breath-of-fresh-air remedies for the all-too-common problem of smelly feet.

Take tea and see. "Using a soak made from tea bags eliminates the odor from smelly feet because the tannic acid in the tea literally tans the hide," says Jerome Z. Litt, M.D., assistant clinical professor of dermatology at Case Western Reserve University School of Medicine in Cleveland. "You take a couple of tea bags and boil them in a pint of water for 15 minutes. Then remove the tea bags and pour the pint of strong, hot tea into a basin or a large pot filled with two quarts of cool water. Soak for 30 minutes daily for a week or ten days and you'll have no smelly, sweaty feet."

Try an acne fighter. "If your feet are *really* smelly—what I call toxic sock syndrome—examine the bottoms," says Rodney Basler, M.D., a dermatologist and assistant professor of internal medicine at the University of Nebraska Medical Center in Omaha. "If you have whitish soles with tiny pits, then you probably have a condition called pitted keratolysis. And since the organism that brings on this condition is the same species that causes acne, you can get relief by using an over-the-counter acne medication with 10 percent benzoyl peroxide, such as Oxy-10."

Use an antiperspirant. You can buy special foot deodorants, but here's a lower-cost alternative: Use an underarm *antiperspirant,* which controls odor *and* wetness, says Stephen Weinberg, D.P.M., a podiatrist who specializes in sports medicine at Columbus Hospital in Chicago. (Deodorants, meanwhile, only control odor.) His advice: Use a roll-on that contains the active ingredient aluminum chloride hexahydrate at least twice daily. Aerosols aren't as effective, since a lot of their oomph is lost in the air.

Forgetfulness

Hmmmm, now what were we going to discuss next? Oh, yeah, how to cure those blasted bouts of forgetfulness. You know, when a name or date is on the tip of your tongue . . . or you can't seem to remember where you parked your car . . . or left your keys.

Frustrating as it is, a memory slip doesn't mean you're edging toward Alzheimer's disease. (Alzheimer's is marked by things such as not knowing the year or forgetting the names of immediate family members.) Everyone has occasional episodes of forgetfulness, so even if you've forgotten the last time it happened to you, here's how to build a better memory.

Get in shape. Scientific research confirms that a healthy body indeed helps breed a healthy mind—memory-wise, at least. Several studies show that people over age 40 who exercise aerobically at least three times a week have 20 percent better memory skills than people who don't exercise. So if you're not a regular exerciser, change those sedentary ways.

"Regular exercise improves blood flow to the brain," explains Richard Gordin, Ph.D., professor of physical education at Utah State University in Logan. "And improved blood flow often means improved thinking and memory."

Tune in talk shows. "The most troublesome tasks for everyone are remembering names and faces and remembering dates and appointments. I recommend you watch TV shows that will help improve those skills," says Douglas Herrmann, Ph.D., a research scientist at the National Center for Health Statistics in Hyattsville, Maryland, and author of *Super Memory*. "Since meeting new people challenges memory, watch talk and game shows, and try to recall each guest's name as the show goes on. A show like 'Wheel of Fortune' is good for improving your vocabulary and recalling word definitions."

Write it down. Putting information in writing also puts it into your memory, says Dr. Herrmann. So try writing down important information in order to remember it more easily later on. Many memory experts suggest you "make lists."

Think in rhymes. Want to *know it?* Become a *poet.* "Make a rhyme for uninteresting things or hard-to-recall facts, or when the information is complicated or highly detailed," says Dr. Herrmann. "Rhymes give us a structure that helps us remember things."

Remember your beta-carotene. Consuming at least one serving daily of foods rich in beta-carotene can improve some aspects of your memory and word fluency or recall, particularly if you're over age 60, according to James G. Penland, Ph.D., research psychologist at the U.S. Department of Agriculture Human Nutrition Research Center in Grand Forks, North Dakota. Dark green vegetables and orange fruits and vegetables are abundant in beta-carotene.

Observe rather than see. Seeing something allows for a momentary experience, which may or may not give you the opportunity to soak up details. But observing means paying attention to detail. For instance, you've seen a $20 bill countless times, but can you remember who's pictured on the front of it? Unless you know it's Andrew Jackson, you're not an observer.

"By noticing special properties or features of commonplace items, you will have a better chance to commit them to memory," says psychologist Robin West, Ph.D., of the University of Florida in Gainesville, author of *Memory Fitness over Forty.*

Play mental games. Playing cards or board games like Scrabble is a good way to practice improving your memory, advises Forrest R. Scogin, Ph.D., associate professor of psychology at the University of Alabama in Tuscaloosa. "But choose the games you like, because it can be very frustrating for someone having memory problems to say 'If I just start playing Scrabble, my memory will improve.'" The process is like building up your stength with exercise. Don't expect too much too soon.

Frostbite

Whoever decided that Jack Frost merely nips on noses must have lived in Florida. Spend enough time outdoors in major frosty weather and you may find that little nip turning into a big bite—frostbite.

Frostbite is what can happen when bitterly cold weather meets a body that's trying to stay warm. Attempting to warm the inner organs, your body cuts back on the circulation to your hands and feet. And if they receive less than their share of warm blood, these parts can freeze.

Severe frostbite may cause permanent damage, but there's no reason why it needs to go that far. From Eskimos to mountaineers, those who venture into the chilliest realms on earth have found ways to prevent lasting damage to toes, noses and fingertips.

When to See the Doctor

When a frostbitten area begins to thaw, you'll feel pain. While some kinds of frostbite are more severe than others, be sure to see the doctor if the pain continues for more than a few hours. And see the doctor as soon as possible if you see dark blue or black areas under the skin or if blistering occurs.

There are four degrees of frostbite, says Carol Frey, M.D., chief of the Foot and Ankle Service and associate clinical professor of orthopedic surgery at the University of Southern California School of Medicine in Los Angeles. Ice crystals on your skin are a sign of first-degree frostbite. When symptoms increase beyond this—for example, if your skin begins to feel warm even though it is not defrosting, or if the skin turns red, pale or white—you should seek a doctor's attention: You have a higher, more dangerous degree of frostbite.

How do you know that you're getting frostbite? Watch the skin, says Carol Frey, M.D., chief of the Foot and Ankle Service and associate clinical professor of orthopedic surgery at the University of Southern California School of Medicine in Los Angeles. There is no standard amount of time within which frostbite can occur, but the ice crystals that form on the skin's surface are the first sign. Here's what you need to do.

Don't rub. "The old adage about rubbing frostbitten areas with snow is false, though it's been perpetuated for years," explains W. Steven Pray, Ph.D., R.Ph., professor at the Southwestern Oklahoma State University School of Pharmacy in Weatherford. "The snow's coldness does not help raise the temperature of the affected area. In fact, any kind of rubbing, with hands or otherwise, only traumatizes it."

Stay put and stay warm. Once you find a warm place and can begin to thaw your frostbite, stay there. If you must leave and there is any chance that your frostbitten area will refreeze, avoid thawing it. According to Dr. Frey, refreezing will cause tissue damage far worse than the original damage from frostbite. Treat your skin gently before and after it has thawed. Avoid hitting or applying pressure to the injured area. If your toes have just been warmed, try to avoid walking (or skiing or skating) for as long as possible.

Thaw in the tub, not by the campfire. Dr. Frey recommends a water bath about 10°F warmer than body temperature for thawing frostbite. A warm-water bath in the range of 102° to 111° is ideal. But avoid the intense, dry heat of a campfire, stove or heater, because you might burn frostbitten areas. (Frostbitten nerve endings don't send a signal to tell you when exposed skin is in danger of becoming burned.)

Avoid contact with metal. Everything from steel-tipped shoes to metal machine controls have caused otherwise prepared people to become frostbitten, according to Thomas Sinks, Ph.D., an epidemiologist with the Centers for Disease Control and Prevention in Atlanta. Take extra precautions when handling snow shovels and tools in cold weather: Wear gloves or mittens.

Warm up your central heater. When you get cold, "the blood has a tendency to leave the surface areas, such as the hands or feet, and go to more central areas," says Dr. Frey. "But by putting on a heavy jacket and keeping your core body temperature higher, sometimes you can decrease the incidence of frostbite." And as an extra precaution when driving during winter, always carry

How to Prevent Frostbite

Staying inside is the only real prevention for frostbite. However, when you must venture into the cold, take these precautions.

Try to walk where the wind is blocked. The wind chill factor is just as important as the temperature, so limit the amount of time you stay in the wind.

Stay dry. Wearing water-repellent clothes and changing clothes when they become wet will help keep your body warm.

Generate your own body heat. If you have no other way to protect your skin, try curling up in a ball or placing your hands underneath your armpits.

"Syn" a little. For outdoor winter clothes, choose synthetic fabrics that act as water barriers, and change your clothes immediately if they become wet.

Wear mittens. Because mittens enclose all the fingers in a single, well-sealed "air pocket," they protect better than gloves. The most effective mittens have inside liners that can be taken out and dried separately from the mittens.

Keep your skin dry. To avoid frostbite, make sure you don't get water, gas or other liquids on your skin in subfreezing weather, warns Thomas Sinks, Ph.D., an epidemiologist with the Centers for Disease Control and Prevention in Atlanta. Gasoline is especially risky, since it evaporates quickly, chilling the skin (a handy thing to remember if you use a self-service gas pump).

extra blankets and clothing in your car, just in case the car breaks down, suggests Dr. Sinks.

Don't drink alcohol. Although it may make you feel warmer, alcohol actually prevents the constriction of blood vessels, increasing heat loss. A swig of brandy *won't* warm your toes and fingertips. In fact, alcohol reduces shivering, which is the body's way of helping you stay warm, according to Murray Hamlet, D.V.M., director of the Plans and Operations Division at the U.S. Army Research Institute of Environmental Medicine in Natick, Massachusetts.

Cover your ears. "Overchilled and windburned ears are best treated by protection as soon as possible," says William Epstein, M.D., professor of dermatology at the University of California, San Francisco, School of Medicine. "In fact, just covering your ear with your hand may be all you need."

Drink plenty of water. Hydration increases the blood's volume, which helps prevent frostbite. Drinking fluids such as herbal teas, hot cider or broth is a good idea. But you should avoid caffeinated beverages, which constrict blood vessels. Drink before leaving shelter, and take a Thermos with you while you are outdoors.

Don't light up. "When you light a cigarette, the blood flow in your hand shuts off," says Dr. Hamlet. Restricted blood flow is a major factor in frostbite, as the body loses its ability to warm itself.

Gallstones

T hink of your gallbladder as a kind of storage tank for your liver. It collects bile, a cholesterol-rich fluid secreted by the liver. When you eat something fatty, your small intestine sends out a biochemical message to the gallbladder—"Hey, squirt out some bile!" The bile interacts with the food, helping to break it down into digestible bits.

Think of gallstones as sand or pebbles in the storage tank. Gallstones form when there is too much cholesterol or pigment in the bile. They start out as tiny globules but can snowball to the size of an egg.

Lots of times, gallstones don't cause any problems at all. People may not even realize they have them until they show up on an x-ray or during an ultrasound examination. When gallstones *do* cause pain, it's usually because one has gotten stuck in a duct, blocking the flow of bile. If that happens, you'll have steady, severe pain in the upper abdomen that lasts at least 20 minutes but may continue up to four miserable hours. You may also feel pain between the shoulder blades or in the right shoulder. Nausea and vomiting are common, too.

Pain-producing gallstones sometimes pass through the duct or drop back into the gallbladder. The pain and the problem are temporarily on hold. When they get stuck in a duct for long, though, they can cause serious problems.

Once you have pain-producing gallstones, you may be able to tame your symptoms by losing weight and going on a moderately low-fat diet, says Henry

When to See the Doctor

Don't assume the pain you're experiencing is your gallbladder acting up. Get a doctor's diagnosis. A variety of tests are available to detect gallstones, including ultrasound and x-rays.

For occasional mild attacks, your doctor may suggest you wait and see if your symptoms become worse before getting treatment. "These days, though, there has been a slight shift toward recommending that something be done earlier than it used to be," says Henry Pitt, M.D., director of the Gallstone and Biliary Disease Center at Johns Hopkins Hospital in Baltimore.

That's because most gallbladders can now be removed with laparoscopic surgery—sometimes called Band-Aid surgery because the incisions are so small. To perform the operation, the doctor makes four hairline slits or incisions, each about an inch long. Through one slit the doctor inserts a kind of periscope into the abdomen. The other slits are just big enough to allow the doctor to work with specially designed surgical instruments and remove the entire gallbladder. The surgery usually involves an overnight stay in the hospital.

Alternatively, a prescription drug, Actigall, can be used to dissolve gallstones, but it isn't for everybody, Dr. Pitt says. "The pills are likely to work in only about 20 percent of patients with gallstones—thinner, younger patients with small- to medium-size cholesterol stones," he explains. The pills take months or years to dissolve the stones, and the stones frequently return when the drug is stopped, Dr. Pitt says.

Two other treatments to remove gallstones, lithotripsy (shock waves that break up stones) and drugs injected into the gallbladder to dissolve stones, are used infrequently.

Pitt, M.D., director of the Gallstone and Biliary Disease Center at Johns Hopkins Hospital in Baltimore.

"Usually the symptoms don't go away, and you may run into complications," he adds. "So your doctor will probably recommend that your gallbladder be removed."

But if you still have a gallbladder and it's giving you gallstone problems, here's what doctors suggest to minimize symptoms.

Shed those few extra pounds. When it comes to developing gallstones, even slightly overweight people have twice the risk of people at their ideal weight. And seriously overweight people run a sixfold risk. Your doctor can check a weight/height chart to determine your ideal weight. If you're overweight, plan a change of diet and exercise to bring down your weight.

But do it gradually. Dropping weight too fast (more than one pound a week) actually *increases* your chances of developing gallstones, which can form within four to six months of beginning a weight-loss program. So stick with a weight-loss program that will let you reduce slowly and steadily, Dr. Pitt recommends.

Avoid no-fat diets. Virtually fat-free weight-loss diets seem to pose a particularly high risk for gallstone formation, according to several studies.

Why? An extremely low-fat diet (less than 20 percent of calories from fat) allows bile to sit and concentrate in the gallbladder, explains Stanley Heshka, Ph.D., a research associate at the Obesity Research Center at St. Luke's–Roosevelt Hospital Center in New York City. Dietary fat stimulates the gallbladder to expel its contents, which reduces the concentration of cholesterol and pigments. "Research suggests that a weight-loss diet of at least 1,200 calories, with 20 percent of calories from fat, may offer protection from gallstones," he says.

But don't go overboard on the fat. Although data are conflicting, many doctors suspect a diet high in saturated fat can contribute to gallstone problems as well as to weight gain, a risk in itself. So stay away from foods that are very high in saturated fat, such as butter, highly processed foods, marbled meats and products containing palm or coconut oils.

Better not count on old-time "cures." Old-time remedies, which involve a three-day fast followed by a whopping dose of olive oil and fruit juice, are said to stimulate your gallbladder so vigorously that it spews out any stones. Some people say they actually see the stones pass in the form of greenish blobs when they try this remedy.

"I am not convinced this works," says Andrew Weil, M.D., associate director of the Division of Social Perspectives in Medicine of the College of Medicine at the University of Arizona in Tucson. "It's possible that the greenish blobs are actually residues of the olive oil, not stones."

Trying this remedy may increase your risk of a major gallbladder attack, with the possibility of stones lodging in the bile ducts, says Johnson Thistle, M.D., professor of medicine at the Mayo Clinic in Rochester, Minnesota.

Genital Herpes

The way someone gets herpes simplex isn't too complex: Come in direct, skin-to-skin contact with an open sore on someone who has the virus and it's possible you'll get infected.

Herpes simplex type 1, usually transmitted through kissing, results in cold sores on the mouth or hands. Herpes simplex type 2—genital herpes—requires more intimate contact such as intercourse.

An estimated 500,000 people a year get genital herpes from having sex with someone who carries it. You may not even know you carry herpes—three of every four people with herpes don't realize they have it. And once you get it, it will stay with you forever in a quiet, or latent, state punctuated by occasional outbreaks. The initial outbreak tends to be the most severe. During an outbreak, burning sores cover the genitals—an uncomfortable sensation that does not exactly put you in the mood for love. (That may be best, since you can infect others with the virus when the sores appear.)

Your doctor will prescribe the drug acyclovir, the only "proven" way to control herpes outbreaks. All first-episode patients should be treated with acyclovir. If your sores are especially tender or uncomfortable, however, you may try the following relief measures.

Take aspirin. "One thing you can do, once you get a herpes outbreak, is take aspirin," says Lawrence R. Stanberry, M.D., Ph.D., a herpes researcher and professor of pediatrics in the Division of Infectious Disease at the University of Cincinnati College of Medicine. "Aspirin works because it's both a pain reliever and an anti-inflammatory. And often you feel pain from genital herpes because the nerve endings in your genitals are infected or inflamed."

Steer clear of ointments. You may be inclined to bombard herpes sores with everything in your medicine cabinet. But mild soap and water is sufficient to keep the area clean, says Dr. Stanberry.

In fact, petroleum jelly and antibiotic ointments can block the air needed for the healing process, cautions Stephen L. Sacks, M.D., professor of medicine at the University of British Columbia in Vancouver and the founder and director of the university's Herpes Clinic. *Never* use a cortisone cream, which can inhibit your immune system and actually encourage the virus to grow.

Put on "drying" lotion. "You don't want to put on anything gooey. But men might find that drying agents like calamine lotion or zinc oxide may speed healing by drying out the lesions," says Dr. Stanberry. He doesn't advise that women try this for vaginal herpes, however, since drying agents should not be used near mucous membranes.

Use a hair dryer. Towel-drying after bathing may prove painful when the terry cloth comes in contact with those tender sores. For a painless way to keep lesions dry, blow-dry the genital area with a hair dryer set on the low or cool setting, says Dr. Sacks. In fact, the air may prove soothing and may help dry out lesions more effectively and with less irritation than traditional towel-drying.

Don't touch! Although the disease is called *genital* herpes, it is possible to pass the virus to other parts of the body by touching an open sore and then bringing your fingers into contact with your mouth, eyes or any break in the skin. For this reason, it is important not to touch your sores, especially during the first episode, says Charlie Ebel, director of publications at the American Social Health Association, with headquarters in Research Triangle Park, North Carolina. If you think you might scratch at night, cover your sores with a protective material that "breathes," such as gauze.

Abstain from sex when you have sores. Besides spreading the disease to others, having sex during a herpes outbreak can actually make *your* outbreak worse. "You can spread more lesions on yourself," says Dr. Stanberry. "During outbreaks, partners should adopt methods of being close that do not include genital sex."

Make stress management a habit. "The best way to *avoid* outbreaks of herpes lesions is to keep yourself in the best physical and mental health possible," Dr. Stanberry adds. Doctors agree that herpes often hits when your resistance is low or when you're overly stressed. So eating right, exercising regularly and managing the stress in your life are the first lines of defense.

Stay comfy with cotton undies. Another way to "air out" is to wear loose-fitting underwear made from cotton, advises Judith M. Hurst, R.N., a staff nurse at the Toledo Hospital and volunteer medical adviser to Toledo HELP, a herpes support group. Avoid wearing synthetic fabrics, because they don't allow skin to "breathe" as easily, she says. She prefers white cotton, because it has no dyes to cause irritation.

Gingivitis

I t seems as though the 300 or so types of bacteria that homestead in our mouths have a biting sense of humor. We fight them tooth and nail to prevent cavities. Then, just as we think we're flossing enough and brushing enough to stop cavities, bacteria burrow into another area—our gums. As we get older, neglect of our gums begins to catch up with us until, when we've reached age 35 or so, our dentist mentions gum disease.

The earliest and most treatable form of gum disease is gingivitis, a buildup of bacterial plaque that causes gums to redden, swell and bleed easily. Although this kind of gum disease is painless, failing to treat gingivitis can lead to periodontitis, a condition that eventually causes tooth loss.

Brushing after meals and daily flossing comprise the one-two punch that can help keep your gums in the pink. But beyond the basics, here are some other ways to help put the bite on gingivitis.

Take your pick. "One of the easiest and most effective ways to prevent gingivitis, especially for people who don't floss regularly, is to use soft wooden toothpicks that you can buy at most drugstores," says David Garber, D.M.D., clinical professor of periodontics and prosthodontics at the Medical College of Georgia in Augusta. These toothpicks have rounded edges and are shaped

When to See the Doctor

What happens if you ignore the sore, bleeding gums that are a sign of gingivitis? You risk more serious periodontal disease and the possible loss of your teeth.

Here are the signs that warn you your gingivitis is getting more serious. If you have any of them, see your dentist immediately.
- You have bad breath that doesn't go away within 24 hours.
- Your teeth look longer—a result of your gums shrinking away from your teeth.
- Your mouth feels out of alignment when you shut it because your teeth come together differently.
- Your partial dentures fit differently.
- Pus pockets form between your teeth and gums.
- Your teeth are loose, fall out or break off near the gum line.

Also, if your gums still bleed when you brush your teeth and continue to be sore and swollen despite your efforts at good oral hygiene, you need to see your dentist again.

to fit between teeth, so you can get into areas where plaque does the most harm, says Dr. Garber. Two popular brands of wooden points are Sanodent and Stim-U-Dent.

Go electric. "Various studies show that you'll remove more plaque with an electric toothbrush than by brushing manually," says Palm Harbor, Florida, dentist Paul Caputo, D.D.S. The Interplak electric toothbrush removes 80 percent more plaque than a regular toothbrush, he says. Other doctors recommend the Rotodent model, but it can be purchased by prescription only. Check with your dentist.

Shoot with a stream. Another helpful device to stop the early stages of gingivitis is a Water Pik or similar device. Just direct the Water Pik's sharp stream of water toward the tiny "moats" between each tooth and the gum line. Bacteria are caught in the stream and washed away when you rinse out your mouth.

Add muscle to your mouth. Just as bones in the rest of your body can get brittle and shrink, so can your teeth and jawbone—making you more susceptible to gingivitis and other dental problems. "Calcium seems to help people with gingivitis," says Dr. Caputo. "It strengthens bones and teeth." Drinking two glasses of skim milk a day provides about 90 percent of your Recommended Dietary Allowance of calcium.

Read the mouthwash label. Score one for truth in advertising. "Research shows that gargling with Listerine really does stop plaque buildup and reduce gingivitis," says Dr. Garber. Studies by other doctors show that Viadent and some other mouthwashes can also help reduce gingivitis. When buying a generic mouthwash, check the label for cetylpyridinium chloride or domiphen bromide, the active ingredients that reduce plaque.

Attack the tartar. There are many toothpastes specifically formulated for tartar control, including Crest, Colgate and Pepsodent. That's important, because tartar, when it hardens, turns into the plaque that causes gingivitis. "They really *are* more effective at preventing gingivitis than other brands that don't claim to fight tartar," adds Dr. Garber.

Time yourself brushing. Sure, brushing and flossing are the best ways to prevent gingivitis, but don't think that a quick 30-second once-over will guarantee you gorgeous gums. "You have a better chance at removing *all* the plaque if you brush for at least five minutes two or three times a day," says Dr. Garber.

Don't forget the gums. Don't be too literal about *tooth*brushing. The usually neglected gum line is where plaque hardens and causes gingivitis, says Vincent Cali, D.D.S., a New York City dentist and author of *The New, Lower-Cost Way to End Gum Trouble without Surgery*. He suggests you place your brush at a 45-degree angle to your teeth, so half of the brush cleans your gums while the other half cleans your teeth.

Knead those gums. Along with extensive gum brushing, a daily gum massage improves blood circulation. That can help make gums more resistant to gingivitis and other gum disease, says dentist Richard Shepard, D.D.S., of Durango, Colorado. Grip an area of your gums between your thumb and index finger (index on the outside) and rub—on the top *and* bottom gums. A few minutes' massage every day, all around the top and bottom gums, should help stop gingivitis.

Brush your tongue. "Your tongue harbors a lot of the bacteria that can cause plaque, so brush it when you brush your teeth," says Dr. Garber.

Brush Up on Your Brushing

There's a simple way to gauge how effectively you are brushing your teeth—and guarding against gum disease.

Most dentists can provide disclosing tablets for patient use. "You simply brush your teeth, take a tablet and chew it up, swish it around your mouth and then rinse with water," says David Garber, D.M.D., clinical professor of periodontics and prosthodontics at the Medical College of Georgia in Augusta. "The tablets color areas on your teeth where you still have plaque, letting you see the areas that require more attention." Modify your brushing to get those areas every time and you'll go a long way toward attacking gingivitis and preventing tooth loss.

Practice with a Proxabrush. This specially designed brush, available at most drugstores, is shaped like a very small bottle brush and is designed to get into hard-to-reach places between your teeth or under a crown or bridge. It's not a substitute for daily brushing with your regular toothbrush, but using a Proxabrush is an extra way to attack hidden plaque, according to dentist Roger P. Levin, D.D.S., president of the Maryland Academy of General Dentistry. You can ask for one at your local pharmacy.

Heal faster with vitamin C. While it won't *cure* gingivitis, vitamin C makes bleeding gums a little less bloody and promotes the healing process. "I recommend vitamin C to my patients," says Dr. Caputo. Oranges and other citrus fruits (as well as citrus fruit drinks) are the star suppliers of vitamin C, and there are great vegetable sources such as broccoli, brussels sprouts, cauliflower and tomatoes. Or, says Dr. Caputo, you can supplement your diet with 500 milligrams of vitamin C daily.

Glaucoma

To anyone who has eye damage from glaucoma, the world is viewed through a long, narrow tunnel.

Chronic glaucoma—the most common type—has been called the "sneak thief of sight." Slowly and painlessly, fluid begins to build up in the eyeball, creating excessive pressure. The delicate nerves inside the eye—nerves that carry visual signals to the brain—are damaged by the pressure. As nerve damage continues, sight deteriorates to the point where you literally have tunnel vision. Unfortunately, unless the pressure is relieved, someone with glaucoma can lose his sight completely.

If you have glaucoma, your doctor probably has already put you on prescription eyedrops to lower the pressure in the eye.

Once on medications, you require routine eye exams two to three times a year to ensure that the damage has stopped. It's the best way to protect your sight. But in between, here's what doctors say you can do for yourself.

Don't skimp on your eyedrops. "To control glaucoma, you must take your medication every day for life, so stick to your schedule," says Kevin Greenidge, M.D., director of glaucoma services at Metropolitan Hospital Center and a member of the glaucoma service at the New York Eye and Ear Infirmary, both in New York City. If you've been advised to use your eyedrops twice daily, it means every 12 hours, says Dr. Greenidge. Four times a day means every 6 hours. But don't double up if you miss a dose, he cautions. If the doses are too large, the medication could cause blurred vision or other side effects.

Close off the drain. You can increase the effectiveness of your eyedrops by pulling down your bottom eyelid, inserting the drops and then pressing your finger against the tear duct in the inner corner of your eye, says Jack Holladay, M.D., professor of ophthalmology at the University of Texas Medical School at Houston. "When you close off the drain, you prevent the medicine from going into your nose and eventually into your bloodstream, where it can

245

When to See the Doctor

If you feel sudden eye pain, it may be a signal that you have an acute form of glaucoma that can lead to blindness. *Acute* glaucoma can occur when the drainage canal from the eyeball is suddenly closed off and the fluid pressure builds rapidly, says Kevin Greenidge, M.D., director of glaucoma services at Metropolitan Hospital Center and a member of the glaucoma service at the New York Eye and Ear Infirmary, both in New York City.

Along with intense pain, you may have blurred vision and see rainbow halos around lights. Some people also experience nausea and vomiting.

This condition may be relieved promptly, but you must get to a hospital as soon as possible. If you are farsighted, a regular eye exam may reveal a tendency toward this condition.

cause side effects," says Dr. Holladay. Then close your eyes for two minutes, he adds. This allows the drug to be completely absorbed.

Avoid eyedrops containing cortisone. Cortisone interferes with the flow of fluid in the eyeball. As a result, it can boost pressure in the eye, according to George Spaeth, M.D., director of glaucoma services at Wills Eye Hospital and professor of ophthalmology at Jefferson Medical College of Thomas Jefferson University, both in Philadelphia.

Choose medicines with care. "If you're farsighted, talk to your doctor before using products such as Contac," says Dr. Spaeth. In some farsighted people, the area where fluid drains from the eye may be quite narrow, he says. Decongestants and antihistamines dilate the pupil, narrowing the drainage canal even further. So you might risk a dangerous buildup of pressure if you take these medications.

Pedal daily to prevent pressure buildup. "Our studies showed that when people who were at risk for glaucoma cycled for a half-hour three times a week for ten weeks, they reduced the pressure in their eyes," says Linn Goldberg, M.D., associate professor of medicine and director of the General Medicine Clinics and Human Performance Laboratory at the Oregon Health Sciences University in Portland. In fact, the study showed that this cycling routine was just as effective as glaucoma drugs. "Heightened pressure inside the eye is to glaucoma what high blood pressure is to heart disease," says Dr. Goldberg. "If you can control the pressure, you can prevent some aspects of the disease." But just because you take up cycling doesn't mean you can drop your drops, cautions Dr. Goldberg. Any change in treatment requires a doctor's okay.

Don't let your eyes catch the flak. *Traumatic* glaucoma occurs in 10 percent of people who have injured the drainage system in their eyes, says Dr. Greenidge. To avoid such injuries, guard against flying mini-missiles. "Anyone involved in carpentry, metalwork, chopping wood, playing racquet sports—any situation where objects could fly through the air and hit the eyes—should wear protective goggles."

Take vitamin C and see. There is evidence that very high doses of vitamin C relieve eye pressure and may also help improve the visual field, according to Jay Cohen, O.D., associate professor at the State University of New York College of Optometry in New York City. However, the amount of vitamin C in

---

Check Out This Sight Test

Only an eye exam by an ophthalmologist (M.D.) can tell whether you have early glaucoma. But you should be alert to any changes in vision such as blurriness or "blanked-out" sight, says George Spaeth, M.D., director of glaucoma services at Wills Eye Hospital and professor of ophthalmology at Jefferson Medical College of Thomas Jefferson University, both in Philadelphia. He's developed this self-test to help you spot warning signs between eye exams.

Sit about a foot away from a large TV set tuned to a channel that has nothing but "snow"—random, blurred spots or lines. Close your left eye and look at the center of the screen with your right eye. Are any areas of the screen blanked out, washed out or less visible? Pay particular attention to the upper left-hand side of the screen: If you have trouble seeing that area, your vision loss may be caused by glaucoma. Reverse the procedure to test your left eye; look at the upper right-hand side of the screen to find out whether you've lost any vision in that eye. If this quick test shows any sight loss, don't wait for your next regular eye exam. Call an ophthalmologist right away.

those studies was too high for practical use. "It appears that vitamin C may help draw fluid out of the eye in some way," says Dr. Cohen.

Dr. Cohen has his glaucoma patients take a maximum of 1,000 milligrams a day. "That amount can't hurt, and it could help," he says. Before trying vitamin therapy, however, get the okay from your doctor.

Gout

Once known as the "kings' disease" because it almost always afflicted the well heeled, this form of arthritis is an equal opportunity deployer: It delivers a *royal* pain to the toe, knee and other joints.

You'll qualify for gout if your kidneys lose some of their ability to flush away excess amounts of a by-product called uric acid. When uric acid crystallizes, it lodges in the joints, causing more than a crystal's worth of pain. "Think of what happens when you put too much sugar in a glass of iced tea," says Jeffrey R. Lisse, M.D., director of the Division of Rheumatology at the University of Texas Medical Branch at Galveston. "The sugar will dissolve up to a point, and the remaining crystals pile up at the bottom."

When that occurs, the joint can get hot, swollen and tender. Sometimes the pain is so bad that it can actually wake you from a sound sleep. "Gout occurs sporadically, but it hits like gangbusters, often in the middle of the night," says Paul Caldron, D.O., a clinical rheumatologist and researcher at the Arthritis Center in Phoenix. "We're talking about pain so intense that the weight of the sheet feels excruciating."

This megagrief can last for hours or days, but a gout bout can vanish almost as swiftly as it comes, leaving you totally pain-free until the next episode. If you've had that experience, here's how to avoid a future round with the crystal attackers.

Lose weight, but not too quickly. The majority of gout patients are overweight— usually 15 to 30 percent over their ideal weights. The greater your girth, the higher your uric acid level. And the more uric acid, the more frequent and more intense the gout attacks. But lose weight gradually: A crash diet can actually raise uric acid levels.

Foods to Avoid

The best way gout patients can avoid a purine-packed flare-up is to avoid foods high in purine. Among the most loaded, containing from 100 to 1,000 milligrams per 3½-ounce serving:

Anchovies	Meat extracts
Brains	Mincemeat
Consommé	Mussels
Gravies	Pork roast
Heart	Poultry
Herring	Roast beef
Kidney	Sardines
Liver	Sweetbreads

The following foods should be limited to no more than one serving daily, since they contain 9 to 100 milligrams per 3½-ounce serving.

Asparagus	Mushrooms
Beans (dry)	Oatmeal
Lentils	Peas (dry)
Luncheon meats	Spinach

Control your blood pressure. Gout patients with hypertension have twice as much to worry about. That's because some blood pressure medications *boost* uric acid levels, says Branton Lachman, Pharm.D., clinical assistant professor at the University of Southern California School of Pharmacy in Los Angeles. His advice: Try to control your blood pressure naturally by decreasing sodium intake, exercising regularly, reducing excess weight and controlling stress.

Live without liver. Foods high in a substance called purine contribute to higher levels of uric acid. "You can't get away from purine, because it's in most foods," says Dr. Caldron. "But it's useful to avoid red meat, especially organ meats, some types of fish and even some dark green, leafy vegetables such as spinach."

Eschew the brew. Alcohol is a double whammy for those with gout, because it boosts the production of uric acid, says rheumatologist John G. Fort, M.D., clinical associate professor of medicine at Thomas Jefferson University Hospital in Philadelphia. Beer is particularly bad, because it has an even higher purine content than wine or other spirits.

But drink lots of water. You can help your kidneys flush excess uric acid from your system by going heavy on H_2O. (Besides, dehydration can trigger an attack.) "Brisk urinary output certainly may help," says Dr. Caldron. To accelerate "urinary output," Robert H. Davis, Ph.D., professor of physiology at the Pennsylvania College of Podiatric Medicine in Philadelphia, recommends no fewer than five glasses of water each day.

Give your sex life a kick. Urinating isn't the only way to get rid of uric acid. One study showed that among men, frequent sexual activity reduces uric acid levels. The study suggests that more sex means less gout—for men, anyway.

Be sweet to your feet. Injure a big toe and you increase gout risk, say researchers. So wear shoes around the house to protect your feet from everyday accidents.

Gum Pain

They say that pain is nature's way of ringing us up to tell us something's wrong. But when it comes to our gums, nature doesn't always use the hotline. More often, the message of gum pain seems to come via the old-time pony express: By the time we get the news, the situation at the point of origin is likely to have gone from bad to worse. So if your gums are hinting that something unusual is going on, it may be an understatement.

But *why* do gums hurt? "The causes could be either serious infections caused by bacteria or a situation where the skin on the gums has something wrong with it," says Kenneth Kornman, D.D.S., Ph.D., clinical professor and former chairman of the Department of Periodontics at the University of Texas Health Science Center at San Antonio. There are many infectious conditions that can cause pain. And every now and then, gum surfaces can be plagued with a maddening host of abrasions, burns, growths and lesions.

But all these problems have one thing in common: If they persist, they can really gum up your life, so don't take any chances when pain makes a rare cameo appearance. Head for the dentist's chair as soon as possible. And meanwhile, take these steps to find some relief.

Brush away gum pain. Removing bacteria with regular tooth care not only prevents gum disease, it can also provide some short-term pain relief, says Dr. Kornman. Proceed with gentle brushing (with a soft brush), flossing and warm-water rinsing. In addition, an over-the-counter rinse like Listerine, diluted or at full strength, may diminish some of the bacteria and ease some pain. (For some people, though, the alcohol content of a rinse may make pain worse. Discontinue using it if that happens.)

Don't rub. Massaging your gums may only cause further irritation, according to Dr. Kornman.

Try a warm saltwater rinse. "Take a few swigs of warm salt water and swish it between your teeth and gums," advises Leslie Salkin, D.D.S., director of postgraduate periodontics and professor of periodontology at the Temple University School of Dentistry in Philadelphia. "It has a general soothing effect. If you have an abscess, the salts will help draw it out and drain it." He recommends one teaspoon of salt in a glass of lukewarm water. (Salt water is also your first line of defense for any gum burn, cut, abrasion or wound.)

Suppress the pain with an analgesic. Any over-the-counter medicine that reduces pain and inflammation could do wonders for your sore gums. It can also help reduce a fever if your pain is caused by an infection. "We're finding that in most cases of dental disease, it is inflammation that causes discomfort," says Samuel Low, D.D.S., associate professor and director of graduate periodontology at the University of Florida College of Dentistry in Gainesville. "Consequently we are recommending anti-inflammatory products such as ibuprofen (Advil)." Or you can take aspirin if you don't have adverse reactions to it (but children should avoid aspirin because of the risk of Reye's syndrome).

Don't put aspirin on your gum. "For some reason, many people have the idea that applying aspirin directly to the affected gum area is beneficial," says Kenneth H. Burrell, D.D.S., director of the American Dental Association's Council on Dental Therapeutics in Chicago. That couldn't be *farther* from the truth, he notes. "Unfortunately, the only thing that happens is that you create a chemical burn in the gum tissue. Don't ever try it."

When to See the Doctor

If you think that a twinge of pain is only the first sign of gum disease, you may be sorely mistaken (no pun intended). Gum disease could already be in the advanced stages by the time you experience pain. So be sure to see a doctor even if the pain seems to go away.

Also, you should visit your dentist when gums are red, tender, discolored or bleeding, *whether or not you feel pain.*

"See your general dentist first before going to a periodontist (a gum specialist)," says Samuel Low, D.D.S., associate professor and director of graduate periodontology at the University of Florida College of Dentistry in Gainesville. "A dentist is equipped to handle many of these problems and then can direct you to a periodontist if needed."

Ice it down. For an all-natural anti-inflammatory, Dr. Low recommends ice. "It really works on swelling," he says, "and also serves as a local anesthetic to dull nerve endings." Apply an ice pack wrapped in a towel to your cheek or lip near the area of pain.

Moisten your mouth. Dr. Salkin recommends sucking on ice chips or a lemon drop if you are suffering from gum irritation due to dry mouth. That should be enough to replenish any missing saliva.

Use peroxide power. Many of the bacteria that cause gum pain cannot survive in oxygen, so some dentists recommend the use of everyday hydrogen peroxide, which you can pick up at any pharmacy and dilute. Dr. Low advises using a rinse of half water, half hydrogen peroxide.

Dab with baking soda. Another way to discourage bacteria is with household baking soda. Just make a paste of baking soda mixed with water and apply it gently on the gums, suggests Dr. Low. But be careful. Overzealous use can abrade gum tissue.

Numb that gum. If you have a burn, a cut, an ulceration or any problem on the skin of the gum, Dr. Kornman says the best thing you can do is apply one of the many over-the-counter gels or ointments that contain benzocaine. Its numbing action delivers instant relief. It also knocks out much of the pain associated with serious gum infections.

Anyone for tea? Some doctors suggest holding a wet tea bag against a gum abrasion or canker sore. Tea leaves contain tannic acid, an astringent that also has some pain-relieving power.

Say no to tobacco. "We see greater gum destruction in smokers," warns Dr. Salkin. He points out that smoking contributes to gum problems and can exacerbate any infectious or ulcerative conditions. Chewing tobacco is another gum irritant and can lead to a variety of gum cancers, according to Dr. Salkin. In addition, smoking often contributes to the onset of trench mouth and worsens the condition if you already have it.

Hangnail

A tiny sliver of skin splits off from your fingernail. And there it hangs, a little skin-thick piece of pain just waiting to happen. The trouble is, when a hangnail catches on something, this most minor of injuries can cause major-league pain.

The best way to avoid hangnails (which have nothing to do with the nails themselves) is by keeping your hands well moisturized. The splits usually occur when the skin around the nails dries up and dies; nail biting is another common cause. Here are some of the best ways to cure them.

Soften before clipping. "A lot of people make the mistake of clipping a hangnail when it's still hard and dry and end up ripping the skin more," says Trisha Webster, a hand model with the Wilhelmina Modeling Agency in New York City whose livelihood depends on perfectly groomed hands. "So before you clip a hangnail, soak it in a little water—or a water-and-oil solution—to soften it." To make the solution, just add two capfuls of mild bath oil or two tablespoons of olive oil to a bowl of warm water.

Clip and cover. "The best thing to do with a hangnail is clip the little piece of skin with a pair of nail scissors—but be sure to wipe the scissors with rubbing alcohol before using them," advises Karen E. Burke, M.D., Ph.D., a dermatologist and dermatologic surgeon in New York City. "Then put on an antibacterial ointment to prevent infection, and cover your finger with a bandage."

Go for soaks. Soaking your nails in a mixture of oil and water on a regular basis is a good way to make sure you don't get future hangnails. Regular water-and-oil soaks replenish lost moisture. "I tell my patients to mix four capfuls of bath oil such as Alpha Keri with one pint of warm water and to soak their fingertips in it for maybe 10 or 15 minutes," says Rodney Basler, M.D., a dermatologist and assistant professor of internal medicine at the University of Nebraska Medical Center in Omaha.

Wrap it up. It's a good idea to bandage your finger after removing a hangnail, but if the bandage falls off (because of the moisturizing soak), wrap your finger in a piece of plastic wrap and secure the wrap with some tape, advises Dr. Basler. "The plastic will keep the moisture in overnight. Just be sure to remove the plastic in the morning, because you don't want to keep it on too long."

Hangover

Maybe you didn't go so far as to wear the proverbial lamp shade last night. But this morning your head feels as though you wore a streetlight—pole and all. So what do you do now? You can't just lie there all day, as lifeless as the worm at the bottom of a tequila bottle. You've got to quiet down those goldfish so that your headache clears (ever notice how their swimming makes the most terrible racket the morning after?) and settle that roller coaster in your stomach . . . and then there's that hairy tongue to shave.

So here's how to get over that hangover the moaning . . . er, morning after.

Run for some Gatorade. Even though now is *not* the time to run a marathon, you can get relief the same way runners do—with Gatorade and other sports drinks that help replace electrolytes (potassium and sodium) and water, says

John Brick, Ph.D., biological psychologist and chief of research in the Division of Education and Training at the Center of Alcohol Studies at Rutgers University in New Brunswick, New Jersey. "Part of the problem of being hung over is that you're dehydrated, and beverages like Gatorade replace the essential fluids you lost from drinking." He suggests consuming sports drinks "the morning, afternoon *and* evening after."

Hit the honey. "You can help a hangover by eating a slice of bread or some crackers spread with honey—or any other food that's high in fructose," says Seymour Diamond, M.D., director of the Diamond Headache Clinic in Chicago and executive director of the National Headache Foundation. "That's because fructose (a natural sugar) helps the body burn off alcohol faster, and honey is the sweetener with the highest concentration of fructose." Other good sources of fructose are apples, cherries and grapes.

Get fruit "juiced." A drink may be the last thing you want to reach for now, but relief will come faster if this time you get juiced on tomato, orange or grapefruit juice. "A large glass of any of these helps in two ways: It's high in fructose, and it's also high in vitamin C, which helps minimize the effects of alcohol," says Dr. Diamond.

Be bullish on bouillon. A bowl or cup of bouillon is the perfect morning-after meal. It's light enough for the way you're feeling, and it can help replenish the salt, potassium and other vitamins and minerals you lose from drinking, says Dr. Diamond.

Avoid coffee. That's right! That jolt of caffeine may be just what you *think* you need, but Dr. Brick says there is no scientific evidence that caffeine helps a hangover in any way. "And since coffee is a diuretic, it may worsen your already dehydrated state," he adds.

Have a water nightcap. "The biggest mistake most people make in treating hangovers is *not* drinking enough water," says Dr. Brick. "Since alcohol is a diuretic that dehydrates the body, I recommend drinking as much as you can before going to bed and then as much as you can the next morning."

Drink it with or without a twist. "Mineral water also works well," according to James Chin, former head bartender at Trader Vic's in San Francisco. "So does soda water with a squeezed lime and a dash of bitters to settle your stomach."

How to Take the Drunk out of Drink

If you *have* to be a party animal, here are some tips on how to avoid feeling like road kill once the festivities end.

Nurse your drink. "It sounds obvious, but the slower you drink, the less you drink," says Seymour Diamond, M.D., director of the Diamond Headache Clinic in Chicago and executive director of the National Headache Foundation. "And the less you drink, the less severe your hangover." His advice? Consume no more than one beverage—beer, wine or cocktail—per hour of indulgence.

Skip the pretzels and nuts. "Salty foods (like those served in most bars) make you thirsty, which makes you drink more," says John Brick, Ph.D., biological psychologist and chief of research in the Division of Education and Training at the Center of Alcohol Studies at Rutgers University in New Brunswick, New Jersey. "The combination of alcohol and salty foods also speeds the dehydrating process, a big factor in hangover."

Go for protein-rich or high-fat foods. "Cheese and other foods high in protein stay in your digestive system longer, so there's something in your stomach to soak up the alcohol," says Dr. Diamond. The result is a less severe state of intoxication—and thus less of a hangover the next morning.

Drink "light." Sometimes it's not the alcohol per se that gets you but rather the additives and impurities—called congeners—formed during the making of the beverage. Generally, for people sensitive to congeners, a good rule of thumb (or of three fingers, as the case may be) is the darker the drink, the cloudier your head will feel the next morning, says Dr. Diamond. Vodka doesn't have that many congeners, but bourbon, scotch, whiskey, red wine and anything aged is loaded with them.

Heel the "hair of the dog." It's demon rum (or gin, bourbon or whatever) that got you this sick, so imbibing more of it the morning after certainly won't help. A morning-after Bloody Mary will only mask the symptoms of your hangover—and will make you feel worse when the masking effect wears off.

Don't take aspirin before you imbibe. Despite popular opinion that taking aspirin *before* you drink will help minimize or avoid a hangover, just the opposite is true. Scientists at the Alcohol Research and Treatment Center at the Veterans Administration Hospital in New York City found that taking aspirin before or during drinking *increases* blood alcohol concentrations to induce a quicker and more severe state of intoxication.

But *do* take it after. If you have a headache or a hangover, you can take aspirin or Alka-Seltzer, but be sure to wait at least four hours after you've finished drinking. "Aspirin is probably still the best way to treat a hangover," says Dr. Brick—but you need to wait a while. Aspirin or similar compounds on a booze-bothered belly can be irritating.

Look for no-smoking zones. Research shows that smoking, or being in a smoke-filled room, while you drink gives you a double whammy of a hangover. Both alcohol and tobacco contain a hangover-causing substance called acetaldehyde, which stresses the liver.

Load up on vitamin C. Taking vitamin C before drinking has been shown to counteract some of the effects of alcohol in some people. "In our tests, people who took vitamin C beforehand weren't as severely affected by alcohol as those who didn't take it," says Vincent Zannoni, Ph.D., a professor of pharmacology at the University of Michigan in Ann Arbor who directed the research. "Vitamin C helps by speeding up alcohol clearance from the body."

Hay Fever

There's no arguing that the thoughts of many knaves and maids turn to love when spring has sprung. But if you're one of those who gets hay fever in this festive season, then your libido isn't the only part of your body in overdrive.

Your nose may be stuffy or runny. Your eyes may itch and water. Your throat may feel irritated. You may even get hives when the bees leave theirs to do some pollinating.

Ah, spring . . . uh, better make that *ahhh-chooo* spring . . . but the truth is, this season has taken a bad rap from snifflers. Hay fever *isn't* solely a rite of spring;

autumn brings its own share of misery. In the fall, when ragweed and other plants are blooming and spreading their windblown pollen everywhere, your respiratory system is one of the miserable landing sites. And while a little congestion and sneezing may be a small price to pay to enjoy the wonders of Mom Nature's handiwork, here's how to get some wholesale relief for your sinuses *and* enjoy the Great Outdoors.

Stay away from melon. Having hay fever can make you more prone to food allergies. Researchers note that many people seem to have an allergic-like reaction after eating certain foods—what's called cross-reactivity. For instance, those allergic to ragweed often experience cross-reactive symptoms when they eat watermelon, cantaloupe or honeydew. And those with birch tree–pollen allergies sometimes react to cherries, apples, pears, peaches, carrots and potatoes. Herbal teas may also produce an adverse reaction in some people.

Ingestion of those foods does not produce hay fever. But it does bring on annoying symptoms such as "itching of the throat and swelling of the lips and tongue," says Robert Bush, M.D., chief of allergy at William S. Middleton Veterans Administration Hospital in Madison, Wisconsin, and professor of medicine at the University of Wisconsin–Madison. "Of course, if eating certain foods produces these or more severe symptoms such as breathing or swallowing problems, the best course is avoidance of the foods."

Make a routine of antihistamine. It's a common mistake: A hay fever sufferer takes *one* over-the-counter antihistamine, feels better and then waits until the symptoms are really bad before taking another one. But this can make you feel like you're on a roller coaster—feeling good one day and bad the next, says allergist William W. Storms, M.D., associate clinical professor of medicine at the University of Colorado School of Medicine in Denver. So if your doctor advises you to go the antihistamine route, it's important to take your medicine every day as a preventive during the allergy season.

Build up gradually. For maximum relief, take an antihistamine 30 minutes before going outdoors, suggests Gerald Klein, M.D., director of the Allergy and Immunology Medical Group in Vista, California. If one kind of antihistamine makes you drowsy, purchase a lower dose and take the lower dose just at bedtime for three days. (Antihistamines are formulated in different concentrations; check the package to compare doses.) During the next few days, gradually increase the dose and also begin taking one tablet in the morning, in addition to your nighttime tablet. "Dosing yourself gradually will help your body build up tolerance to the side effects, so you won't get so sleepy," explains Dr. Klein. (He also suggests asking your doctor about nonsedating antihistamines, available by prescription.)

Don't be an early bird. Pollen counts tend to peak between 5:00 A.M. and 10:00 A.M., so limiting outdoor activity during the morning hours can help keep your allergies to a minimum. That means limiting exercise and other activities until mid- to late afternoon, when pollen is at its lowest, advises Dr. Klein. (You can also check prevailing winds and pollen counts in the newspaper, and they're mentioned in some radio and television weather forecasts.)

Go easy on the nasal sprays. Despite the temptation, don't use over-the-counter nasal sprays for longer than three days in a row. After that, they can actually increase congestion—and can even lead to addiction. "What happens with continued use is that the nose tissue becomes irritated and swollen and you feel even more stuffed up," explains Charles H. Banov, M.D., clinical professor of medicine and microbiology/immunology at the Medical University of South Carolina in Charleston and past president of the American College of Allergy and Immunology. "So you require more and more of the medicine for the tissue to shrink."

A safe, nonaddictive alternative for fighting nasal congestion is to inhale salt water, says Dr. Banov. Use one teaspoon of salt to one pint of water, plus a pinch of baking soda, and stir until both dissolve. Then place a few drops in a small spoon and sniff it up each nostril.

Run the air conditioner. Keep your house and car windows closed and your air conditioner on during spring, summer and fall months, advises H. James Wedner, M.D., chief of clinical allergy and immunology at Washington University School of Medicine in St. Louis. "If you don't want cooled air, at least flip on the fan setting. The fan will filter out the offending pollen." He also suggests, "During the pollen season, you should clean your air conditioner filter approximately once a month."

Use your clothes dryer. "Wind-dried clothes can become pollen catchers," says Dr. Klein. And when you wear them, you get a full dose. But drying clothes in a dryer, or hanging them inside to dry, will keep them pollen-free.

Lather your locks. After being outside for a long time during the day, wash your hair to avoid inhaling pollen that falls from your hair onto your pillow, suggests Robert Scanlon, M.D., clinical professor and director of the Allergy

Clinic at Georgetown University Medical Center in Washington, D.C. If it's not possible to take a shower every evening, at least try to thoroughly wash your face, hands and eyes.

Headache

L ife is often a pain in the neck, right? And stress keeps going up, right? Then it stands to reason that the stresses of your neck-paining life have but one place to go—*up* into that already fragile space between your ears.

That means headache. And you know what *that* means, because headaches affect almost everyone. In fact, Americans spend more than $400 million a year on over-the-counter pain relievers, says Seymour Diamond, M.D., executive director of the National Headache Foundation and director of the Diamond Headache Clinic in Chicago. But before you spend yet another buck on pills that put down pain, here's how to head off headaches the drug-free way.

Apply ice to your head. Placing ice on your head while it hurts is one of the fastest and most effective ways to end a headache. "In fact, if you can get the headache when it's a dull throb, close to 80 percent of people can abort their headaches," according to Fred Sheftell, M.D., director of the New England Center for Headache in Stamford, Connecticut, and coauthor of *Headache Relief.* To put the deep freeze on your headache, he recommends placing an ice pack wrapped in a towel, a bag of frozen vegetables or a specially made product called an ice pillow (available at most drugstores) on your forehead or on top of your head when you first notice any pain.

Try some heat on your neck. When neck muscles tighten because of stress and reduced blood flow to the brain, the result is tension headache. Heat helps by soothing muscles and increasing blood supply. "Placing heat on the back of the head is great for relieving the pressure that accompanies tension headaches," says Glen Solomon, M.D., a headache specialist at the Cleveland

Clinic Foundation in Cleveland and associate professor of medicine at Ohio State University in Columbus. He recommends a heating pad, a long hot shower (turn the spray to the back of your neck) or a hot bath.

Take a load off. "Probably the simplest thing you can do to feel better is go to a dark, quiet room and lie down," adds Dr. Solomon. "That's because any kind of movement can aggravate a headache, and anything you can do to keep those neck muscles from tightening will help." Why a dark and quiet room? Because headaches—even small ones—make you more sensitive to light and noise. "In fact, most people seem to prefer total silence to even soft, soothing music," says Dr. Solomon.

Give yourself a scalp massage. To soothe that aching head, try massaging your scalp with your fingertips as if you were washing your hair. Another technique: Place a natural-bristle hairbrush at your temple, just above the eyebrow, and slowly move it toward the back of your head in slow circles. This massage helps ease tension and bring relief.

Dim the lights. Often headaches are caused by eyestrain that people get from watching a lot of television or staring at a computer screen. If your eyes get a real workout during the day, take this tip from Dr. Sheftell: "Every few hours, take off your glasses or contact lenses and place your palms over your eyes to completely block out the light. Look at that darkness for 30 seconds." Before you take your hands away, close your eyes. Then lower your hands and slowly reopen your eyes.

How to Fly without Headache

Air travel can take you to new heights of headache. The pain is often caused by the hours of sitting in an awkward position and stressing your neck muscles. But here's how to avoid it.

"I personally use one of those inflated neck pillows whenever I travel," says Seymour Diamond, M.D., executive director of the National Headache Foundation and director of the Diamond Headache Clinic in Chicago. "They're great for protecting against the headache you can get from sitting in an uncomfortable airline seat—and they cost only about $10."

Head for the gym. Although it's not advised to exercise once a headache starts, "many find they avoid headaches or lessen their severity with a regular exercise program," says Dr. Diamond. That's because exercise is an excellent stress reducer. (If you find that exercise induces headaches, however, be sure to see your doctor.)

Press on. "You can 'massage' away headaches by pressing on certain acupressure spots," says Dr. Sheftell. "One way is to squeeze the web of skin between your thumb and forefinger. Another area is the tiny ridge between your neck and the back of your head (approximately parallel with your earlobes)."

If you don't get relief after 10 or 15 minutes of rubbing those areas, try rubbing some other parts of your body: the top of your foot, in the area between your big and second toe; the outside area of your shin, just below the knee; or your Achilles tendon.

Roll your noggin. Dr. Sheftell suggests starting off each day by doing ten slow neck rolls in each direction. "Just let your neck muscles go limp and let your chin hit your chest," he says. "Then just rotate your head all around to loosen up your neck muscles." But be gentle: Doing it too fast or too vigorously could cause additional strain.

Or roll in the hay. "Not tonight, I have a headache" should be "Yes! Tonight! I have a headache!" Research done at Southern Illinois University School of Medicine shows that women can get full or partial headache relief from having intercourse. (Sorry, guys, but researchers don't have data on how it affects you.)

Sleep on your back. "Headaches can be caused by sleeping in an awkward position—even on your stomach—because the muscles in your neck contract," says Dr. Diamond. "Sleeping on your back is the best thing you can do, but many of my patients who are restless sleepers find relief with a Walpin pillow (named for its inventor), which is hollowed in the middle to help your neck." The Wal-Pil-O, a standard-size pillow designed to relieve neck stress, is available at some drugstores and surgical supply stores.

Lighten up your lighting. It could be that the cause of your headache is over your head—literally. That's because fluorescent lights—the most popular choice of lighting in most offices (and gaining popularity in homes)—appear to be "on" all the time, but they actually flicker about 60 times a second. This constant flickering, though not noticeable, fatigues the brain, causing headaches,

When Caffeine Helps a Headache

Having a cup of coffee or tea *with* your aspirin provides better relief than aspirin alone. In fact, caffeine can boost the pain-relieving powers of aspirin by about one-third, according to research published in the medical journal *Archives of Internal Medicine.*

"Caffeine can be very helpful, because it constricts blood vessels," says Fred Sheftell, M.D., director of the New England Center for Headache in Stamford, Connecticut, and coauthor of *Headache Relief.* "In fact, most aspirin products have a fair amount of caffeine in them." But Dr. Sheftell recommends limiting your intake of caffeine to about 200 milligrams a day—the amount in two five-ounce cups (not mugs) of coffee. And avoid using more than two aspirin tablets a day.

And if you're a coffee drinker during the week, don't stop drinking it on weekends or you'll risk a real head splitter. "That's because even one day of skipping is enough to trigger a caffeine withdrawal headache," according to Glen Solomon, M.D., a headache specialist at the Cleveland Clinic Foundation in Cleveland and associate professor of medicine at Ohio State University in Columbus.

according to Robert A. Baron, Ph.D., an industrial psychologist and professor at Rensselaer Polytechnic Institute in Troy, New York, who has done extensive research on how lighting affects mood and health. If you think fluorescent bulbs might be causing your headaches, try out a table lamp with an incandescent bulb for a couple of days. If that makes a big difference, replace fluorescent lights with incandescent lighting or table lamps.

Stand tall. Posture plays a key role in tension headaches. "It's the same problem as sleeping in an awkward position," adds Dr. Diamond. He recommends that you avoid leaning or tilting your head to one side, since your neck muscles contract when you're in these positions.

Avoid high-altitude headache. If you're headed for a vacation in the high Rockies or Peruvian Andes, you may be at risk for high-altitude headache. You may help *avoid* a headache by taking 3,000 to 5,000 milligrams of vitamin C the day before you leave and one each day when visiting, advises Seymour Solomon, M.D., director of the Headache Unit at Montefiore Medical Center and professor of neurology at Albert Einstein College of Medicine of Yeshiva University, both in New York City. Also, take two aspirin tablets each day, beginning the day you depart (but remember not to give aspirin to children because of the risk of Reye's syndrome).

Head Lice

About the only positive thing you can say about head lice is that they've made contributions to our vocabulary. The insult *nitwit* originates from the myth that head lice infect only poor, uneducated children. In reality, lice affect people of *all* income levels and social classes. And *nit-picking* started out as a reference to the tedious removal of lice from the scalp.

At this very moment, an estimated ten million Americans are scratching their heads because of lice. All that itching is the result of the lice's saliva entering tiny holes in the scalp created as the insects feed on human blood.

"You can't really prevent lice. They are transmitted from child to child from a common resting place, like a mat at school," says Mitchell C. Sollod, M.D., a pediatrician in San Francisco. "You don't even need head-to-head contact."

Once they grab a head-hold, female lice lay up to ten new eggs every day. These babies, called nits, are white, football-shaped critters that look like dandruff but hang on to hair strands with the same intensity as a pit bull on a mail carrier's leg. Left untreated, head lice can lead to local scalp infection. Here's how to send them packing.

Wash them away. Most doctors suggest using a lindane-based shampoo available only by prescription (Kwell is the most popular brand). These shampoos can be dangerous to children under five and shouldn't be used by pregnant or nursing women or anyone with cuts on his hands or arms. Safer options are available. "There are several over-the-counter shampoos that are also effective against lice, but I think one by the name of Rid probably works the best," says Dr. Sollod.

Take your time shampooing. "No matter what shampoo you use, the trick in making it work is to leave it on for no less than two minutes and preferably ten

When Head Lice Head South

Y ou need to use your head when head lice invade hair on other parts of your body. "For lice on your eyelashes, rub a thin coating of petroleum jelly on your lashes twice daily for eight days," advises Karen E. Burke, M.D., Ph.D., a dermatologist and dermatologic surgeon in New York City. This smothers the nits, so you can easily remove them.

And don't forget that clothing worn while you're battling lice should be either dry-cleaned or washed in a hot cycle and followed with a thorough ironing—especially at all seams, says Dr. Burke.

minutes," says Dr. Sollod. "That gives enough time for the active ingredient to penetrate through the eggshells of the nits, so they can be killed before they hatch in your scalp."

Use a vinegar "conditioner." After shampooing, you can remove stubborn hangers-on with a rinse made of equal parts white kitchen vinegar and water, suggests Karen E. Burke, M.D., Ph.D., a dermatologist and dermatologic surgeon in New York City. "The vinegar helps dissolve the dead nits and wash off their remains." An added bonus: A vinegar rinse helps hair look thicker and more shiny.

Disinfect combs. Another way to get rid of remaining lice, says Dr. Burke, is to comb your hair with a fine-tooth comb that's been soaked in Lysol disinfectant or a lice-killing shampoo (such as Kwell) for one hour. But, she warns, don't pour Lysol directly on your scalp. A more tedious but more exact way is to thoroughly examine the hair and remove lice with an emery board or Popsicle stick. Don't use your fingers, because nits that are still alive might settle under your fingernails.

Forget about a haircut. A seemingly easy solution to head lice is to give your child a haircut. "Unless you're going to shave the head, that won't get rid of the nits, because they usually settle about ¼ inch from the scalp," says Dr. Sollod.

Hearing Problems

When someone tells you there's a fast bat flying out of the barn and you think he's saying a fat cat is flying over the corn, you might as well face it: Your hearing is going. And it didn't just walk out the door today.

"The type of hearing loss experienced by most adults probably started when they were kids," says Robert E. Brummett, Ph.D., a pharmacologist at the Oregon Hearing Research Center in Portland. "Most people's hearing gets worse so slowly that they don't realize what's happening until they have severe hearing loss."

Most adults over age 60 do have *some* hearing loss. But any hearing problem can be greatly reduced by working with an audiologist or an otolaryngologist (ear, nose and throat doctor), according to Denise Wray, Ph.D., associate professor of speech/language pathology at the University of Akron. While hearing loss is usually irreversible, you owe it to yourself to take advantage of technology. "That means getting yourself outfitted with the best hearing aids and assistive listening devices possible," says Sam Trychin, Ph.D., director of a Coping with Hearing Loss Program at Gallaudet University in Washington,

When to See the Doctor

If you have dizziness, pain, nausea, sudden ringing in the ears or sudden hearing loss, you should see your doctor. This is especially important if the impairment is in one ear. It could be as simple as wax in the external ear, but it might be a more serious problem that requires immediate medical attention, according to Robert E. Brummett, Ph.D., a pharmacologist at the Oregon Hearing Research Center in Portland.

Assistive Listening Devices

If words sound *garbled* rather than too soft, you might be helped by an assistive listening device," according to Michael P. Sabo, director of audiology at Good Samaritan Regional Medical Center in Phoenix. For example, an assistive listening device for TV is a hand-held or headset receiver that picks up sound transmitted directly from the television speaker to your ear.

Other devices are specially designed for amplifying telephone conversations, according to Cynthia Compton, director of the Assistive Devices Center in the Department of Audiology at Gallaudet University in Washington, D.C. Also, look for assistive listening devices in public places, such as churches and theaters. They are sometimes provided to hard-of-hearing attendees as a public service.

D.C. But whether or not you have a hearing aid, here are some hear-better strategies that will make everyone more audible.

Make some sound choices. "Whenever you walk into a room, make a quick appraisal of what might present problems," Dr. Trychin suggests. Reduce the background noise as much as possible by turning off the TV or radio when you have a conversation, adds Sharon A. Lesner, Ph.D., professor of audiology at the University of Akron. "And if the noise around you is out of your control, move to another room to talk," she suggests.

Dine away from din. "In a restaurant, position yourself away from the kitchen and away from the entrance," says Dr. Lesner.

Ideally, choose a booth with a high back, so you can hear the person sitting across from you. Or sit with your back against a wall, so there's a "sounding board" behind you.

Look to listen better. You'll be able to understand more if you can *see* more. "Make sure light is on the face of the person you're trying to listen to. And if you wear glasses, make sure your vision is as good as possible," says Dr. Lesner. You don't have to be an expert lip-reader to pick up on visual signals that help people communicate. But you do hear better if you watch lip movement and expressions.

Speak up for yourself. "Be assertive about what you need speakers to do so that you can understand them," says Dr. Lesner.

"For example, you might politely tell a person to slow down. Ask her to rephrase—not repeat—what she said. Or tell her what you believe she said and ask her if that is correct."

Block that clatter. Even if you already have hearing loss, you can further damage your hearing if you are in noisy situations. "Tie a pair of ear plugs or an earmuff-type hearing protector to any noisy equipment you might use," suggests Dr. Brummett. These personal "mufflers" will remind you to protect your ears.

Double the noise stoppers. "If you're going to be in a very noisy situation— using a power saw, for instance—wear *both* foam earplugs and earmuff-type protectors," Dr. Brummet suggests. The more protection, the better.

Heartburn

What can you do when that burning sensation right under your rib cage won't go away? You belch. But there's no Ladder Company Number 9 to put out this fire. This is the inferno of that after-dinner bother—heartburn.

The cause of this post-dining fire storm is actually the hardworking sphincter in your lower esophagus. This is a muscle that relaxes to let food pass into your stomach, then quickly closes. But when it doesn't close properly, the contents of your stomach can back up—a condition known as esophageal reflux—creating burning or irritation under your rib cage. Hello, heartburn.

In pregnant women, and in everyone over age 40, the esophageal sphincter is likely to weaken a bit. Not much you can do about that. But the main causes of heartburn are usually obesity, stress and the wrong diet. And those things (unlike age) you *can* do something about.

There's other good news. Your esophagus can heal from the burning caused by stomach acid within seven weeks with proper care, decreasing your chances of recurring episodes. So here's some body-plumbing help that will give your pipes a soothing rest.

When to See the Doctor

If you have heartburn daily or even several times a week, see your doctor, says William J. Ravich, M.D., associate professor of medicine in the Division of Gastroenterology at Johns Hopkins University School of Medicine in Baltimore. Frequent or repeated symptoms *could* be an indication of esophagitis, or inflammation of the esophagus.

Other warning signs may indicate an ulcer. According to *Seven Weeks to a Settled Stomach,* by Ronald L. Hoffman, M.D., director of the Hoffman Center for Holistic Medicine in New York City, sometimes the first indication of an ulcer is a lot of belching and bloating, which might lead you to think you have severe gas pains. The pain may be worse between meals when your stomach is empty, and you may feel better after you eat something. If these symptoms sound like yours, consider the possibility of an ulcer and see a doctor.

If you are experiencing what you think may be heartburn accompanied by any of the following symptoms, you should be checked out by a physician *fast.*
• Difficulty or pain when swallowing
• Vomiting
• Bloody or black stool
• Shortness of breath
• Dizziness or light-headedness
• Chest pain or pain radiating into the neck and shoulder

According to Samuel Klein, M.D., associate professor of medicine in the Division of Gastroenterology and the Division of Human Nutrition at the University of Texas Medical School at Galveston, these symptoms indicate problems far more complex than heartburn, ranging from obstruction of the esophagus to a heart attack.

Watch out for repeat offenders. Coffee, alcohol, spicy foods and citrus fruits often bring on a five-alarm blaze, according to John Sutherland, M.D., clinical professor of family practice at the University of Iowa College of Medicine in Iowa City and director of the Waterloo Family Practice Residency Program in Waterloo. And watch out for fried and fatty foods as well as tomatoes and chocolate. Any of these can "irritate your esophageal lining or relax your

---

Don't Forget Antacids

You can reach for relief with antacids, but timing is important, says Dennis Decktor, Ph.D., scientific director of the Oklahoma Foundation for Digestive Research in Oklahoma City. "Use antacids after you eat but before heartburn occurs. Food and drink wash them away."

It appears to be the coating action rather than the acid-neutralizing action of antacids that matters, according to Dr. Decktor. For this reason, he advises, "don't drink water with an antacid or you may wash the coating away."

Tablets, pills or liquid? Take a chewable, Dr. Decktor recommends. When you chew, you create saliva, which helps neutralize some of the "burning" acid.

---

sphincter muscle, triggering reflux," says Ronald L. Hoffman, M.D., director of the Hoffman Center for Holistic Medicine in New York City.

Obliterate that onion. Do you suffer after spicy meals with onions? The onions, not the spices, may be the cause, says Melvin L. Allen, Ph.D., a gastroenterology researcher at the Presbyterian Medical Center of Philadelphia. It helps to refrigerate raw onions before you slice them. It reduces their potency. Better yet, cook them!

Or opt for a *different* onion. "There are three types of onions that don't cause heartburn," says Stephen Brunton, M.D., director of family medicine at Long Beach Memorial Medical Center in Long Beach, California. "Try the Texas sweet onion, the Maui and the Walla Walla varieties." (You may not find these in your grocery store unless it has a large and diverse produce section, but be persistent and check your local farmer's market or food co-op.)

Try less on the plate. "Eat small meals to avoid heartburn," advises William J. Ravich, M.D., associate professor of medicine in the Division of Gastroenterology at Johns Hopkins University School of Medicine in Baltimore. It's best to eat more frequent meals of small portions, instead of three "normal" meals a day. And try to have your last meal of the day at least three hours before bedtime, since you're more likely to get heartburn when you're lying down.

Drink water with your meals. Drinking water will wash stomach acids from the surface of the esophagus back into your stomach, says Dr. Hoffman. The saliva you swallow with the water will help neutralize the acid.

Four after-dinner no-no's. Your after-dinner habits may be causing your heartburn. For greater comfort, avoid drinking, smoking, napping and strenuous lifting. After-dinner drinks tend to bring on nighttime reflux, Dr. Hoffman says, and "smoking may weaken your lower esophageal sphincter." Avoid lying down after dinner, because gravity helps food stay in your stomach where it belongs. ("Try to resist the after-dinner nap, especially after eating a heavy meal," says Dr. Sutherland.) And as for taking out the garbage after dinner, lifting heavy things after eating can also bring on heartburn, Dr. Ravich says.

Sleep on a slope. "Place the head of your bed on six-inch blocks," advises Dr. Hoffman. "This seems to reduce heartburn by minimizing the flow of reflux from your stomach into your esophagus at night." Also, if you're in the habit of lying on your right side, try sleeping on your left side instead, suggests

Hiatal Hernia Isn't the Problem: Heartburn Is

Nearly one in every three people has a hiatal hernia, a condition where the upper portion of the stomach protrudes upward through an opening in the diaphragm into the chest. This usually occurs as a result of weakening of the tissue around the diaphragm.

Although hiatal hernia causes no pain and produces no symptoms, it's often confused with heartburn, says William B. Ruderman, M.D., chairman of the Department of Gastroenterology at the Cleveland Clinic–Florida in Fort Lauderdale. That's because people who have reflux heartburn often have a hiatal hernia as well.

But if you're *not* prone to heartburn, having a hiatal hernia usually means little, says Dr. Ruderman. In fact, many people are completely unaware they have a hiatal hernia—even though it affects half of all people over age 50. "The bottom line is that it isn't necessary to do *anything* about a hiatal hernia," says Dr. Ruderman. "But it is necessary to take care of heartburn if you're feeling pain."

William B. Ruderman, M.D., chairman of the Department of Gastroenterology at the Cleveland Clinic–Florida in Fort Lauderdale. "The stomach is lower when you're lying on your left side," observes Dr. Ruderman. In that position, stomach acid is less likely to make its way up into your esophagus.

Run not, burn not. Although exercise is a great habit, running can cause "runner's reflux," says Dr. Hoffman. If that's a problem, try other forms of exercise that don't jostle the body as much—such as bicycling or working out with weights. (But avoid doing any form of exercise except a relaxed stroll right after a meal.)

Review your Rx. Some medications lead to heartburn. For example, "make sure your stomach doctor knows what your heart doctor has prescribed," says John Horn, Pharm.D., associate professor at the University of Washington School of Pharmacy in Seattle. "Certain medications for high blood pressure, particularly calcium channel blockers, can cause reflux."

Try the vomit nut. It's unappealingly named, but the so-called vomit nut, or nux vomica, is a homeopathic remedy that relieves heartburn, says Dr. Hoffman. Check your local health food store for availability and follow the directions on the bottle.

Heart Palpitations

There's nothing like an off-beat ticker to scare the daylights out of you. Some irregularities in heartbeat are considered harmless and self-correcting. You may sense that your heart has skipped a beat, a condition known as ectopic (from the Greek *ektopos*, "misplaced") atrial heartbeat. Or your heart may suddenly speed up, a condition called tachycardia. Sometimes this kind of arrhythmia passes quickly, with no serious effects.

But—and this is a big but—only a doctor can say with certainty that your heart palpitations are nothing to worry about. "If you have any question about what you are experiencing, the safest thing is to have it checked out," says Jeremy Rushkin, M.D., director of the Cardiac Arrhythmia Service at Massachusetts General Hospital and associate professor of medicine at Harvard Medical School, both in Boston. That advice holds true whether you're young or old. (And even if other heart problems are ruled out during an exam, the doctor may want to prescribe medication specifically for arrhythmia.)

You may think of your heart simply as a muscular pump, but the fact is, this organ is very sensitive to many things going on in the body. A near accident, cigarette smoke, drugs (both prescription and nonprescription), emotional upsets and overindulgence in food, alcohol or caffeine can all upset the carefully orchestrated pattern of electrical charges that leads to a normal heartbeat.

"People are often unaware of how they are setting themselves up for an arrhythmia problem," says Stephen Sinatra, M.D., chief of cardiology and director of medical education at Manchester Memorial Hospital in Manchester, Connecticut, and assistant clinical professor of medicine at the University of Connecticut School of Medicine in Farmington. "They need to address a number of things that could be contributing to their problem."

Here are some steps to consider.

If you smoke, stop. "Smoking is an extremely dangerous activity if you have cardiac arrhythmia," Dr. Rushkin says. "It can undo even the best of medical care."

Warm up and cool down. If you exercise, add at least ten minutes to the beginning and end of your routine to give your heart time to change pace gradually. And no 50-yard dashes to the bus stop or sudden sprints up the stairs, unless you've warmed up first with a few passes around the block.

"Sudden exercise is a very common trigger in people prone to arrhythmia," Dr. Rushkin says. Cooling down is equally important, especially if you've been running, cycling or doing other exercises that involve your legs, Dr. Rushkin says.

Save skydiving for another lifetime. If you've never had arrhythmia, chances are you won't develop it pursuing even the most daring of avocations. "But if you're prone to arrhythmia, we suggest you not put yourself into such stressful circumstances," Dr. Rushkin says. That goes for occupational stress, too. A firefighter or policeman may need to switch to a less hair-raising job.

Stick with noncompetitive sports. "I have the opportunity to take care of a number of competitive athletes with heart arrhythmias, and they tend to have problems only when they are in a competitive situation," says Dr. Rushkin.

When to See the Doctor

A single skipped heartbeat or an extra beat sensed occasionally throughout the day usually is no cause for concern, according to Jeremy Rushkin, M.D., director of the Cardiac Arrhythmia Service at Massachusetts General Hospital and associate professor of medicine at Harvard Medical School, both in Boston. "Almost everyone experiences these, especially as we get older."

But if you feel more than that, such as a string of skipped beats, or if your heart seems to race without provocation, you should see a doctor right away. You should also see the doctor if you have additional symptoms of dizziness or faintness.

"The combination of competition and physical stress is a much more powerful trigger of arrhythmias than is either one alone, and that's not surprising."

Restrain yourself at all-you-can-eat buffets. Stuffing yourself to the gills—what doctors politely call metabolic overload—can bring on heart palpitations in those prone to them, Dr. Rushkin says. So eat lightly.

Go easy on alcohol. "Some people with arrhythmias are extremely sensitive to alcohol, and they usually know it—they sometimes get palpitations after just one drink," Dr. Rushkin says. "We advise them to be very cautious and moderate in their drinking. I prefer that they not drink at all."

Say no to joe. Coffee, tea, chocolate and certain drugs that contain caffeine, such as diet pills, can exacerbate arrhythmia problems in some people. "I recommend that people who have a history of arrhythmias should avoid caffeine as much as possible," says Dr. Rushkin.

Give your medicine chest the twice-over. Quite a few drugs can cause heartbeat problems, including those sometimes prescribed to correct arrhythmia. Culprits include digitalis, beta blockers, calcium channel blockers, all anti-arrhythmic drugs, tricyclic antidepressants and cimetidine (Tagamet), a popular ulcer drug.

"A doctor can sometimes tell early on that a drug is going to cause problems, and that's why many of these drugs are started in the hospital," Dr.

Rushkin says. "But some effects may occur later and may occur unexpectedly." Contact your doctor immediately if you think you're having a problem.

And be especially wary of decongestants. Even popular over-the-counter drugs can cause problems, says Dennis Miura, M.D., Ph.D., director of cardiac arrhymthias and electrophysiology at Albert Einstein College of Medicine of Yeshiva University in New York City. "Decongestants and asthma sprays that contain ephedrine or pseudoephedrine are the most common offenders," he says. They can cause a faster and somewhat more forceful heart rate and, in some circumstances, can cause or exacerbate serious arrhythmias. If you're already prone to arrhythmia problems, don't use these drugs without your doctor's okay.

Breathe calmly and fully. If you tend to hold your breath, as some people do when they're frightened, tense or straining in some physical activity, or if your breathing is shallow and rapid, you can upset your heart's natural rhythm, says Robert Fried, Ph.D., director of the Biofeedback Clinic at the Institute for Rational Emotive Therapy in New York City and author of *The Psychology and Physiology of Breathing in Behavioral Medicine.* So pay attention to your breathing. Allow yourself to exhale fully, then relax your belly and give your lungs time to fill before you exhale again.

Roll with the punches. "I am convinced that stress can be a powerful factor in enhancing or increasing susceptibility to arrhythmia," Dr. Rushkin says. "I would certainly endorse any program or activity that reduces stress. People simply need to find what works best for them." Meditation, biofeedback, yoga, prayer, music—all can ease tension.

Fill up on fish. Preliminary studies from researchers in Australia suggest that omega-3 fatty acids from fish such as salmon and mackerel may help reduce arrhythmias. The researchers think these fats may alter the composition of heart muscle cells, making them less prone to rhythmic disturbances.

Heat Exhaustion

You carry around your own air conditioner, and most of the time it works like a charm. All that pollution-free liquid evaporating from your skin (better known as good old sweat) cools your body without depleting the ozone layer one bit. The trouble is, if you spend too much time in the sun and not enough time drinking to replace fluids lost by sweating, you're subject to heat exhaustion.

Since dehydration is usually the cause, the first symptom of heat exhaustion is extreme thirst. But there are other symptoms as well, including loss of appetite, headache, fatigue, dizziness and nausea or even vomiting. Other signs of heat exhaustion: Notice if your heart races and you have trouble concentrating after spending a long time outdoors in hot weather. The first thing you should do whenever you start to feel *any* of these symptoms is rest in a nice shady spot—or, even better, get indoors. Then follow up with some tactics that will help your body beat the heat.

When to See the Doctor

If someone has trouble walking, standing, answering questions coherently or staying conscious after long heat exposure, experts suggest that you get the person to a doctor as soon as possible. Those are all symptoms of heatstroke, a potentially fatal condition in which the kidneys shut down and the body goes into shock.

If you even suspect that a person has heatstroke, call for emergency assistance. If you have to wait for a ride or an ambulance, cool the person as quickly as possible by whatever means possible. Some ways include splashing cool water on him, wrapping him in soaked towels, moving him to an air-conditioned room or immersing him in cool, shallow water.

Drink Up—But Not Alcohol

Want to celebrate summer with a cold beer and fun in the sun? Well, all that beer may lead to one big case of heat exhaustion, say experts.

Beer, like other alcoholic drinks, can actually promote heat exhaustion by "fast-forwarding" dehydration, says Danny Wheat, head trainer for the Texas Rangers professional baseball team. (The team often plays in 100°F-plus conditions in Arlington, Texas.) Since beer is a diuretic that causes excessive urination, it should be avoided even *before* you venture into the hot sun. Wheat stresses to his players that "the night before a day game, they should limit their alcohol consumption."

Instead of beer, stick to drinking water, fruit juices or sports drinks like Gatorade. If you feel symptoms of heat exhaustion, Pedialyte and other rehydrant formulas for infants are also effective. (The Texas Rangers give them to their players in extremely hot weather, Wheat says.)

Fill to the top with fluids. "The key is to keep properly hydrated," says Peter Raven, Ph.D., professor of physiology at Texas College of Osteopathic Medicine in Fort Worth and past president of the American College of Sports Medicine. That means drinking enough fluids to feel full before you venture outdoors—particularly if you'll be doing anything strenuous. Most experts recommend that you drink *at least* 8 ounces (one large glass) before going outdoors. Even better, drink up to 20 ounces (or enough water that you have to urinate). "Ideally, you should drink another cup of water every 10 to 15 minutes *while* you're outdoors," adds Dr. Raven. "I suggest you carry a water bottle with you, so you can take frequent drinks."

Keep your shirt on. Going bare-chested makes you more susceptible to heat exhaustion. "You pick up more radiant heat exposure with your shirt off," says Lanny Nalder, Ph.D., director of the Human Performance Research Center at Utah State University in Logan. "Once you start perspiring, a shirt can act like a cooling device when the wind goes through."

Eat lots of fruits and vegetables. "They have a fairly high water content and good salt balance," says Richard Keller, M.D., an emergency room physician at St. Therese Medical Center in Waukegan, Illinois. Another bonus: They also replace vitamins and minerals lost in sweat.

Forget salt tablets. Although dehydration can also result from a lack of salt, don't think you're doing your body a service by taking salt tablets. "They do the opposite of what they're supposed to do," says W. Larry Kenney, Ph.D., associate professor of applied physiology in the Laboratory for Human Performance Research at Pennsylvania State University in University Park. "The increased salt in the stomach keeps fluids there longer, which leaves less fluid available for necessary sweat production."

Weigh yourself. Before you venture outdoors, weigh yourself—and then weigh yourself again when you return. "All of that lost weight is water loss, so drink that much back," adds Dr. Raven. Keep in mind that one pound equals two glasses of water.

Heat Rash

Sure, the aerobics class was fun, and you worked up a nice sweat. But now it seems you've developed a rash, and your skin feels prickly all the time. Probably both the rash and the pricklies come from sweating—and that means you have heat rash, also known as prickly heat. Heat rash occurs because sweat ducts become plugged and sweat leaks into the skin instead of out of it. But the good news is that it's easy to treat.

How do you know that your rash is prickly heat, as opposed to eczema, an allergic reaction or hives? "If you look at it very closely, you'll see little red dots," says W. Larry Kenney, Ph.D., associate professor of applied physiology at the Laboratory for Human Performance Research at Pennsylvania State University in University Park. "These are sweat glands that have become inflamed at the opening. With further exposure to heat, there will also be a prickly 'pins and needles' sensation on the skin, which is why it is called prickly heat."

Cool off. "Since prickly heat occurs when the sweat ducts are blocked and sweat leaks into the skin, the only way to reverse it is to be in a situation where there is no sweating for a while," says Norman Levine, M.D., chief of dermatology at the University of Arizona College of Medicine Health Sciences Center in Tucson. Cool off, he suggests, by spending as much time as possible in an air-conditioned building for a day or two.

Wear loose clothing. Be selective about the clothing you wear and heat rash may vanish, according to Dr. Kenney. "Anything that will wick moisture away from the body and keep the skin dry will discourage heat rash." Whether you're recovering from heat rash or trying to avoid it, Dr. Kenney suggests that you "choose loose clothing made from cotton or polypropylene and avoid nylon, polyester or any tight-fitting clothes." This is especially important during the summer months.

Wash with mild soaps. To avoid the worst of heat rash, "wash with a mild, antibacterial soap," suggests Rodney Basler, M.D., a dermatologist and assistant professor of internal medicine at the University of Nebraska Medical Center in Omaha. "I would recommend Dial or Lever 2000, followed by a thorough rinsing and drying."

Take a baking soda bath. A baking soda bath can also be beneficial, Dr. Basler says. This will ease the itching and make you feel more comfortable while your heat rash is healing.

Just add a few tablespoons of baking soda to your normal bath water and stir it to dissolve completely.

Soothe with lotion. A number of over-the-counter skin lotions are designed to take the pricklies and itch out of heat rash. Warren Epinette, M.D., a dermatologist at Westwood-Squibb Pharmaceuticals in Buffalo, New York, recommends nonprescription lotions such as Moisturel that contain dimethicone. Calamine, the traditional poison ivy lotion, can also ease the itching and irritation caused by heat rash.

Give it the dust-off. Want to prevent the return of heat rash in hot summer months? Besides wearing loose cotton clothing, you can also dust yourself with absorbent powders. Richard Berger, M.D., clinical professor of dermatology at the University of Medicine and Dentistry of New Jersey Robert Wood Johnson Medical School in New Brunswick, recommends the medicated powder Zeasorb-AF, available in most pharmacies. Cornstarch or talcum powder will also do.

Watch your weight. Just when you thought you knew all the reasons for weight loss, here's another one: Obesity often causes folds in the skin, which can become sweaty and irritated, says Melvyn Chase, M.D., a dermatologist in Phoenix. "People who are overweight tend to sweat more and generate more body heat, so they are more likely to have heat rash."

Heel Spurs

Heel spurs are bony protrusions on the bottom of the foot, caused by continuous pulling of the ligament that runs across the sole. Runners and others who are hard on their feet are very likely to get them, especially if their feet turn *in* (pronation) when they run. (That excess movement just adds to the ligament pulling.) Those with high arches are also more likely to develop spurs.

"A lot of people think that because they have heel pain, it's a spur," says Terry Spilken, D.P.M., a podiatrist and adjunct faculty member at the New York College of Podiatric Medicine in New York City. "But we also have to rule out other conditions such as arthritis and bursitis. The only way to properly diagnose a heel spur is with an x-ray." Once that's done, here's how to take the hurt out of your spur.

Don't walk au naturel. "Walking barefoot is the *worst* thing you can do if you have heel spurs," says William Van Pelt, D.P.M., a podiatrist in Houston and former president of the American Academy of Podiatric Sports Medicine. "Walking barefoot stretches out the ligament on the bottom of the foot even farther, and being barefoot results in a less stable walk."

Wear the footgear of a cowboy. Instead, you should wear a shoe with a ¾- to 1½-inch heel, like a cowboy boot. That's because the heel moves the front of the foot forward, taking some pressure off the heel.

Enlist sponge rubber support. Over-the-counter arch supports and heel cups, which are sold in most drugstores and sporting goods stores, help those with heel spurs in two ways: "They support the arch, which controls excess foot rolling or movement, and they help elevate the heel a bit, which takes some of the pressure off the spur," says Dr. Van Pelt. He recommends that you first try a pair of sponge rubber arch supports. If they don't bring relief, try a heel cup.

Give yourself a massage. "A regular massage of your entire foot, and particularly the heel, also helps a lot," says Dr. Spilken. The best way to do the massage? "Rub across the aching area with your thumb in order to get more pressure."

Apply ice for pain. When your heel spur is acting up, apply an ice pack wrapped in a towel to stop the pain, advises Dr. Spilken. Keep it under ice for ten minutes, then remove the pack for another ten. Repeat this procedure several times, or until the throbbing subsides.

Use heat for maintenance. Doctors recommend applying heat on a daily basis in order to bring more blood to the area and break up inflammation. A 15- or 20-minute session with a heating pad is usually enough.

Hemorrhoids

It's easy enough to see a bulging varicose vein in your leg. But when a vein bulges where the sun doesn't shine, you're more likely to *feel* it than see it. A hemorrhoid is exactly that: a varicose vein in the anus or rectum that can cause considerable discomfort—itching, burning and, occasionally, throbbing pain.

Hemorrhoids can bleed when they are scraped by a hard bowel movement. Your first symptom may be an alarming streak of bright red blood on the feces or drops of blood on the toilet paper. (The bleeding usually stops by itself in a few minutes.)

If the doctor says you have hemorrhoids, you probably know what causes them, too. Hemorrhoids are most often caused by constipation, or "straining at stool." Just as the veins in your temples pop out when you're trying to lift something heavy, the veins in your anus can pop out when you try too hard, for too long, to have a bowel movement.

It's true that hemorrhoids do tend to shrink when the pressure's off, but daily straining can make them continually protrude (or prolapse), bleed and hurt. But here are some ways to ease the discomfort and help heal the hidden annoyance.

Clean with care. While it's important to keep your bottom clean, vigorous wiping will only aggravate your hemorrhoids, says Max M. Ali, M.D., director and president of Hemorrhoid Clinics of America in Oak Park, Michigan. Wipe first with moistened toilet paper, or use a premoistened wipe. Then pat with dry toilet paper. Or try using a plastic squeeze bottle of water to gently "shower" your bottom, then pat dry with toilet paper. Avoid using scented or colored toilet paper containing chemicals that irritate tender tushies. If you must use soap to clean, use an unscented, hard-milled bar such as Ivory.

Dab on petroleum jelly or zinc oxide paste. In studies, both of these low-priced drugstore items worked just as well as more expensive creams. You can try either, or both, to reduce the pain and swelling of hemorrhoids. After wiping, dab a small amount of the cream or paste on a cotton ball and apply to the anal area.

Sit in a sitz. "Of all the things you can do when your hemorrhoids are sore, sitz baths are the best, in my opinion," says Lester Rosen, M.D, chairman of the National Standards Task Force of the American Society of Colon and Rectal Surgeons and associate clinical professor of surgery at Hahnemann University School of Medicine in Philadelphia.

"Warm water relaxes the anal sphincter muscle," Dr. Rosen explains. A relaxed anal sphincter muscle takes the squeeze off tender protrusions.

Fill your bath with three to four inches of warm (not hot) water. Don't add anything to the water—not Epsom salts, bubble bath or bath oil, Dr. Rosen says. Sit in the tub for 15 minutes or so.

Pay heed when nature calls. "Try to tune in to the stomach/bowel reflex that should occur twice a day, within 20 minutes after breakfast and dinner," says Sidney E. Wanderman, M.D., author of *The Hemorrhoid Book* and former senior clinical instructor in surgery at Mount Sinai School of Medicine in New York City. The reflex is a signal that feces have moved into your colon and are ready to come out. Schedule your day to give yourself time to go when the urge strikes, Dr. Wanderman suggests. "You'll have less straining if you work with nature on this one."

Get up and moving. "It really works," Dr. Rosen says. Exercises such as walking, running, biking and swimming make food move through your bowel faster. That helps prevent constipation and hemorrhoids. "Good overall muscle tone and a firm tummy also let you respond decisively to nature's call," Dr. Wanderman says.

When to See the Doctor

It's best not to assume that bleeding during a bowel movement is caused by hemorrhoids until a doctor verifies that's the case. Intestinal polyps, anal fissures, even colon cancer can also cause rectal bleeding.

"Everyone, even people with diagnosed hemorrhoids, should get regular examinations for bowel cancer and should see a doctor if there is a change in bowel habits," says Max M. Ali, M.D., director and president of Hemorrhoid Clinics of America in Oak Park, Michigan.

Go or get off the pot. If you want to go, should you sit and wait?

Some people believe that having good reading material handy makes for a leisurely, relaxing (even enjoyable) excretory experience. "I personally believe that if you sit on the toilet long enough to read an entire magazine article, you're there too long, and you are probably constipated," Dr. Rosen says. "Several minutes should be enough to evacuate your bowels."

Eat foods that fight hemorrhoids. Include in your diet high-fiber foods that naturally produce softer stools that move easily past tender spots. Try oats, oat bran or barley, suggests dietician Patricia H. Harper, R.D., of North Huntingdon, Pennsylvania. Aim for several servings a day of fruits and vegetables. In addition, if you can eat a cup or so of beans, chances are your hemorrhoids will shrink to a mere memory.

If chewing is a problem for you, get your fiber by eating applesauce mixed with oat bran, hot oat or rice cereals, mashed carrots or sweet potatoes and creamy vegetable or bean soups, Harper suggests.

Drink up. It's equally important to get plenty of fluids. Try to get a minimum of six to eight glasses of water or other fluids a day, Harper suggests. Since some kinds of fiber absorb fluids, the more you drink, the more you'll help keep stools soft.

Hiccups

Hippocrates said that sneezing would bring relief. Plato swore the answer was to hold your breath and gargle. For centuries, the world's greatest minds have pondered long and hard the cures for this most perplexing medical mishap.

Which seems like a real waste of great-mind time. C'mon, we're only talking about *hiccups,* guys.

Why all the pondering? Maybe it's because almost everyone has a super-favorite, nothing-like-it, can't-be-beat, surefire cure. And many of them work. "Any time someone suggests something and the hiccups disappear, they assume it's a remedy, so just about anything could qualify as a remedy," says John Renner, M.D., a consumer health expert and clinical professor of family medicine at the University of Missouri at Kansas City. "That's because most hiccups disappear on their own in a few minutes. Just wait long enough, and in most cases, doing *nothing* will cure hiccups. But right now, there are people who swear that wearing stockings or smelling perfume will cure hiccups."

The *cause* of hiccups is simple: Usually something has triggered involuntary contractions in the diaphragm. You may have swallowed air when you were eating fast or taking a shower or when you suddenly got excited. You can get hiccups from eating an "irritating" food (usually gas inducers such as vegetables or beans) or from eating both hot and cold foods at the same time. Drinking alcohol or carbonated beverages can also set off those involuntary (*hic!*) contractions. In short, just about anything can cause hiccups, says James Lewis, M.D., vice president for medical development at Glaxo Pharmaceuticals in Research Triangle Park, North Carolina, and an authority on hiccup causes and cures.

But whatever the cause, quicker relief is in sight if you:

Hear no evil, have no hiccups. Plugging your ears with your fingers for about 20 seconds can halt hiccups, says Dev Mehta, M.D., a gastroenterologist at Hahnemann University Hospital in Philadelphia. This remedy, reported in

When to See the Doctor

Persistent hiccups that last for several days *without* improvement might indicate a serious medical problem and require medical attention.

"If you have hiccups that you can't get rid of for three or four days, see your doctor," says John Renner, M.D., a consumer health expert and clinical professor of family medicine at the University of Missouri at Kansas City. "It may mean you have a gastrointestinal disorder, a problem in your nervous system or an infection of some kind."

Of course, bouts of hiccups that last for several days are highly unusual. But according to Dr. Renner, if you *repeatedly* get hiccups, you should let your doctor know about it. "It could mean more than the regular muscle spasm that causes most hiccups," he says.

the medical journal *Lancet,* operates on the theory that sticking fingers in your ears temporarily short-circuits the vagus nerve, which controls hiccuping. That, in turn, interrupts the hiccup cycle.

Drink pineapple juice . . . or just about anything else. "This is a popular folklore remedy, but we use it in my house when someone gets hiccups, and it works great," says Dr. Renner. "It's the acidic content of pineapple juice that's said to do the trick, but the truth is, drinking just about any liquid will have the same effect. Drinking requires a lot of swallowing, and doing a lot of swallowing is probably the best way to stop hiccups."

Breathe into a brown paper bag. If swallowing isn't your style, do what the pros do: "The first thing we do when someone comes into the hospital with hiccups is have him breathe into a brown paper bag," says Dr. Mehta. "We're not exactly sure why it works, but we think that breathing more carbon dioxide affects the diaphragm in a way that stops hiccups."

Act like a brat. "Sticking your tongue out is another proven remedy," adds Dr. Renner. "It stimulates the glottis, which is the opening of the airway to the lungs"—and a closed glottis causes hiccups.

Rub the roof of your mouth with a cotton swab. It tickles a bit, but Dr. Lewis says it's another way to stimulate the glottis—without looking childish.

Try This Bartender's Remedy

If there's anyone who knows more about hiccups than doctors, it's bartenders. After all, drinking is a leading cause of hiccups. So what's their secret cure?

"You tell them you have a surefire way to cure hiccups, but they have to follow your instructions—with no questions asked," says Tony Liott, a longtime bartender in Palm Beach, Florida. "Then you take a glass of water, stick a metal spoon in the glass and tell them to drink it very fast, guzzle it without stopping."

Why the spoon?

"It takes their mind off their hiccups, I guess," says Liott. "I don't know what other reason it serves, but I've never seen anyone continue to have hiccups after trying it."

Hold your breath. This age-old remedy really does work, says Bahman Jabbari, M.D., chief of neurophysiology in the Department of Neurology at Walter Reed Medical Center in Washington, D.C. "It probably works in the same way breathing into a paper bag does."

Try a tongue pull. One theory says that any time you touch the back of your throat with your finger, a cotton swab or anything else, it stimulates the nerve to stop the diaphragm from hiccuping. Of course, the "gagging response" can also induce vomiting, so here's another way: Gently yank at your tongue! That causes the same reflex, but without the unpleasant gagging sensation.

"Squeeze" the hiccups out. While sitting in a chair or on the floor, compress your chest by pulling your knees up to your chest and leaning forward, advises Dr. Lewis.

Get your "gulper" working. When you swallow hard or quickly, all that gulping action could put an end to your hiccups. So what should you swallow? "A tall glass of ice water always works for me," says Dr. Jabbari. "Drinking vinegar is a popular choice," says Dr. Renner, "because it takes a lot to get it down and requires a lot of swallowing. The same goes for dry bread or crackers." Dr. Lewis also suggests sucking on lemon wedges soaked in angostura bitters—it's such a palate displeaser, you'll get that juice down *pronto!*

Swallow some sugar. This is especially popular for children who have hic-cups. "Since a child isn't about to suck on bitter lemon wedges or drink vine-gar, I suggest placing some sugar on the back of the tongue and swallowing it," says Dr. Mehta. *Good news:* It works just as well for adults.

High Blood Pressure

Poor diet, lack of exercise, heavy-duty weight training, even innocuous-sounding activities such as public speaking can make your blood pressure leap. But when your blood pressure goes up and stays up, there's cause for concern: Of all the risk factors for heart attack, high blood pressure remains the most accurate predictor of who will get cardiovascular disease after age 65.

Anyone with high blood pressure needs to be under a doctor's care—not only for regular monitoring but often for medication as well. The good news is that many of the 60 million Americans with high blood pressure can do something about it without drugs. If you're among them, your doctor has no doubt mentioned the importance of regular exercise, avoiding smoking, managing stress and changing your diet to put limits on alcohol, salt and fat. But here are some lesser-known factors that can take your blood pressure down a notch or two and significantly slash your risk of heart failure, stroke and kidney disease.

Munch on celery. Celery and its oil have been used in oriental folk medicine for centuries to treat high blood pressure and circulatory problems, and now the West may know why. University of Chicago researchers have found that a compound in the vegetable helps lower blood pressure by relaxing muscles lining the arteries. This allows the muscles that regulate blood pressure to dilate.

Best of all, it doesn't take much to reap the rewards. Eating the equivalent of only four stalks a day can lower blood pressure in rats an average of 13 percent, reports William Elliott, M.D., Ph.D., assistant professor in the Department of Preventive Medicine at Rush–St. Luke's–Presbyterian Medical Center in Chicago.

And gobble down garlic. The reason isn't as well established, but garlic is another blood pressure buster. "We know that eating garlic can lower your blood pressure, but we're still trying to learn exactly why," according to Yu-Yan Yeh, Ph.D., associate professor of nutrition at Pennsylvania State University in University Park and a researcher on the healing properties of garlic. "Eating as little as one clove a day—either raw or used in cooking—seems to have a beneficial effect."

Note: In animal studies, garlic has also been shown to lower cholesterol and triglycerides—other factors that have an impact on heart disease. And it doesn't matter whether you eat fresh garlic or take it in a capsule: In either form, it has the beneficial effect.

Get a pet. "We know that when people touch or pet their animals, there's almost always a small but significant drop in blood pressure," according to Alan Beck, Sc.D., coauthor of *Between Pets and People* and professor of ecology at Purdue University School of Veterinary Medicine in West Lafayette, Indiana. "Even just *looking* at an animal, such as a fish in a tank, results in a consistent drop in blood pressure. Being around animals seems to put people at ease and help reduce their stress."

Speak softly. According to some studies, speaking loudly and rapidly can significantly raise your blood pressure during normal conversation. And if

Home Treatment Helper

Perhaps the best thing you can do for yourself once you've been diagnosed with high blood pressure is to invest in a home blood pressure monitor. A daily measurement of your blood pressure can indicate whether your medication and home remedies are actually working to lower your blood pressure.

But even if you notice an improvement, don't stop taking a doctor-prescribed medication unless you have your physician's approval, advises David Spodick, M.D., director of clinical cardiology at St. Vincent Hospital at the University of Massachusetts Medical School in Worcester. You'll be most likely to remember your medication if you establish a routine, such as taking it immediately before breakfast or right after you walk your dog each morning.

people do this while engaged in emotional exchanges, especially angry ones, their blood pressure can shoot up even higher, says Aron Siegman, Ph.D., professor of psychology and director of the Behavioral Medicine Program at the University of Maryland, Baltimore County, in Catonsville.

Chronic anger-produced elevations in blood pressure may be a serious risk factor for coronary heart disease, according to Dr. Siegman. "As people raise their voices, it increases their blood pressure, and as their blood pressure goes up, they tend to raise their voices further in an ever-increasing cycle that tends to turn anger into rage," he says. The good news is that speaking softly and slowly, even about the most anger-provoking events, totally eliminates the cardiovascular upheaval.

Don't lie around. Besides speaking softly, speak the truth. Lying has been found to boost blood pressure, because it requires more brain function. The more you lie, the more you add stress (and, hence, increase your blood pressure), says David Robertson, M.D., director of the Clinical Research Center at Vanderbilt University School of Medicine in Nashville, Tennessee.

Make your exercise aerobic, *not* isometric. While regular exercise is one of the best ways to lower blood pressure, it has to be the right kind. Isometric exercises in which you clench and hold, such as weight lifting, should be avoided, says David Spodick, M.D., director of clinical cardiology at St. Vincent Hospital at the University of Massachusetts Medical School in Worcester. That's because heavy weight lifting can cause blood pressure to temporarily skyrocket, especially if you hold your breath while lifting (as most people do).

Have a few laughs. Laughter *is* the best medicine—or at least it's as good as relaxation therapy, exercise or other methods used to combat stress, says Steve Allen, Jr., M.D., son of the famous comedian and clinical assistant professor of family medicine at the State University of New York Health Science Center at Syracuse College of Medicine.

"When you laugh, you decrease adrenaline and cortisone production," says Dr. Allen, who specializes in laughter therapy. (Adrenaline and cortisone are both hormonal compounds that have an adverse effect on blood pressure.) "My prescription is that you should do something silly at least twice a day or as needed."

While laughter can help everyone, Dr. Allen points out that people with high blood pressure who are particularly angry, frustrated or unhappy often benefit the most from laughter therapy. "Laughter is one of those ways that's cheap as well as effective," says Dr. Allen.

Hives

Different parts of your body react to allergens (allergy-causing substances) in different ways. The throat scratches. The nose drips. The eyes water. And your skin may react by breaking out in blotches of red and itchy welts. Both the redness and itchiness are major clues: You probably have hives.

Hives are caused when cells release histamine, which is the typical body response when cells are exposed to allergens. Histamine makes blood vessels leak fluid into the deepest layers of the skin. It's also quite possible to get hives even if you don't have allergies: Hot weather, food ingredients, cold weather and even plain water cause hives in some people.

While allergies or irritations may be the original cause, hives are exacerbated by stress. So worrying about hives, or anything else, is likely to just make them worse.

What's the best treatment? Many doctors recommend over-the-counter antihistamines such as Benadryl or Chlor-Trimeton. And applying calamine lotion or alcohol lotions can certainly soothe your itching. But whatever you find at the pharmacy, here are some other worry-free ways to reduce the itching and swelling of hives.

Quash that histamine. Applying a cold compress or even rubbing an ice cube over hives helps shrink blood vessels. That keeps them from opening, swelling and allowing too much histamine to be released, says Leonard Grayson, M.D., a clinical associate allergist and dermatologist at Southern Illinois University School of Medicine in Springfield. "It's only temporary," he says. But if you're one of the few people who get hives from cold and ice, you'll need to try some other treatment, says Dr. Grayson. *Note: Don't* use a hot-water compress; that only makes the itching worse.

Order an herbal brew. To calm your nerves (which will calm your hives), you may want to try drinking herbal tea, says Thomas Squier, president of Botanico

When to See the Doctor

Although hives are usually a surface problem, they can be life-threatening if they interfere with your breathing. If you get hives in your mouth or throat, call an emergency number immediately, says Leonard Grayson, M.D., clinical associate allergist and dermatologist at Southern Illinois University School of Medicine in Springfield. For people who have severe hives, most doctors will prescribe medication to have on hand for emergencies.

Also, you should see the doctor if you have hives that last longer than six weeks or cause intense discomfort, according to Dr. Grayson.

Educational Services in Aberdeen, North Carolina, and a Cherokee herbologist. He recommends peppermint or passionflower teas. Chamomile, valerian and catnip are other common sedative herbal teas.

Try the alkaline answer. "Anything that's alkaline usually helps relieve the itch," says Dr. Grayson. So try dabbing milk of magnesia on your hives. "It's thinner than calamine lotion, so I think it works better," he says.

Give it the squeeze. Some people have reported success at getting rid of hives by trying acupressure. To get relief this way, you need to deeply massage your trapezius muscles on each side of your neck. The trapezius muscle runs between the neck and shoulder. The point you want to massage is located midway on the muscle, just an inch or so over the back side of the ridge. "If it doesn't hurt somewhat, you haven't found exactly the right point," says Michael Blate, founder and executive director of the G-Jo Institute in Hollywood, Florida, which promotes the use of acupressure. For maximum effectiveness, massage the point for up to 30 seconds—usually until you feel a slight clamminess or perspiration. Repeat several times a day until the hives start to clear up.

Hot Flashes

As a woman reaches menopause—usually around age 50—hormone levels fall rapidly as the ovaries halt production of the hormone estrogen. Sensing this, the body's internal thermostat tends to react quite strongly. Blood vessels on the skin's surface open up like a radiator, enveloping you in intense heat and flushing your face. About 80 percent of all women experience these hot flashes as they go through menopause.

Your doctor may prescribe estrogen tablets if your hot flashes are severe. But many women find they can deal with milder symptoms with home treatments.

Track those flashes. Hot flashes may occur more predictably and less randomly than you think, studies show. To prove it, take note of the date, time, intensity and duration of the hot flash, suggests Linda Gannon, Ph.D., professor of psychology at Southern Illinois University at Carbondale. Also record the circumstances preceding it—what you ate or drank, how you felt emotionally.

"Some women find that hot flashes worsen when they drink alcohol or coffee, smoke cigarettes or encounter stressful situations that elicit strong emotions," says Dr. Gannon. Your hot flash diary can show you what triggers you need to avoid to keep cool.

Lower the temp. Keeping cool is important for menopausal women, since many of the precipitating factors in hot flashes are related to heat, says Sadja Greenwood, M.D., assistant clinical professor of gynecology at the University of California, San Francisco, Medical Center. She suggests sipping cool drinks and wearing natural fabrics that "breathe." And one study at Columbia University in New York City showed that menopausal women had fewer and milder hot flashes in cool rooms than in hot rooms. So turn on the fan or the air conditioner to keep the temperature down. And when you're going out, carry a fold-up fan with you, Dr. Greenwood advises.

Keep a cool head—meditate. Some brain research has shown that hot flashes are stimulated by a brain chemical (neurotransmitter) known as norepinephrine, which influences the temperature-regulating center in the brain, says Dr. Greenwood. "This may explain why daily stress reduction practices such as meditation, deep breathing and yoga, which result in lower levels of norepinephrine, help some women reduce their hot flashes," she says.

In one study, menopausal women with frequent hot flashes were trained to slowly breathe in and out six to eight times for two minutes. These women had fewer hot flashes than women trained to use either muscle relaxation or biofeedback.

Douse it with vitamin E. "This nutrient often does a commendable job of relieving the severity and frequency of flashes. Lots of my patients have good luck with it," says Lila E.Nachtigall, M.D., associate professor of obstetrics and gynecology at New York University School of Medicine in New York City. She recommends starting with 400 international units twice a day (a total of 800 international units).

But check with your physician before beginning vitamin E supplementation. While the vitamin is generally considered safe, it can have a blood-thinning effect. Meanwhile, try to include more vitamin E–rich foods in your diet: wheat germ, wheat germ oil, safflower oil, whole-grain breads and cereals, peanuts, walnuts, filberts and almonds.

Sip some sarsaparilla. For centuries, herbalists have used special "women's herbs" that have a weak regulating effect on estrogen and may help control hot flashes, according to Susan Lark, M.D., medical director of the PMS and Menopause Self-Help Center in Los Altos, California. The herbs include sarsaparilla, dong quoi, black cohosh, false unicorn root, fennel and anise.

These herbs are available combined in ready-made formulas, or they can be used alone, says Dr. Lark. To make a tea, empty one herb capsule into a cup of boiling water and let it steep for a few minutes. Don't drink more than two cups of herbal tea (along with meals) daily. Discontinue the herbs if you notice nausea or other symptoms, says Dr. Lark. And talk to your doctor before taking these herbs if you're at risk for cancer or other conditions that rule out estrogen replacement therapy.

Get up and go. In one Swedish study, severe hot flashes and night sweats were only half as common among physically active postmenopausal women as among bench warmers. "Possibly, exercise elevates the level of endorphins, the feel-good hormones that drop when there is an estrogen deficiency," says Timothy Yeko, M.D., assistant professor in the Department of Obstetrics and Gynecology, Division of Reproductive Endocrinology, at the University of South Florida in Tampa. The endorphins affect the thermoregulatory center—your thermostat, says Dr. Yeko. Regular physical activity may increase endorphin activity and therefore diminish the frequency of hot flashes.

Don't aim to be a skinny-mini. "Estrogen is actually manufactured in body fat from other hormones after menopause," says Dr. Greenwood. "A very thin woman will have less natural estrogen in her system, which may give her more problems with hot flashes."

Hyperactivity

Mention that your child *won't* sit still or pay attention and most folks would say you've got a typical, red-blooded, all-American kid. Say that Junior *can't* seem to and he might be diagnosed with the most common psychiatric condition of childhood.

Attention deficit hyperactivity disorder (ADHD)—better known as hyperactivity, with or without the classic busy-bee behavior—affects about two million children in the United States, most of them boys. Yet even though ADHD is so widespread, scientists are only beginning to learn more about it. For years, the popular opinion was that these fidgety, incredibly impulsive kids were just brats—and that upbringing (or the lack of it) was the likely cause.

"Now we know that ADHD is not the fault of the parents but rather the result of an insufficient amount of one or more of the chemicals in the nervous system responsible for concentration and attention," says Ellen Gellerstedt, M.D., assistant professor of pediatrics at the University of Rochester School of Medicine and Dentistry in Rochester, New York, who specializes in developmental and behavioral pediatrics. "It's not that these kids are stupid or brats. They *know* the rules. They just are so impulsive that they act before they think."

Raising a hyperactive child is no easy task, but that doesn't mean it's a lost cause. "The symptoms always appear before age seven, so raising a hyperactive child is a real challenge," says Dr. Gellerstedt. "What may seem to be a disability in school often becomes a gift in adulthood. The kids often grow up to become adults who have incredible amounts of energy, are usually very creative and can often see things in ways that others can't."

Some prescription medications such as Ritalin can help reduce overactivity and focus attention. But here are some other ways to help children who have been diagnosed with hyperactivity.

Make *everything* step-by-step. "Hyperactive kids need an extreme amount of structure and organization, and if they get it, they usually calm down and do a lot better," says Ben J. Williams, Ph.D., a child psychologist who is the former director of the Hyperactivity Assessment Program at Baylor College of Medicine and Texas Children's Hospital in Houston.

"To do that, I encourage parents to break every activity into a six- or seven-step process, whether it's getting up, eating meals, watching TV, doing homework—virtually *every* aspect of the child's life. It's not enough to say 'Get ready for school.' It has to be 'First get out of bed. Then go to the bathroom to brush your teeth. Then wash your face.' And so on." Such regimentation may seem like belaboring the obvious, but Dr. Williams says it's necessary for hyperactive children, whose attention often lapses after just a minute or two.

Chart their progress. Another good way to give hyperactive kids the structure they need is with a daily calendar or chart outlining what's expected of them. "It's good to operate on a point system. By fulfilling their obligations, kids earn points, which are used for special privileges such as going out for ice cream or going to the movies," says Dr. Williams. "You should back up this structure with logical punishment—taking away privileges, for instance, rather than giving them spankings when they fail to meet their obligations. It's best to spell out everything on the chart, so there are no arguments later."

Be a "parrot" parent. "Since these kids act on impulse, you have to be prepared to remind them 5,000 times about what they're supposed to be doing," says Dr. Gellerstedt. "And not just for a day or two. For always. It's *very* important for parents to discipline themselves to remind kids again and again and again they have to brush their teeth or shut off the TV, even when it seems perfectly obvious."

Get them involved in the *right* activities. "Hyperactive kids tend to be above average in activities involving large-muscle movements but slower than average in sports that require hand-eye coordination. So they will do very well in

What about Diet?

Although studies have not proven that certain foods and ingredients (such as sugar) cause hyperactivity, the diet connection has been explored often and debated even more. While most doctors say there is no solid medical evidence that shows that diet plays any role in hyperactivity, many parents of hyperactive children believe otherwise.

One such parent is Jane Hersey, mother of a hyperactive child and national director of the Feingold Association of the United States, a group in Alexandria, Virginia, that believes food additives and even common fruits and vegetables trigger certain reactions in chemically sensitive people—including those with hyperactivity. "Many parents tell me they see a drastic change almost immediately when they change diet," says Hersey. "My daughter showed improvement in her behavior very quickly and dramatically once she started the Feingold diet."

The Feingold diet—started by a noted allergist and pediatrician, the late Ben Feingold, M.D.—helps parents find out whether a child is sensitive to food additives. The Feingold Association has a shopping list of foods that do not contain artificial colorings, flavorings or the preservatives BHA, BHT and TBHQ. If a child shows a lot of improvement while consuming the acceptable brand-name foods, he or she is probably chemically sensitive and should stay on the diet, according to Hersey. "Besides the food additives, a large number of common fruits and some vegetables appear to have compounds in them that can also trigger reactions," says Hersey. Among them are berries, cherries, apricots, apples, grapes, peaches and tomatoes.

activities such as swimming and soccer but will probably become very frustrated playing Little League baseball," says Dr. Williams.

"Outside of sports, it's good to get hyperactive kids involved in activities that have a good parent/child ratio, such as Cub Scouts or the YMCA Indian Guide Program. And try to arrange for the hyperactive child to sit either next to or directly across from the leader for maximum eye contact and involvement."

Have family rap sessions. Sibling rivalry is often a problem in families with hyperactive children—particularly when the hyperactive child torments a younger sibling. "One of the best ways of dealing with that, outside of professional counseling, is to have regular family meetings where everyone discusses his feelings—not just about that but *everything*," says Dr. Williams. "This allows the younger child to express his feelings, and the family will usually come up with solutions." It's better to "talk out" than to "act out" or be hyperactive.

It's also helpful because many hyperactive children often have trouble identifying with role models. Hearing his father talk about how he deals with life's everyday stresses, for instance, may teach a hyperactive boy important lessons. "In fact, one of the best things you can do for a hyperactive child is give a lot of quality time with the same-sex parent," adds Dr. Williams.

Give kids responsibilities. To channel these children's attention, many experts suggest providing them with household chores to foster responsibility. "You can incorporate the chores into the point system from about second grade on," says Dr. Williams. "I recommend a procedure where the child has four chores a day that are tied in to his allowance and special privileges. He gets a base allowance regardless but has an opportunity to make more money based on what he does with regard to grades, behavior, chores and other responsibilities. Generally these kids make excellent workers, because they have so much energy."

Hyperventilation

Fast, shallow breathing is a typical response in a so-called fight-or-flight situation. Back in the days when humans regularly met up with saber-toothed tigers—and had other life-or-death encounters every day—that fast breathing probably helped us survive. We got more oxygen in, more carbon dioxide out. And when you have to run for your life, that's just the extra oomph you need for headlong flight.

But these days, saber-toothed encounters are rare, and fast and shallow breathing is usually unnecessary for survival. In fact, its uselessness is implied by its modern name: *hyperventilation.*

Anyone who suffers from anxiety (and that's *everyone*) can suffer from hyperventilation. When you're frightened, you breathe rapidly and deeply, even

When to See the Doctor

Although uncommon, hyperventilation may be related to lung disease, pneumonia or a blood infection, according to doctors. Also, in certain cases, it could be a sign of a heart attack, since hyperventilation and cardiac arrest have similar symptoms. If your doctor has ruled out these causes, it may be that your hyperventilation is part of a panic attack, and you may wish to see a mental health professional for treatment.

though you don't need more oxygen. This causes you to exhale a large amount of carbon dioxide. Besides heavy breathing, you may also experience chest pain; light-headedness; tingling or coldness in the fingers, face or feet; excessive yawning or sighing; belching; and/or fatigue.

The classic "cure" is to breathe into a paper bag, so you breathe *in* some of the carbon dioxide that's normally "blown off" when you're hyperventilating. But this is an inefficient way to counter the problem, according to David H. Barlow, Ph.D., director of the Center for Stress and Anxiety Disorders at the State University of New York at Albany. Beyond paper bags, here's how to avoid future attacks and take the punch (and worry) out of hyperventilating.

Time your breathing. Don't overcompensate for hyperventilating by taking exaggerated breaths. The best way to restore normal breathing is to consciously slow the pace until you're taking about one breath every six seconds. In fact, if you're prone to hyperventilating, it's a good idea to practice this technique twice daily for ten minutes per session, according to Gabe Mirkin, M.D., associate clinical professor of pediatrics at Georgetown University School of Medicine in Washington, D.C., and sports medicine practitioner at the Sportsmedicine Institute in Silver Spring, Maryland.

Take a yoga class. Many deep-breathing techniques learned in yoga classes can help prevent hyperventilation or help you slow your breathing once hyperventilation has already started. Dr. Barlow suggests that you can learn how to do yoga-style deep breathing with this practice-at-home technique: Lie on your back with a book placed on top of your belly. Try to raise the book with each inhalation. Once you learn "belly breathing" in this prone position, you're ready to graduate to upright-style again. Practice it for ten minutes daily while sitting in a comfortable chair. With practice, it shouldn't be long before you can do belly breathing anytime and anywhere, even in the middle of a tension-filled board of directors' meeting.

Walk a few miles. Any kind of exercise decreases anxiety and helps people cope better—especially if you get your heart rate up. Besides helping you cope with stress, regular exercise improves breathing technique.

Slice your vices. Caffeine and nicotine are both stimulants, which are potential triggers for hyperventilation, says Dr. Barlow. Keep in mind that besides coffee, other caffeine sources include tea, cola and chocolate.

Impotence

Yeah, yeah, it happens to *all* men. Sure, sure, it's as much a part of being male as an Adam's apple or refusing to ask for directions. But when the very *symbol* of maleness lets you down, don't be surprised if you feel some embarrassment and humiliation. Many men do. And many fear that their rock 'em, sock 'em sex lives have been reduced to mere memories—all because they are unable to achieve or maintain erections.

But before you start playing taps for your bedroom abilities, understand that being impotent doesn't mean you have to stay that way. Whether you feel let down by a onetime episode or think you have a long-term problem, here's how to turn the tables and achieve healthy erections once again.

Try it standing up. If your trouble is *maintaining* an erection, then the problem is likely due to insufficient blood flow—either getting the blood into the penis or keeping it there. It's a normal part of the aging process and a large reason why one in four men over age 65 is impotent at least occasionally.

"Certain sexual positions can help men who suffer from decreased blood flow," says J. Francois Eid, M.D., director of the Erectile Dysfunction Unit at The New York Hospital–Cornell Medical Center in New York City. "Try having sex standing up, because standing facilitates blood flow." If standing isn't for you, try intercourse lying on your side, or enter your partner from behind, he advises.

Are Your Drugs to Blame?

Medications used to treat conditions such as high blood pressure, anxiety and depression can cause impotence and also make an impotent condition harder to treat.

"Many widely prescribed drugs—Valium included—can cause impotence," says Sheldon Burman, M.D., founder and director of the Male Sexual Dysfunction Institute in Chicago, the country's largest treatment center for male sexual problems. While you should never stop taking a medication simply because you fear impotence, do talk to your doctor about changing your medication or therapy.

"Sometimes you can treat depression, anxiety and high blood pressure without drugs—so speak to your doctor to see if you qualify for drug-free treatment," says Dr. Burman. Or ask your doctor about medications that don't inhibit your ability to have an erection.

Try hashing it out. "Impotence often occurs when men hold in negative feelings—anger, stress, frustration, irritation or hurt," says Alvin Baraff, Ph.D., director of MenCenter in Washington, D.C., and author of *Men Talk: How Men Really Feel about Women, Sex, Relationships and Themselves*. He encourages men to tell more, especially to their partners.

"The problem is that most men don't feel comfortable expressing their feelings or even realize that feelings have anything to do with their impotence," says Dr. Baraff. "Holding in negative feelings toward their partner is often the culprit in impotence. A good starting point is to talk about the impotence itself—how they feel about it, why they think it has occurred."

Eat low-fat. Just as a high-fat, high-cholesterol diet can play havoc with your heart, it can do similar damage to your penis. "Plaque from a bad diet and sedentary lifestyle can line the walls of the arteries in and to your penis, reducing blood flow and causing impotence," says Mark H. Cline, Ph.D., a psychologist and researcher at the Male Health Center in Dallas.

The good news is that adopting a healthy lifestyle may *reverse* this situation, adds Sheldon Burman, M.D., founder and director of the Male Sexual Dysfunction Institute in Chicago, the country's largest treatment center for male sexual problems. "Lose weight if you need to, exercise regularly, control your cholesterol and triglyceride levels, and the amount of blood flow in your penis's arteries can increase for better erections."

Cut back on caffeine. Although a cup or two a day is fine, serious coffee drinking may lead to serious problems. "Caffeine releases adrenaline in your body, and one of the things that adrenaline does is shut off arterial flow to the penis," says Dr. Cline. The problem is that the effects of caffeine can last 12 hours or longer after you drink it. So if you are having trouble with erections and drink a lot of coffee, maybe you ought to cut back or switch to decaffeinated, suggests Dr. Cline. Caffeinated tea and cola and chocolate are other sources of caffeine to avoid.

Stay smoke-free. If you smoke, stop. "Quitting is one of the most important things you can do to avoid the early onset of impotence or help reverse it," says Dr. Burman. Smoking is harmful because it hampers circulation and blood supply and contributes to hardening of the arteries, and if less blood reaches the penis, it's more difficult to get an erection.

When Erections Won't End

Although some might not consider it a problem, occasionally one must deal with an erection that simply won't quit. Usually this occurs among men who use doctor-prescribed pumps and vacuums to achieve erections.

"The erection may last hours, and after a while, it can really hurt," says Sheldon Burman, M.D., founder and director of the Male Sexual Dysfunction Institute in Chicago, the country's largest treatment center for male sexual problems. The answer: Take a couple of tablets of Sudafed, an over-the-counter sinus and hay fever medication. "Sudafed has an adrenaline-like substance in it that should help end your erection quickly," Dr. Burman explains.

"We tell patients to do ten deep knee bends, take a cold shower, then apply an ice bag (wrapped in a towel) to the penis. If at the end of three hours the patient has a sustained erection that looks like it won't quit, he must immediately get medical help. There is danger to the penis if it remains erect longer than that."

Avoid the avid smokers. For those who *don't* smoke, it's smart to stay away from those who do. "Secondhand smoke—what you breathe from other people's cigarettes—can be even worse," says Dr. Cline. That's because sidestream smoke from the tip of your neighbor's cigarette doesn't pass through a filter before it reaches your lungs.

Don't exercise right before sex. Along with diet, regular exercise is part of a healthy lifestyle that can prevent or remedy impotence—as long as you don't work out right before sex. "Whenever you exercise, the body directs blood to the group of muscles that is being used—and away from your penis," says Dr. Burman. This diversion of blood may stop you from getting or maintaining an erection.

Skip the happy hour. You *don't* need a stiff drink. Serious alcohol consumption can also cause impotence. That's because booze is a nervous system depressant, inhibiting your reflexes and arousal. You may be drinking to "relax," but getting *too* relaxed can adversely affect sexual performance.

Ingrown Hairs

If you have ingrown hairs, a morning shave can be "shear" agony. This painful condition—doctors call it pseudofolliculitis barbae—occurs because shaving puts hairs under tension and cuts them at an angle. When the sharp tips of the hairs become embedded, they irritate, inflame and scar the skin. The problem mostly affects those with coarse, curly hair; black men are particularly vulnerable.

"Ingrown hairs are a difficult problem with one easy solution—grow a beard," says David Feingold, M.D., chairman of the Department of Dermatology at Tufts University School of Medicine in Boston. But if growing a beard is not a practical solution for you, or if you're a woman who's had ingrown hairs on your legs or underarms, here's how to keep skin free from hair *and* pain.

Rough up your skin. "One of the best ways to prevent the hairs from embedding in your skin is to take a dry washcloth and rub it over your skin before you shave," advises Dr. Feingold. "That way, you'll help 'loosen' embedded hairs from their follicles for a less irritating shave."

Don't double up. Using twin-track razors can give you a double dose of agony. That's because the first blade pulls the hair while the second cuts it below skin level, often at a sharp angle that can embed back into your skin. Jerome Z. Litt, M.D., assistant clinical professor of dermatology at Case Western Reserve University School of Medicine in Cleveland, says you're better off using a single-track razor and settling for a less close shave.

Pivoting-head razors like the Gillette Sensor cause less friction (and irritation) and do a better job than fixed-head types, adds John F. Romano, M.D., a dermatologist and clinical assistant professor of medicine at The New York Hospital–Cornell Medical Center in New York City.

Change your shaving routine. Sometimes you can lessen ingrown hair pain simply by changing your shaving direction. "I try to get my patients to shave with the grain, whereas most people go against the grain," says Dr. Feingold. While you're at it, you may also want to change your choice of shaving gear. "If you now shave with a blade, try an electric razor. If you now use electric, go manual."

Play Sherlock Holmes. "Make a regular routine of examining your face very carefully with a magnifying glass, to look for hairs that are caught in the follicle," says Dr. Feingold. These troublemakers should then be removed with tweezers that have been sterilized in rubbing alcohol.

Ingrown Toenails

I t takes six to nine months for a toenail to grow out. But when that growing toenail takes a wrong turn, you can't wait a minute for relief. That's because ingrown nails, which usually occur in the big toe, cause big-time pain. The nail actually cuts into soft tissue around the top of the toe, and that cutting action produces swelling and redness. Infection sometimes follows.

People with curved toenails are particularly prone to the problem. But whatever the shape of your toenail, you can aggravate the problem by wearing shoes that are too tight around the toe. Even stockings can sock it to you by pressing the nail until it cuts into the tissue. But here's how to nail those nasty ingrown nails and prevent a recurrence.

Cut the nail straight across. Leave the half-moons for cloudy nights. "The *best* way to cure an ingrown nail and prevent new ones from forming is to always cut your nail straight across, not slightly curved or in a half-moon shape as most people do," says William Van Pelt, D.P.M., a Houston podiatrist who is former president of the American Academy of Podiatric Sports Medicine. "You should cut the nail so that it's just over the crease of the nailfold."

Give it a soak before a trim. Before cutting—and you should use good-quality, long-handled scissors or nail clippers—soak your foot in warm water to soften the nail and lessen your pain, says Frederick Hass, M.D., a general practitioner in San Rafael, California, and author of *The Foot Book*.

There are products available over the counter that are made to soften ingrown nails, but read the label before using them. Some cannot be used by those with conditions such as diabetes or impaired circulation.

File the corners. While the nail should be cut straight across, nail *corners* should be filed and buffed. This eliminates sharp edges. It reduces the pain you get from an ingrown nail cutting into your toe, and it prevents new ingrown nails from forming, says Dr. Van Pelt.

Cut a V and Harm You'll See

It's time to divorce yourself from that old wives' tale that you can treat an ingrown nail by cutting a V-shaped wedge out of its center. (The theory behind this fallacy is the misconception that ingrown toenails are the result of a nail being too big.)

This practice *won't* prevent an ingrown nail, as some believe. "Chances are the only thing you'll do is hurt yourself," says Houston podiatrist William Van Pelt, D.P.M., former president of the American Academy of Podiatric Sports Medicine.

Protect your nail with cotton. An alternative to filing corners is to take a very thin strip, not a wad, of cotton and place it beneath the burrowing edge of your nail, advises Dr. Hass. The cotton helps lift the nail slightly, so it can grow past the tissue it's digging into.

Shun bad shoes. Tight shoes and pointy-toed styles can cause an ingrown toenail and make existing ones worse—especially if your nails tend to curve, says Suzanne M. Levine, D.P.M., clinical assistant podiatrist at Wycoff Heights Medical Center and adjunct clinical instructor at New York College of Podiatric Medicine, both in New York City. You're better off wearing open-toed shoes or sandals—*especially* when you have an ingrown nail.

Use common sense. When working around the house, wear substantial but comfortable shoes, since accidents can also cause ingrown nails, says Dr. Hass. Steel-toed boots should be worn by those doing lots of lifting. And avoid tight panty hose or socks, which can also cause ingrown nails.

Inhibited Sexual Desire

You've lost that loving feeling. It's gone, gone, gone, and nothing you do seems to get it back.

Well, there's no reason to believe it's gone forever. Usually the lack of sexual interest is only temporary. In fact, it's a normal reaction to stress, illness, hormonal swings or emotional upset.

But what happens when there's not even a flicker of renewed interest? That's a condition psychologists call inhibited sexual desire.

"People with inhibited sexual desire lack the desire to have sex, even though they have opportunities to do so," explains Shirley Zussman, Ed.D., a marital therapist and a director of the Association for Male Sexual Dysfunction in New York City. "In some instances, they completely lose interest in sex." Or their interest in sex may change dramatically over a period of months.

Of course, not everyone considers a low libido a problem. But some do, and more than a fair number of people with a low sex drive have spouses who consider it a *big* problem, says Peter A. Wish, Ph.D., director of the New England Institute of Family Relations in Framingham, Massachusetts.

If you're among them, here are some tips that may help you rekindle your flame and help you and your mate adjust to each other's differing appetites.

Shake your booty. Regular, strenuous exercise may be a potent aphrodisiac, helping to boost your sex life. Two studies that included healthy men on regular exercise programs showed that the exercisers enjoyed sex more often than nonexercisers.

"The exercise may have sparked an increase in testosterone in the more active men," speculates David McWhirter, M.D., professor of psychiatry at the University of California, San Diego. Testosterone is the hormone that controls the male sex drive. "Exercise may also help people feel better about themselves and the way they look," he says.

But don't overdo it. Training *too hard* may lower testosterone levels and decrease sex drive. In one study where men doubled their daily exercise, testosterone levels dropped significantly, and all the men reported declines in sexual interest. So if you're working out more but enjoying sex less, you may want to consider a change of pace.

Make a date. "No time for sex is a frequent complaint, so make it a priority by making time," Dr. Zussman suggests. Be playful and creative, and start "dating" again. Go to a drive-in movie on a hot, humid night. Watch the sun

---

When To See the Doctor

If you find you can't even broach the subject with your mate, or if sex isn't the only thing you are no longer able to enjoy, you may benefit from discussing your problem with a professional. You can ask your family doctor, a gynecologist or a urologist for a referral.

Doctors recommend that you address both the psychological and physical aspects of inhibited sexual desire. Individual therapy or a medical checkup might be advised before marital therapy. Inhibited sexual desire can be a symptom of depression. It can also be due to low hormone levels, which are best diagnosed and treated by an endocrinologist, who specializes in the body's internal secretion system.

set. Snuggle up together under the blankets with a good book. Hide from the kids the same way you used to hide from your parents when you were teenagers. Leave notes, send cards, give gifts, bring home flowers just for the joy of it.

Eat lean and mean. A steady diet of cheeseburgers, french fries and other fatty foods may curb the production of testosterone, researchers have found. "It may be that fatty acids act on the cells that make testosterone, cutting down on production," observes Wayne A. Meikle, M.D., professor of medicine in the Division of Endocrinology and Metabolism at the University of Utah in Salt Lake City. For a man who likes thick steaks and fatty shakes, a change to lean rations may be the best aphrodisiac.

Catch some rays. There's no doubt that a day of sunshine can lift your spirits. But did you know that exposure to the sun may be sexually stimulating, too?

Researchers at the University of Texas Health Science Center at San Antonio found that a person who gets a lot of sunlight has a stronger sex drive. Not only that, sunlight increases ovulation in women and sperm production in men. "Get out in the sunlight for a half-hour or so at midday during the winter months," suggests Russell J. Reiter, M.D., Ph.D., professor of neuroendocrinology at the health science center.

And keep your living space bright by opening the curtains to let in natural sunlight and using high-wattage bulbs.

Try to work it out. "Many sex drive problems are really intimacy problems," Dr. Wish says. "There might be anger, unresolved conflicts or any one of a number of things that are incomplete." He emphasizes that it's important to talk about these things in a supportive way.

Accentuate the positive. Pick a place far removed from the bedroom to have a discussion, suggests Dr. Zussman.

"Start out not in an angry way but by affirming what's positive about the relationship," she suggests. "You may want to begin with 'We have so many good things between us, and this seems to be one area that just isn't working right.' People are very vulnerable about their lack of sexual interest, and it does no good to attack them for it."

Discover the whole body. Couples who concentrate on just reaching orgasm deprive themselves of prolonged pleasures. Do more touching, hugging and hand-holding, Dr. Zussman suggests.

Read the fine print on drugs you're taking. Some drugs crimp not only sexual performance but sexual desire as well. Common lust busters: anti-anxiety and sleep-inducing drugs and some blood pressure medications. Ask your doctor about side effects. He may be able to substitute a drug with fewer desire-dampening effects.

Insect Bites

F lies. Mosquitoes. Gnats. Fire ants. Many names, many species. But *all*, you'll notice, share one common nickname—*bug!* Why? Because they "bug" the living begeebers out of us, especially when they bite.

Although insect bites rarely require medical attention, they are bothersome. (Few people are allergic, but if you are—and you'll know by vomiting, fever and other severe reactions—refer to "When to See the Doctor" on page 36.) Most people get nothing more than some swelling and itching and sometimes ugly welts that are tender to the touch. Since an ounce of prevention is worth its weight in future scratching, here are some tried-and-true ways to squash the pain (even if you can't do the same to the cause of it).

Treat it like a tough steak. Rubbing on a meat tenderizer containing papain can take the ouch out of that bite, suggests Arthur Jacknowitz, Pharm.D., professor and chairman of clinical pharmacy at West Virginia University School of Pharmacy in Morgantown. He says Adolph's or McCormick works fine, but don't try this with highly spiced Ac'cent. "The best way is to make a paste with water and the meat tenderizer and apply it directly on the bite area as soon as possible," explains Dr. Jacknowitz. For severe itching and swelling, apply some calamine lotion.

Try some mud relief. "Do what I did as a kid: Pack mud on the bite," suggests Rodney Basler, M.D., a dermatologist and assistant professor of internal medicine at the University of Nebraska Medical Center in Omaha. "I'm not sure *why* it works, but it works."

Get help from your kitchen. For a variety of household itch and pain reducers, Claude Frazier, M.D., an allergist in Asheville, North Carolina, suggests checking out your kitchen cabinets. You can make a paste by mixing table salt with water and applying it to the bite. Another way: Place ice packs wrapped in towels on the area for 10 minutes. Or dissolve one teaspoon of baking soda in a glass of water, dip a cloth into the solution, and place it on the bite for 20 minutes.

Clean the bite thoroughly. Of course, flies and mosquitoes can spread disease. So to prevent further infection, wash the bite thoroughly with soap and water and apply an antiseptic, advises Dr. Frazier.

Apply the real McCoy. Yes, you can also apply bona fide insect repellent to repel insects. According to Philip Koehler, Ph.D., an entomologist at the U.S. Department of Agriculture Laboratory at the University of Florida in Gainesville, the best known and most effective repellent is DEET (diethyl-toluamide). Products containing DEET have a number of different trade names. Be sure to read the label: You should use DEET sparingly on exposed skin, and keep it away from your eyes.

Start relying on thiamine. People who have diets high in thiamine (vitamin B_1) report fewer insect bites than others. "That's because the vitamin gives off an odor when you perspire that is unattractive to insects but undetectable to

---

When Baby Butterflies Are a Bother

Butterflies never have exactly struck fear in the hearts of man or beast. So you might figure that about the only thing *less* threatening than a butterfly is a caterpillar.

Think again.

"You can get 'stung' by caterpillars," says Philip Koehler, Ph.D., an entomologist at the U.S. Department of Agriculture Laboratory at the University of Florida in Gainesville. "The stinging occurs because some caterpillars have hollow hairs that have irritating prickers inside—and those prickers can cause irritation if you brush against them."

Dr. Koehler suggests this quick fix: "Before doing anything, put a piece of transparent tape over the affected area and remove it gently to pull out the hairs," he says. "Then wash the area with soap and water to clean it and prevent any infection."

humans," says John Yunginger, M.D., professor and pediatrics consultant at the Mayo Clinic in Rochester, Minnesota. Good sources of thiamine include whole grains, organ meats and brewer's yeast.

Don't hold the onion. Consuming a lot of onions or garlic is a nutritious way to help keep bugs away. "Eat a couple of raw onions daily during the summer, or use a lot of garlic in your cooking, and mosquitoes and other insects will usually avoid you," says Jerome Z. Litt, M.D., assistant clinical professor of dermatology at Case Western Reserve University School of Medicine in Cleveland. That's because, like thiamine, both these heart-healthy foods give off an unpleasant odor to insects when you perspire.

Lotion 'em away. Another effective insect repellent is skin lotion. Avon's Skin-So-Soft is recommended for keeping off gnats and mosquitoes, according to Dr. Koehler. "People report good luck at keeping insects away when they apply it to their skin before going outside." Others claim similar success with Alpha Keri lotion.

Dress down. Bees aren't the only pests attracted to brightly colored clothing and perfumes. Dressing in more subdued colors—khaki or white in particular—and *not* wearing fragrances can help keep bugs away, adds Dr. Koehler.

VapoRub 'em. Applying strong-smelling Vicks VapoRub to your skin is another way to keep pests away, suggests Herbert Luscombe, M.D., professor emeritus of dermatology at Jefferson Medical College of Thomas Jefferson University and senior attending dermatologist at Thomas Jefferson University Hospital, both in Philadelphia.

Insomnia

You think you've got insomnia problems? Pity poor Mrs. Socrates. Seems *Mr.* Socrates, the famed philosopher, had so much trouble getting shut-eye that he would keep his wife up all night—*every* night—expounding his views on the nature of the universe. That is, until one night when she took revenge—by dumping the contents of their chamber pot (the ancient Greeks' version of a toilet) on his head.

That, no doubt, led to further philosophic discussion.

Why are we telling you this? Because if you're cursed with insomnia, you might take some solace in knowing that at least you're in good company. You're sharing this ailment (along with the late, late show) with some 120 million other Americans—among them many hard-driving achievers who can't sleep well because their minds continue to stay active long after their bodies punk out.

If you're among them, don't lose sleep over losing sleep. Here's what you can do to make sure you rest soundly.

Take a whiff of lavender. Many people can't fall asleep because they can't relax. But certain smells have been proven to induce a deep sense of relaxation, which can help some people get the shut-eye they need. "A lavender fragrance, for instance, is very effective at inducing a more relaxed state," says Alan R. Hirsch, M.D., a psychiatrist and neurologist who heads the Smell and Taste Treatment and Research Foundation in Chicago. "Other aromas that work very well at lowering stress include spiced apple dishes and other baked desserts as well as the aroma of the salty air of the seashore."

Switch to linen sheets. Researchers at the University of Milan in Italy report that people who sleep on linen sheets fall asleep faster and wake up in a better mood than those using cotton or other fabrics. The researchers believe it may be because linen sheets feel different against the skin and disperse body heat better than other fabrics.

Get a heating blanket (with a timer). "Using a heating blanket will help you get to sleep by relaxing the muscles and increasing brain temperature—two factors that induce sleep," says psychiatrist Henry Lahmeyer, M.D., professor of psychiatry and behavioral sciences at Northwestern University Medical School and co-director of the Sleep Program at Northwestern Memorial Hospital, both in Chicago. "But if you use the blanket all night, you will probably wake up early in the morning. So if you're going to use a heating blanket, use one with a timer, so it will shut off just after you fall asleep."

Say no to nightcaps. "Alcohol *does* help people get to sleep, but its sleep-inducing effects wear off very quickly. Often people who have taken a nightcap wake up in the middle of the night and then cannot get back to sleep," says Alex Clerk, M.D., director of the Sleep Disorders Clinic at Stanford University

Color Away Insomnia

If you've tried everything and still have insomnia, maybe you ought to try repainting your bedroom. Why? Because color behaviorists say that color can subconsciously influence our mood, our behavior and even our sleeping patterns.

If that's the case, here are some hues you can use when you decorate for super slumber.

Green evokes peacefulness and serenity and helps lower the heart rate. "Green is comforting to most people and a good color for stress reduction," says color expert Carlton Wagner, director of the Wagner Institute for Color Research in Santa Barbara, California.

Blue is another good choice for the bedroom, since it causes the brain to secrete tranquilizing hormones. "Blue encourages fantasizing and daydreaming," says Wagner.

Violet and other purple shades calm nerves and slow muscular response.

Pink has a calming effect—particularly to the high-strung and easily angered. But different shades appeal to different sexes, says Wagner. "Men prefer yellow-based pinks like apricot and peach, while women go for blue-based pinks like bubble gum."

in Stanford, California. "Even when it doesn't cause you to wake up, studies show that alcohol fragments your sleep, so you don't wake up refreshed. A third problem with alcohol as a sleep inducer is that when it's used over time, you develop tolerance, so you need more of it to get to sleep—and that can lead to abuse problems."

Schedule your bath. "Taking a warm bath an hour or two before bedtime increases the deep stages of sleep," adds Dr. Lahmeyer. He speculates that the warming effect of the bath, like that of a fever, triggers the same sleep-inducing mechanism in the brain. "But timing is very important," Dr. Lahmeyer points out. "Taking a bath *right before* bedtime is too stimulating and will keep you awake rather than help you sleep."

Take up a hobby. "Stress can cause insomnia," says Dr. Clerk. "Taking up a hobby or doing anything else to distract you from your troubles is a great way to overcome stress-related sleep problems."

Try a "white noise" machine. "You can get a white noise machine at Sears or other department stores. The machine emits a sound that helps people get to sleep," adds Dr. Lahmeyer.

Have a midnight snack. If you're having problems hitting the hay, hit the fridge. "A light bedtime snack with protein and sugar increases brain neuro-transmitters to induce sleep," says Dr. Lahmeyer. "The classic bedtime snack of a bowl of cereal with milk or a glass of milk with some cookies is perfect." But doctors advise going easy on your noshing, because a heavy meal will disrupt your sleep.

Don't push it. One common mistake is to assume you *need* the sleep you're missing. "We all need sleep, but we don't all need the same amount," says Ernest Hartmann, M.D., director of the Sleep Disorders Center at Newton-Wellesley Hospital in Boston. "A lot depends on your personality and what kind of life you lead." Busy people tend to *need* less sleep. And the older we get, the less sleep we seem to need: Those over age 50 average only about six hours a night.

Intermittent Claudication

Think of this condition as heart disease in your legs. The same circu-latory problem that can restrict blood flow to your heart—athero-sclerosis, or hardening of the arteries—is blocking the blood flow in your calves, thighs, feet or hips. The result: When you walk too far, you have severe pain in your legs, usually centered in the calves.

If you have intermittent claudication, you're a prime candidate for a heart attack or stroke, and you should be under a doctor's care. But there are several day-to-day things you can do to slow the progression of this peripheral circulatory problem—or perhaps even rid yourself of it completely.

Eat low-fat. "The oxygen in your blood isn't reaching your legs because of the plaques that line artery walls, causing atherosclerosis. And what causes those plaques is fat in your diet," says Arthur Jacknowitz, Pharm.D., professor and chairman of clinical pharmacy at West Virginia University School of Pharmacy in Morgantown. "So eliminating excess fat from your diet is essential for preventing or treating intermittent claudication."

Another benefit: A low-fat diet helps you lose weight, which is helpful for intermittent claudication as well as scores of other ailments.

Choose fish. Perhaps no food is better for those with intermittent claudication than fish—especially cold-water fish such as salmon, herring and mackerel. Besides being low in fat and high in nutrition, fish helps boost your levels of high-density lipoprotein (HDL), the so-called good cholesterol that scours fatty deposits from artery walls. "Tuna, sardines and some shellfish such as clams and mussels are also excellent choices," says Dr. Jacknowitz.

Take aspirin. Studies show that taking low-dose aspirin every other day helps reduce complications of peripheral vascular disease. Researchers believe that aspirin helps thin the blood, preventing circulation to the farthest parts of your body from getting worse.

Trash all tobacco. It's no mere coincidence that up to 90 percent of those with intermittent claudication are smokers. In fact, smoking is the single highest risk factor for peripheral vascular disease. Cigarette smoke increases the potential damage from the disease by substituting carbon monoxide for oxygen in the already oxygen-starved muscles of your legs. And nicotine constricts blood vessels, which further restricts blood flow. This can damage the arteries and may make blood cells more rigid, leading to blood clots. (Worst-case scenario: Clots can result in gangrene and make amputation necessary.) "Unless you stop smoking, you won't receive any benefits from the other aspects of your treatment," warns Dr. Jacknowitz.

"Stopping smoking is the most important thing to do if you have intermittent claudication—period," notes Robert Ginsburg, M.D., director of the Unit for Cardiac Intervention at University Hospital in Denver and professor of medicine at the University of Colorado in Boulder.

Drink only now and then. Alcohol initially dilates blood vessels, which helps increase blood flow, but then has a rebound effect and constricts them (although not as much as smoking). An occasional beer or glass of wine is fine, but if you have intermittent claudication, it's *not* a good idea to drink regularly, experts say. In fact, people who drink chronically often develop intermittent claudication.

When to See the Doctor

Everyday foot problems may be minor inconveniences for people who have healthy circulation, but those problems can turn into major infections if you have impaired blood flow to the limbs.

"Any time there's a break in the skin on the feet, you have to be on guard that it heals up in short order," says Michael D. Dake, M.D., chief of cardiovascular and interventional radiology at Stanford University Hospital in Stanford, California. "Nonhealing foot problems that get infected are probably the leading cause of amputation."

So if you get a cut, scrape or blister that becomes red, swollen and painful, see your doctor immediately. You're likely to have fewer problems with proper care of the toenails, early treatment of athlete's foot and avoidance of extremely hot or cold temperatures. If you have intermittent claudication or other circulation problems, be sure to inspect your feet carefully every day. Get prompt medical attention whenever you see any signs of injury or infection.

Hit the road. Although any type of regular exercise is good, the *most* helpful is walking. That's because walking improves blood flow to your legs and gives your circulatory system a boost where it needs it the most. "Get out every day for at least an hour of walking exercise," suggests Jess R. Young, M.D., chairman of the Department of Vascular Medicine at the Cleveland Clinic Foundation in Cleveland.

Dr. Young says you don't have to walk that hour's worth all at once, "but for the walking to do any good, you have to bring on the discomfort of intermittent claudication." In other words, walk until you bring on the pain. But don't stop at the first sign of pain. "Wait until it gets moderately severe," says Dr. Young. "Then stop and rest a minute or two until it goes away, then start walking again."

Repeat that pain/walk cycle as often as you can during your 60 minutes of daily walking, he advises. And don't give up after a few weeks. Improvement will take several months.

Ban the heat. Because the blood flow in the legs is restricted, people who suffer from intermittent claudication often suffer from cold feet, too. If you're among them, *don't* warm your feet with a heating pad or hot water bottle. "You need increased blood flow to help dissipate that heat," Dr. Young explains. "If the blood flow is limited, however, it can't get down to where you're putting the heat, and you'll burn the skin." Instead, warm your tootsies with loose wool stockings.

Iron-Deficiency Anemia

Are you fatigued? Short of breath? Chilly?

If so, worries about your health and state of mind have probably led you to the doctor's door already. And if you're a woman in your thirties or forties, there's a good chance the doctor told you that you have iron-deficiency anemia. That's the kind of anemia that occurs when the iron supply, which usually carries oxygen and carbon dioxide through the body, is depleted.

Not *all* premenopausal women suffer from iron-deficiency anemia, but they are more likely to have this problem than younger women—and *much* more likely than men, says M. T. Atallah, Ph.D., associate professor of nutrition at the University of Massachusetts Department of Food Science and Nutrition in Amherst.

Nutrition research has also shown that women usually need higher than usual doses of iron when they are menstruating, pregnant or lactating. But all of us tend to require more iron as we get older than we did as youngsters.

So even if you don't have full-blown iron-deficiency anemia, you may need more iron to ward off the feelings of chilliness or fatigue that people often get when the iron supply in their bodies is depleted.

Eating food that's high in iron is not the entire answer, however. You need to get iron in a form that is absorbable by the body, which means you need to be choosy about your food sources.

Some foods have a good supply of *heme* iron, which is readily absorbable. But in other foods, iron is in the *nonheme* form, which the body has trouble absorbing. Yet here's the twist: Even nonheme iron can be absorbed more readily if it's eaten with certain foods.

Hard to absorb that information? No harder than the iron itself if you heed these tips from the experts.

Eat more lean meat. "The basic answer to anemia is to eat a balanced diet while increasing the amount of meat, which is high in heme iron," says John Beard, Ph.D., professor of nutrition at Pennsylvania State University in University Park.

Make OJ part of your meals. For better absorption of the nonheme iron that's contained in plant foods such as vegetables and grains, add citrus juice to your meals. Though absorption of iron from plant sources or iron-fortified cereals is normally between 2 and 10 percent, you can almost *double* that rate if you consume a vitamin C–rich food or drink at the same time. So a glass of orange or grapefruit juice with your iron-fortified breakfast cereal means more iron for your body, according to Dr. Atallah.

Look for the iron bonuses. Iron-fortified cereals such as Cream of Wheat, raisin bran and wheat and bran flakes are excellent sources of nonheme iron, though you will need vitamin C for optimum absorption. Legumes such as soybeans are also high in nonheme iron. Carrots, potatoes, broccoli and tomatoes are other excellent plant sources of iron.

Steer clear of the iron-blocking veggies. Some vegetable sources contain a large amount of iron but also a substance called phytate, which blocks iron's ability to be absorbed. The high-phytate crowd includes butter beans, lentils, beet greens, spinach and other leafy vegetables. So if it's iron you need, don't eat these veggies with your chicken and burgers. The amount of phytate will block the heme iron absorption.

Avoid coffee or tea during meals. "It's best not to have coffee or tea with a meal if you are trying to prevent iron deficiency," says Gregory Landry, M.D., associate professor in the Department of Pediatrics at the University of Wisconsin Medical School in Madison and the head medical team physician at the university's sports clinic. These beverages contain chemicals that block iron absorption.

Be choosy with supplements. Look for an iron supplement that's made from ferrous gluconate instead of ferrous sulfate. It's easier on the stomach, says Dr. Landry. And avoid taking calcium supplements along with iron. "All-in-one supplements containing iron are *not* recommended," says Dr. Beard, "because the other vitamins can interfere with your body's ability to absorb iron." If you take both calcium and iron supplements, take the calcium in the morning, and take the iron supplement at night.

Take supplements with citrus sips. If you're taking an iron supplement, do your body a favor and wash it down with citrus juice, which helps the body absorb it.

Look for reduced iron. Reduced iron is often added to processed foods, such as cereals. But in spite of its negative name, it's actually a plus. "Generally, reduced iron would have *higher* availability to the body than regular iron," says Dr. Atallah.

Keep warm. According to a study conducted by Dr. Beard, women who have sufficient iron supplies tend to feel warmer than those who do not. Wearing an extra sweater when you are iron-deficient may not cure the problem permanently, but it will help you stay comfortable.

Cook spaghetti sauce in an iron pot. When you use an iron pot for cooking, some of the iron will migrate into the food—and into your body. But not all foods have an ironclad guarantee of mining iron from the pot. The key is acidity. "If you are cooking tomato sauce, the amount of iron you'll get is high because of the acidity of the sauce," says Dr. Atallah.

Irritable Bowel Syndrome

Maybe it was the innocent ingestion of the "wrong" food that started your colon kvetching. Or perhaps your bowel complaint got started with stress, and all the everyday irritants only make your bowels more irritable. Doctors don't know all the "whys" of irritable bowel syndrome (IBS). What they do know is that some people have more or less constant problems with constipation, diarrhea, bloating, heartburn and nausea, singly or in combination, usually accompanied by abdominal pain.

If this describes your misery, you have good company. Some doctors believe that IBS may be nearly as widespread as the common cold. But naturally, people don't mention IBS as much. Doctors suspect that many people suffer in silent embarrassment and don't even tell their own physicians.

The good news is that IBS is not fatal and doesn't lead to more serious medical complications. (If your symptoms are accompanied by bleeding, fever or weight loss, doctors warn that you may have something more serious than IBS.)

But if you do have IBS, or if you suspect you have it, you should definitely tell your doctor. And meanwhile, there are plenty of things you can do to take some of the irritability out of your bowels.

Don't be too sweet on sweets. Controlling your sweet tooth is one of the best ways to put the bite on IBS-triggered diarrhea. "You have to be careful with sugars if you have IBS, especially fructose and the artificial sweetener sorbitol," says Stephen B. Hanauer, M.D., professor of medicine in the Section of Gastroenterology at the University of Chicago Medical Center. That's because sugars, which are not easily digested, are a leading cause of the runs. His advice: Avoid candy and gum, which contain these sweeteners, and read food labels on other products.

Munch when you're mellow. Another often-overlooked factor of IBS is *how* and *where* you eat. "You should eat slowly and in as relaxed an environment as possible," suggests Arvey I. Rogers, M.D., chief of the Gastroenterology Section

Get Rid of Gas with Beano

Beans, cabbage and carbohydrates from veggies can cause gas. And for someone with irritable bowel syndrome (IBS), eating a simple meal can lead to uncomfortable aftereffects.

But there is a way to have your chili and eat it, too. "An over-the-counter product called Beano does reduce the gas caused by many foods and certainly can help those with IBS," says gastroenterologist Stephen B. Hanauer, M.D., professor of medicine in the Section of Gastroenterology at the University of Chicago Medical Center. "The key is to look at all the things that might be causing your IBS symptoms. Then if you're going to eat these foods, put in a few drops of Beano before you eat to halt any potential problems."

To help narrow down your list of possible offenders, note that IBS sufferers often have problems with spicy foods such as chili; gas-producing vegetables such as broccoli, cabbage and cauliflower; *all* types of legumes; fatty foods, which are hard to digest; and even carbohydrates such as bread and pasta.

at the Veterans Administration Medical Center in Miami and professor of medicine at the University of Miami School of Medicine. By eating relaxed, you avoid swallowing air, which can aggravate abdominal pain and other IBS symptoms. And you provide time for digestive juices to start flowing before the food passes by.

Get a juicer. Most store-bought juices contain high amounts of sorbitol—especially fortified apple, peach, pear and prune juices, adds Dr. Rogers. Since fruit juices are an excellent source of nutrients, you can make your own—with reduced sorbitol content—by using a commercial juicer that can be bought at most department stores.

Minimize milk. Milk isn't much better for people with IBS, since many may have lactose intolerance, which can mimic IBS. If in doubt, eliminate dairy products for a while and see if your condition improves. Generally, however, limit dairy products whether or not you are lactose-intolerant (unless they are being relied upon as a major source of calcium).

Bulk up. Eating a high-fiber diet—between 35 and 50 grams daily, compared with the average 11 grams most Americans eat—is perhaps the best way of taking the irritability out of your bowels. "Fiber increases stool production and reduces pressure in the intestines, which is good for both constipation and diarrhea," says Dr. Hanauer. "It also allows for more regular bowel movements."

Since increased fiber usually causes more gas and can temporarily worsen symptoms, the slow and steady route is strongly recommended. "I advise my patients to start with ½ cup of oat or wheat bran high-fiber cereal (or three tablespoons of pure bran) every day at breakfast. I suggest they have a green leaf salad with lunch and dinner and plenty of fresh fruits and vegetables throughout the day," advises Alex Aslan, M.D., a gastroenterologist and staff physician at North Bay Medical Center in Fairfield, California. "Continue to slowly add the bran over a six-week period until you have 1 to 1½ cups each morning, while having two salads and lots of fruits and vegetables." Adequate fluid intake is also very important.

Meditate. Even when you're not eating, controlling the stresses in your life is a key factor in controlling IBS. "Being under stress will definitely make IBS worse," says Dr. Hanauer. "And *not* being under stress can help." You may benefit from relaxation techniques such as meditation, self-hypnosis, biofeedback, regular exercise or even keeping a "stress diary" to determine what's causing you (and your bowels) grief.

But don't medicate. You won't help yourself by relying on medicines to control diarrhea, constipation or other gastrointestinal problems. "Laxatives and antidiarrhea medications should be used only on a short-term basis—if at all," says Dr. Hanauer. The exceptions: Natural psyllium-based laxatives such as Metamucil or Citrucel can be taken daily to boost your fiber, and they actually cause *less* gas than bran.

Give pain the "heat-ho." For the abdominal pain of IBS, nothing beats a heating pad. Turn it on low heat and rest it on the painful area. Another warm-up strategy: Take a warm bath, says Dr. Rogers.

Don't be a coffee achiever. Coffee and other caffeinated drinks play a significant role in IBS—and it's not a beneficial one. "For one thing, caffeine, even in very small amounts, stimulates motility. And that's bad news if you're prone to diarrhea," says Dr. Aslan. "Even if you're not, there's an unknown chemical in coffee that can cause cramping." His advice: Either cut back or cut out coffee and limit intake of tea, chocolate, cola and other caffeinated substances.

Jet Lag

Funny thing about air travel: You spend a few hours high in the sky, and you wind up feeling as low as some airline stocks after you land. Blame it on jet lag, that less than uplifting response to time-zone changes that your body doesn't appreciate.

Usually our body clock operates on a 24- to 25-hour cycle that keeps time by stimuli such as eating and sleeping habits, exercise patterns, reactions to light and darkness and other triggers. But when you put yourself in a new time zone—as you do with long-distance travel—you change the normal time of these triggers, which puts your body clock out of sync. The result: headache, earache, fatigue, lethargy, irritability, trouble concentrating and making decisions . . . sometimes even loss of appetite and diarrhea.

And the more time zones you cross, the worse your jet lag. "Basically, the rule of thumb is that after you land, it takes one day to recover for *each* time zone you go through," observes jet lag researcher Charles F. Ehret, Ph.D., senior scientist emeritus at the U.S. Department of Energy Argonne National Laboratory in Argonne, Illinois, and author of *Overcoming Jet Lag.* "So if you're traveling coast-to-coast, that translates to about three days, because you're crossing three time zones," says Dr. Ehret, who is a leading authority on jet lag. "If you cross 15 time zones, as going from New York to Japan may entail, full recovery may take considerably more than a week."

There's also a directional factor, according to Dr. Ehret: "Jet lag usually is worse when you're traveling west to east, since you're 'losing' time due to the way the time zones are." So flying from Japan to New York may be even harder than the New York to Japan flight. It's easier to slow down the biological clock than to speed it up.

The good news is, you don't *have* to go Greyhound to keep your mood sky-high. Avoiding or remedying jet lag is as easy as making a few minor but significant adjustments in your lifestyle—before leaving, in the air and once you arrive at your destination. Here's how.

Book your flight so that you arrive at night. To help your body adjust to the change in time zones, try to arrange your flights so that you *land* sometime in midevening. That gives you enough time to unwind, eat a good meal and get to bed by 11:00 P.M. *destination time,* says Timothy Monk, Ph.D., associate professor of psychiatry at the University of Pittsburgh School of Medicine and director of the Human Chronobiology Research Program there. Since eastbound travel is most likely to deprive you of adequate shut-eye, researchers at the Royal Air Force Institute of Aviation Medicine in Farnborough, England, suggest this rule: When flying east, fly early; when heading west, fly late.

Get enough sleep the night before. "Just before trips, many people go to a lot of bon voyage parties, do extra shopping or do other activities that rob them of sleep," says Dr. Ehret. He advises that you maintain a consistent sleep pattern before the flight.

Avoid in-flight alcohol. Airplane cabins are notoriously dry, and a lengthy trip can dehydrate you faster than a weekend in the Sahara. Dehydration *worsens* jet lag, and alcohol consumption worsens dehydration. "Alcohol is one of the most potent dehydrators there is," says Howie Wenger, Ph.D., an exercise consultant to the globe-trotting Canadian Olympic Team and professional hockey's Los Angeles Kings. Instead of ordering an alcoholic beverage, do what the pros do—load up on fruit juices, water and sports drinks like Gatorade while airborne.

Exercise *on* the plane. Since a 727 isn't exactly designed for long-distance running, Dr. Ehret suggests these on-board exercises *just before* you land to keep you refreshed in your new time zone: Walk up and down aisles; squeeze a ball in the palm of each hand for five minutes; press your hands together in front of your chest; stretch your body as best you can; do deep knee bends (in the back of the plane).

Follow the sun. "I always make it a point to sit on the side of the airplane that's exposed to the most amount of sunshine, so I can take charge of when I want to enjoy or avoid exposure," says Dr. Ehret.

After you arrive, don't play catch-up. Trying to overcompensate for the sleep you've lost will only make matters worse. "If you lose some sleep because of the

---

Eat to Beat Jet Lag

A few days of readjusting your eating habits before departing can save you a week or more of agony when you arrive. But following the "anti–jet lag diet" devised by jet lag researcher Charles F. Ehret, Ph.D., when he was senior scientist at the U.S. Department of Energy Argonne National Laboratory in Argonne, Illinois, has helped many travelers avoid or lessen the symptoms of jet lag.

- Three days before departure: *Feast day!* "Have a relatively high-protein breakfast and lunch and a supper high in complex carbohydrates to stimulate the body's daily cycle of activity and inactivity," advises Dr. Ehret. Good choices include eggs, cottage cheese, fortified cereals, yogurt, lean meats and green vegetables.
- Two days before departure: *Fast day!* "This is a day to lessen calorie intake, but fasting doesn't mean you shouldn't eat anything," according to Dr. Ehret. Stick with "light" foods such as fruits, soups and broth, skimpy salads and small pieces of unbuttered toast. The key is to keep calories *and* carbohydrates to a minimum.
- The day before departure: Another feast day, with a high-protein breakfast and lunch and a supper high in complex carbohydrates.
- The day of departure: Another fast day. Once you arrive at your destination, put on the feedbag to "break" the fast with a regular meal or full-size breakfast at the appropriate local time.

change in time zones, *don't* try to make up for it the next morning," says Maria Simonson, Ph.D., Sc.D., professor emeritus and director of the Health, Weight and Stress Program at Johns Hopkins Medical Institutions in Baltimore and medical adviser to the International Flight Attendants' Association. "Instead, get up at your usual hour—say, 7:00 A.M.—but that hour in your new time zone, in order to get your body clock synchronized."

Head for the gym, not the mattress. Unless you're landing late at night, have a short but invigorating workout soon after arrival. "After sitting in the plane for five hours, a good workout gets the metabolism up," says Frank Furtado, athletic trainer for the Seattle Supersonics professional basketball team. But don't overdo it late at night or you might have trouble falling asleep.

Visit the Great Outdoors. "When you're in a new time zone, one of the most effective treatments for jet lag is exposure to sunlight or any bright light early in the morning," says Walter Tapp, Ph.D., a jet lag researcher and neuroscientist at the Veterans Administration Hospital in East Orange, New Jersey. "The more time you spend in the sunshine at your new destination, the better off you'll be."

Jock Itch

That new workout program has done wonders to whip your wimp image: Now you have bigger biceps, daunting deltoids and a stomach that looks like a washboard. Trouble is, you've also got a Hulk Hogan–size case of jock itch.

Don't feel like a dumbbell. There's a fungus among us, namely *Trichophyton rubrum,* that thrives—along with assorted fungal and bacterial brethren—in the hot, moist and dark areas of the groin. Constant rubbing and chafing only worsen the situation.

"The main point is that the fungus needs certain conditions to start—anyplace that's warm and moist," says Michael Ramsey, M.D., clinical instructor of dermatology at Baylor College of Medicine in Houston. "I see it more in people who work outdoors all day or truck drivers who are going 12 to 14 hours a day without a shower."

But you can bench jock itch for good by taking action at the first sign—and then taking measures to prevent its return. So before you burn your athletic supporter in effigy, try these strategies.

Hit the shower. Wash the infected area thoroughly with an antibacterial soap such as Dial, Safeguard or Lever 2000 and then rinse well, suggests Dr. Ramsey.

Blow away jock itch. If you've got the itch, you need to keep the crotch area as dry as possible. Use a hair dryer after showering, recommends Dr. Ramsey. "Just make sure it's on the coolest setting. Otherwise, the heat could make you perspire—and that defeats the purpose of drying the area."

Grab a towel. If you don't have access to a hair dryer, towel-drying is just fine—if you do a thorough job. Be sure to dry your groin area very well, suggests Dr. Ramsey.

Get creamed. After you've dried yourself completely, use an over-the-counter cream containing the ingredients miconazole and clotrimazole (found in Lotrimin and Micatin). If you use the cream daily, following directions on

Jock Itch—Without the Jock

Despite its locker room image, jock itch doesn't just plague cup-wearing male athletes—women can get it, too.

But as you might expect, the affliction isn't exactly the same in both. For one thing, tinea, a fungus nourished by sweat and heat, generally does the damage in men, while a yeast infection called *Candida albicans* is usually the culprit in women.

"Candida usually starts as vaginitis (infection and inflammation of the vagina) and progresses to the outside skin," says Marilynne McKay, M.D., associate professor of dermatology and gynecology at Emory University in Atlanta.

Both men and women can get ringworm, an oval ring of red pustules in the groin area. But female candida can be more extensive and inflamed. Despite these differences, however, treatments for men and women are the same, says Dr. McKay.

the tube, you can knock out a mild case in about two to four weeks, according to Dr. Ramsey. More serious infections, however, will require a prescription.

Baby yourself. "By covering the groin area with baby powder, you'll help prevent the moisture that leads to jock itch," says Andy Clary, head trainer for the University of Miami football team in Coral Gables, Florida. Just sprinkle on a light dusting of powder whenever you change your underwear.

Wear shorts under your support. Athletic supporters irritate the groin area. This irritation provides an environment for the fungus to grow. One of the best ways to guard against jock itch is to put on a pair of clean, all-cotton shorts before pulling on your athletic supporter, says Clary. "The jock doesn't rub the skin nearly as much, and the cotton pulls some of the moisture and the perspiration from the area by absorbing it."

Shed those sweaty workout clothes. It's virtually impossible to keep the groin sweat-free while working out, but once the whistle blows, switch into an "insta-change" mode, says Clary. "A lot of people sit around in their workout clothes after they exercise, but that's one of the best ways to get jock itch. You need to get out of your workout clothes as soon as possible." And don't put those sweaty workout clothes back on or back in your locker for tomorrow.

Lose weight. If you're a man or woman carrying extra pounds, you may be at increased risk of getting the itch, says Dr. Ramsey. "The patients with jock itch that I see tend to be a little more obese and, as a result, perspire more and have more skin-to-skin contact."

Kidney Stones

Anyone who has passed a kidney stone can verify that this is an experience he never wants to repeat.

The stone has to travel down a passage—the ureter—that easily carries liquid but has a terrible time with a small, grainy, calcified object like a kidney stone.

When it's all over, the stone passer (who is most often male) will breathe a huge, well-deserved sigh of relief. The trouble is, relief may last only for a while.

Usually, once you've had one stone, you're at a higher risk of getting another, says Leroy Nyberg, M.D., director of the urology program at the National Institute of Diabetes and Digestive and Kidney Diseases at the National Institutes of Health in Bethesda, Maryland. And then the risk can *double* after a second stone.

What causes these pebbles of pain? When the concentration of stone-forming minerals such as calcium or oxalate in your urine is too high, you begin to get a buildup of crystals of calcium salts and other minerals that are normally flushed away during urination. The buildup of these crystals in the kidneys eventually begins to form into a hard deposit, similar to a rough pebble. Besides the pain stones cause, you may detect blood in the urine. Only time—and a heck of a lot of water—will help flush a kidney stone. Sometimes a stone must be surgically removed.

Your doctor will need to determine by chemical analysis what kind of kidney stones you have and which treatments are appropriate. But here are some ways you can reduce your chances of forming another pain-producing stone.

Drink a lot of water. By increasing fluid intake, you raise urine volume and decrease the concentration of stone-forming elements in the urine. But how much is enough? "I tell my patients to drink enough fluid that they have a urine volume at least equivalent to a two-liter soft-drink bottle every day," says Brad Rovin, M.D., a kidney specialist and assistant professor of medicine and nephrology at Ohio State University College of Medicine in Columbus. To do that, you may have to drink almost a gallon of water a day—especially if you spend a lot of time exercising outdoors.

When to See the Doctor

Once you pass a stone (thank goodness!), your doctor needs to evaluate it, so you can take measures to reduce your risk of developing another. You should also see your doctor if you're experiencing pain in the groin, lower back or testicles or if you see blood in the urine. Any of these signs may indicate that you're getting another stone.

"It's even more important for people with stones, or who are prone to them, to keep properly hydrated," says Dr. Rovin. And it *is* important to gauge your urine output. Dr. Rovin suggests using an empty milk carton for measuring, until you find out how much you have to drink to get at least two liters' worth of urine.

Get plenty of exercise. Regular exercise helps put calcium back into your bones, where it's most needed. "People who are inactive tend to accumulate calcium in the bloodstream," says Dr. Nyberg. A daily workout for at least 30 continuous minutes is advised.

Watch your calcium. Most stones are calcium-based, so it's essential that you avoid excessive intake of milk, butter, cheese and other calcium-rich dairy foods. "If you've had a kidney stone, you shouldn't have more than one gram of calcium a day—the equivalent of about three glasses of skim milk," says Dr. Rovin.

Monitor protein. But calcium isn't the only no-no. Protein can also raise calcium levels, and it may increase the presence of uric acid and phosphorus in the urine—which may lead to stone formation. So if you've had uric acid or cystine stones, don't exceed six ounces of meat, fish or other protein-rich foods daily.

Bypass oxalates. If you've had a calcium oxalate stone (your doctor can tell you), then oxalate-rich foods can cause you trouble. So limit your intake of beans, beets, blueberries, celery, chocolate, grapes, nuts, rhubarb and spinach.

Contain condiment consumption. Table salt and condiments high in sodium should also be avoided. Salt restriction will help decrease the concentration of calcium in the urine. You should reduce your sodium intake to two to three grams per day, according to the National Kidney Foundation. Besides limiting high-salt seasonings such as ketchup and mustard, reduce consumption of processed and pickled foods, luncheon meats and snack foods such as chips and pretzels.

Beware of stomach antacids. Some antacids are enormously high in calcium, warns Peter D. Fugelso, M.D., medical director of the Kidney Stone Department at the Hospital of the Good Samaritan and clinical professor of urology at the University of Southern California, both in Los Angeles. If you've had a calcium stone, and if you are taking an antacid, check the ingredients listed on the side of the box, and make sure the antacid is not calcium-based. If it is, choose another brand.

Be a careful vitamin shopper. Ask your doctor about using certain vitamins to prevent future stones. A daily supplement of magnesium helped stop stone recurrence in nearly all those included in one Swedish study—so it's a good bet that magnesium supplements are beneficial. Also, vitamin B$_6$ is believed to lower the amount of oxalate in the urine. (But your doctor will probably tell you to avoid supplements that also contain vitamins C and D, since these nutrients increase the risk of calcium-based stones.)

Knee Pain

M odern warriors from the mighty fullback to the weekend fast walker have made knee pain one of our most frequent health complaints. An estimated 50 million Americans suffer from some sort of knee pain or injury.

Any continuous pressure on the kneecap can cause pain. And that pressure increases when your leg muscles aren't prepared to do whatever you're trying to *make* them do.

"In my opinion, a lot of knee pain is caused by muscle weakness in the thighs and hamstrings," says Andy Clary, head trainer for the University of Miami football team in Coral Gables, Florida. "We've seen a lot fewer knee problems with our athletes when they've been able to strengthen their lower bodies."

But whether you're a running back or a mall walker, doctors say you can beat knee pain. Here are some routes to relief, along with some tips to prevent knee pain in the future.

Know when to fold them. If you get a sudden twinge in your knee that makes it "lock up," restricting full motion, get off your feet, says Clary. You may be able to move again cautiously after a few minutes. But begin gently: Don't resume heavy or strenuous activity, Clary advises.

Press on some ice. For any knee pain, applying ice will help force your body to flush the knee with blood and oxygen, elements vital for repair. Ice also acts as an anesthetic to soothe the ache, says Patrice Morency, a sports in-jury management specialist in Portland, Oregon, who works with Olympic hopefuls.

Use an ice pack or ice cubes inside a plastic bag. Just make sure the ice pack is wrapped in a towel, so it doesn't come in direct contact with your skin. Apply ice to the sore knee no longer than 20 minutes every hour, says Morency.

Try an anti-inflammatory. You can calm inflammation and soreness with over-the-counter remedies that contain the anti-inflammatory ingredient ibuprofen, according to Paul Raether, M.D., a marathoner who is a physical medicine specialist at the Kaiser Permanente Medical Center in Portland, Oregon. Nuprin, Advil and Motrin are among the brands of over-the-counter anti-inflammatories. (You can also find low-priced versions marked "ibuprofen" in most pharmacies.)

Taken as directed, ibuprofen is also a painkiller, so it's important *not* to be lulled into a false sense of security when the pain eases. When you resume your activity, try it when you're not taking an anti-inflammatory, so you can feel the pain if your knee sends out warning signals.

Make a beeline to bromelain. Made from pineapple, bromelain is touted as a natural anti-inflammatory that is thought to speed healing, according to Morency. It is sold in tablet form in some health food stores. "I've used it personally and know that it works," says Morency. According to the directions, you can take up to three tablets a day until the knee pain subsides. Then start to resume your activities with caution. (The only drawback is that bromelain can cause dermatitis in some people, so you should stop taking it if your skin begins to feel itchy.)

Unbrace yourself. Wearing a knee brace may be a short-term solution after a particularly painful bout of knee pain. But try to go without that brace as soon as possible to prevent becoming psychologically attached, suggests Dr. Raether.

Avoid the knee bashers. Some activities, such as running and hiking over hilly terrain, put a greater demand on the kneecap than others. "These force the kneecap strongly against the end of the thigh bone," says Dr. Raether. If you're having knee pain, minimize those activities until you've had time to strengthen your leg muscles, he says.

Check out new workouts. Knee problems often occur when someone starts a workout program without first understanding how to properly perform ex-

When to See the Doctor

Any time you notice that there is pain or weakness or that your knee is swelling (especially after an injury), you should see the doctor, according to Paul Raether, M.D., a marathoner who is a physical medicine specialist at the Kaiser Permanente Medical Center in Portland, Oregon. Swelling could be a sign of serious internal knee damage, including bleeding or torn cartilage.

ercises or an activity. "You need to know the precautions before you launch into a new exercise routine," says Mike Nishihara, director of athletic development for the National Institute for Fitness and Sports in Indianapolis.

Runners and walkers, check your soles. If you're a frequent runner or walker, you need stable shoes if you want to avoid knee injury. Examine the shoes you have been wearing to see whether it's time for a new pair, suggests Dr. Raether. One way to check is to place them on a table at eye level to see whether the shoes stand straight up. (If the soles have worn down unevenly, the shoes will tip out or in.) Also examine around the midsole and sides to spot excessive wear. "Many shoes will begin to severely break down after 300 miles," says Dr. Raether.

Buy shoes with your knees in mind. If you have kneecap-related pain, there's a good chance that you're a pronator—someone whose foot turns toward the inside with every step. When you examine your shoes, notice whether your right shoe is caved to the left or your left shoe is caved to the right, suggests Dr. Raether.

When shoes are worn down this way, it's a sure sign that you are a pronator. Ask for a stable shoe when you're buying running or walking shoes.

Muscle up your leg muscles. To strengthen the quadriceps, the thigh muscles that hold your knees in place, start with straight leg raises, says Dr. Raether. Lie on your back with your right knee straight and your right foot angled about 20 degrees toward the outside. (To keep your spine in a neutral position, you can place a rolled-up towel under the small of your back.) Keeping the foot angled, slowly lift your leg a few inches off the floor. Hold your leg in place for a count of three and then lower it. Repeat with the left leg.

This exercise should be repeated about 50 times. "It's one of the best quadriceps strengtheners around," says Dr. Raether.

Work your hamstrings. To rehabilitate an injured knee, it's essential to build up strength in the hamstring muscles on the back side of the thighs. Dr. Raether recommends the following exercise to work the hamstrings.

Strap on some ankle weights and lie on your stomach with your legs outstretched. Bend your knees slowly to lift the ankle weights. Lift both legs to a 90-degree angle (your feet are over your knees), then slowly lower your feet to the floor again. Repeat 12 times.

Note: Begin with very light ankle weights. You can gradually increase the weight as long as it doesn't cause a flare-up of knee pain.

Lose some weight. Every time you run or walk, the force of your feet hitting the ground is felt in your knees. "For someone who's 20 pounds overweight, that's a tremendous blow," says Clary. Less weight on your frame simply means less damage with each step, he says.

Master the stair-climber. If you use a stair-climbing machine, reduce stress on your kneecap by taking short steps and maintaining good posture. "By taking shorter steps, you will prevent the knee from going out over the ankle," says Clary. "This reduces the stress on the knee joints."

Lactose Intolerance

Dare to eat dairy? For those with lactose intolerance, it can be a gamble. If you're among them—and up to 70 percent of the world's population has some, if only minor, symptoms of lactose intolerance—then you probably know that eating anything from Elsie the cow can be a *moo*ving experience. Maybe you feel a little bloated after a bowl of ice cream or a glass of milk—or perhaps your stomach rumbles enough to register on the Richter scale. Other symptoms include diarrhea, flatulence, stomach cramping and similar unpleasantries.

"Lactose intolerance varies from person to person, so there's no clear-cut advice on how to treat it," says Dennis A. Savaiano, Ph.D., a nutritionist and associate dean of the University of Minnesota College of Human Ecology in St. Paul. "You can find your limits by experimenting with differing amounts of dairy products."

Whether you're severely lactose-intolerant or just merely "annoyed" by dairy products, it's because your small intestine doesn't produce enough lac*tase,* the enzyme needed to digest lac*tose,* the natural sugar found in milk.

Still, there are ways to have your dairy and eat it, too—without having to rely on milk substitutes. And here they are.

Be a cocoa nut. Early research suggests that cocoa may reduce symptoms of lactose intolerance—one reason why many lactose-intolerant people get no severe reactions when drinking chocolate milk. "I suspect that the cocoa helps slow stomach emptying, which reduces the rate at which lactose reaches the colon," says Dr. Savaiano. "If you must have milk, one of the easiest things to do is to make it *chocolate* milk." But use powdered cocoa, which has no fat, instead of chocolate syrup, which is high in fat.

Put some enzymes in your milk. You don't necessarily have to drink chocolate milk, though. You can simply use enzyme tablets like Lactaid, sold in most drugstores and health food stores. "Even if you're severely lactose-intolerant, you can enjoy milk without any of the symptoms," says Manfred Kroger, Ph.D., professor of food science at Pennsylvania State University in University Park. "Just sprinkle powdered Lactaid into a glass of milk the night before, and the next morning, half the lactose in the milk is gone—and that's enough to prevent any symptoms. Besides, the milk will taste sweeter, because the lactose, which isn't sweet, will break down to glucose, which is."

Combine dining with dairy. "Some people find their symptoms disappear if they take their dairy products with meals," says Theodore Bayless, M.D., director of clinical gastroenterology at the Johns Hopkins Hospital in Baltimore. That's because one of the key factors in lactose intolerance is the rate at which the stomach empties. "If you can slow the stomach's emptying, you can reduce or prevent symptoms," adds Dr. Savaiano. "And having a complete meal slows the rate at which your stomach empties." However, it's not advisable to load up on several dairy products at one meal.

Feed on fermented fare. Not only are fermented dairy products such as yogurt, buttermilk and hard cheese calcium-packed (the *real* reason for eating dairy in the first place), they don't carry the punch of regular milk for the lactose-intolerant. For instance, the organisms that make yogurt what it is also

Try These Alternatives for Calcium

The best reason for consuming dairy products in the first place is to get calcium—essential for building strong bones and preventing diseases such as osteoporosis. But that's about the only reason.

After all, whole milk, cheese and ice cream are high in fat. And because they originate from cows, *all* dairy foods contain cholesterol.

But what about that calcium? Well, you don't necessarily need dairy to get it. In many cultures (the Chinese and Eskimos, for instance), people rarely (if ever) drink milk yet have surprisingly low rates of osteoporosis. How can *you* get the calcium you need without dairy?

Eat your greens. Green leafy vegetables such as spinach are rich in calcium, says Manfred Kroger, Ph.D., professor of food science at Pennsylvania State University in University Park. "And you'll benefit from vegetables even more if you have them with orange juice. That's because your body absorbs calcium better when there are acid conditions in your intestines." He recommends three glasses of orange juice each day for optimum intestinal acidity.

Go fishing. Sardines, anchovies and other fish with soft, edible bones are a calcium gold mine. "That's why Eskimos never get osteoporosis—because they eat fish bones," says Dr. Kroger. The soft bones of sardines and anchovies are easy to digest, unlike bones of other fish. Besides, these fish are rich in omega-3 fatty acids, which help boost "good" cholesterol.

Try antacids . . . now and then. Tums and other antacids are rich in calcium. But don't rely on them as your primary source, since excessive use can interfere with your stomach's natural acidity.

produce lactase to digest the lactose—which is why most lactose-intolerant people can eat yogurt with no problem, says Naresh Jain, M.D., a gastroenterologist in Niagara Falls, New York.

But one cautionary note: Frozen yogurt will produce the same reaction as ice cream or ice milk. That's because once yogurt is frozen, it loses its "helpful" bacteria.

Buttermilk is also "pretty tolerable," adds Dr. Jain (and despite its name, it usually has *less* fat and cholesterol than 2 percent milk). And calcium-rich hard cheeses have less lactose than milk. "Swiss and extra-sharp Cheddar contain only trace amounts of lactose and are thus less likely to produce digestive upset," says Seymour Sabesin, M.D., a gastroenterologist and director of the Section of Digestive Diseases at Rush–St. Luke's–Presbyterian Medical Center in Chicago.

Laryngitis

You may have lost your voice. But all is not lost. Laryngitis is nature's husky way of saying . . . er, *signaling* that your vocal cords need a break. Sometimes extreme hoarseness is the result of a cold or infection, and your voice will return when the cold leaves. Usually, though, laryngitis is more like an injury caused by overusing your vocal cords. Maybe you went for too many high notes in the shower or you rooted for your favorite team a little too enthusiastically. But whether the cause is an infection or a heck-raisin' holler, here's how to rein in the hoarseness and quickly get your voice back to normal.

Don't gargle. A good gargle may seem like an obvious remedy, but it will actually do more harm than good. "Gargling doesn't seem to reach down into the larynx where the irritated or inflamed tissue is," says Robert J. Feder, M.D., a Los Angeles otolaryngologist who teaches singing at the University of Southern California School of Music. "More important, if you make noise as you gargle, the vibration can actually harm inflamed vocal chords."

Stay *completely* quiet. And that means avoiding whispering, too. It's a given that talking should be avoided: It strains your vocal cords, prolonging or worsening laryngitis. But it's a little-known fact that whispering can be just as bad, or even worse. "Whispering causes you to bang your vocal cords together as strongly as if you were shouting," explains George T. Simpson II, M.D., chairman of the Department of Otolaryngology at the State University of New York at Buffalo School of Medicine and Biomedical Sciences.

Lead your hoarse to water. Downing at least eight glasses of water a day— and preferably ten—ensures that your larynx stays moist, a key step in curing

When to See the Doctor

If your voice loss is accompanied by pain so bad that you have trouble swallowing, you need to see a doctor immediately, says George T. Simpson II, M.D., chairman of the Department of Otolaryngology at the State University of New York at Buffalo School of Medicine and Biomedical Sciences. It may be the result of swelling in the upper part of your larynx that could be blocking an airway—a life-threatening situation that requires immediate medical care.

You should also see your doctor if you cough up blood or hear severe wheezing or other "noises" when you breathe. Also, if your laryngitis doesn't improve after five days of persistent voice rest (and you don't have a cold or another infection), you should see your doctor.

laryngitis. The water should be warm or room temperature—not overly hot or cold. And don't add salt or alcohol. (Forget about hot toddies: They're too drying.) If water isn't your favorite beverage, Dr. Feder says you can also drink juice and (warm) tea with honey. *Note:* Drink even *more* if you're flying, because the air you breathe in planes is very drying.

Avoid aspirin. If you've lost your voice because you were yelling too loudly, you've probably ruptured a capillary. So stay away from aspirin, advises Laurence Levine, D.D.S., M.D., associate clinical professor of otolaryngology at Washington University School of Medicine in St. Louis. Aspirin increases clotting time, which can impede the healing process.

Choose cough drops wisely. Avoid mint and mentholated products, which are too drying, says Dr. Feder. Stick with honey- or fruit-flavored soft cough drops instead. But keep in mind that cough drops are basically just candy. They don't have any healing effect.

Get steamed. Hanging your head over a steaming bowl of water for five minutes two to four times a day can restore lost moisture in your throat and quicken healing time. If you have a cold-air humidifier, that also does the trick, adds Scott Kessler, M.D., an otolaryngologist in New York City who specializes in performing arts medicine and a physician for many of the performers at the Metropolitan Opera and the City Opera and on Broadway.

Leg Cramps

L eg cramps are an equal opportunity annoyer—they can strike when you're running, walking, riding a bike, standing up, even sleeping. But what could prompt such intense pain at such diverse times?

If you're a runner, muscle fatigue can be a factor. If you catch a cramp when you're resting, however, poor circulation could be the culprit.

But you don't have to let leg cramps hamper your style. Consider these home remedies.

Pinch away pain. Ready for instant relief? Try this acupressure technique. Grab your upper lip between your thumb and index finger, and squeeze for about 30 seconds.

"It's hard to believe, but it works great," says Patrice Morency, a sports injury management specialist in Portland, Oregon, who works with Olympic hopefuls. Although there's no definite explanation for *why* acupressure works, it's a pain relief technique many athletes have found to be effective.

Let your fingers do the massaging. You can use the direct approach, too: Grab the cramping muscle tightly, pushing your fingertips deep into the cramp for about 10 to 15 seconds, then release. You can repeat as often as necessary to relieve the cramp, says Morency.

Contract and relax. Contracting any muscle that opposes a cramping muscle forces the cramped one to relax, says Morency. When you suffer a severe leg cramp in the calf muscle, for example, flex your shin muscle (which opposes your calf muscle) by pulling your toes toward your knee.

Better yet, while you're pulling your toes up, have a friend gently press the top of your foot the other way to provide resistance, says Morency. That maxes out the tension on your shin muscle, which should cause the cramped calf to release.

Stretch toward comfort. After the cramp is gone, stretch out the muscle—but begin slowly and without bouncing on it, says Andy Clary, head trainer for the University of Miami football team in Coral Gables, Florida. Here's a stretch that will ease the hamstring, which lies under the thigh, almost behind the knee: To begin, sit down on the floor and extend the leg. Then reach out and gently pull your toes toward your knee. That applies pressure over the belly of the hamstring muscle, stretching it comfortably. "You simply want to elongate the muscle," says sports injuries specialist Craig Hersh, M.D., of the Sports Medicine Center in Fort Lee, New Jersey.

Water your pain. Drinking a cup of water (about eight ounces) every 20 minutes before, during and after exercise will help keep your system from dehydrating. And when you prevent dehydration, you prevent cramping, says Dr. Hersh.

Give your electrolyte balance a boost. "People who are maintaining their weight and seem to be well hydrated but are getting recurrent cramping may have an electrolyte imbalance—too little sodium or potassium in the blood," says Dr. Hersh. He recommends any sports drink that replenishes sodium or potassium. "But you should probably have a blood test to make certain that's the problem," Dr. Hersh adds.

Train harder. Longer runs and walks will teach your muscles to better tolerate fatigue, says Morency.

Low Blood Pressure

If you've ever experienced low blood pressure after standing up, you probably know the symptoms: You climb out of bed feeling perfectly fine—and then, an instant later, you feel as though you might pass out.

This is because when you stand up suddenly, there's a brief period (about a minute or so) when your circulatory system has to adapt to a new body position and may not be sending enough blood to your brain. That's what accounts for the momentary light-headedness, which usually corrects itself after you've been on your feet and moving around a bit.

Low blood pressure symptoms sometimes can also occur after eating a meal or after standing for a long period of time. Under any of these circumstances, if you get light-headed, you are at risk for falls or fainting, according to Scott L. Mader, M.D., assistant professor of medicine at Case Western Reserve University in Cleveland. If this occurs frequently, you should definitely get a doctor's advice.

Another reason to see the doctor: If you're taking medications for other conditions, these drugs may be *causing* low blood pressure. "Tell your doctor about your symptoms," suggests Mark J. Rosenthal, M.D., associate professor of medicine and geriatrics at the University of California, Los Angeles, School of Medicine and a staff physician at the Geriatric Research, Education and Clinical Center at the Veterans Administration Medical Center in Sepulveda. It may be possible to reduce your dosage or to switch to a drug with fewer side effects.

In the meantime, here are some other ways to get the pressure up.

Fill 'er up with water. Dehydration reduces blood volume, which can lead to a drop in blood pressure. "I tell my patients to drink liberally," Dr. Rosenthal says. He recommends drinking about one glass (eight ounces) per hour; other doctors suggest eight glasses a day.

Pump your calves. When your blood pressure is low, gravity gets the upper hand. There's too much blood pooling in the lower part of your body. How can you keep it moving?

"If you're standing or sitting for long periods of time, keep blood from pooling in your legs by flexing and pointing your toes, stepping in place and rhythmically contracting and relaxing your calf muscles," Dr. Rosenthal suggests.

Adopt a flex stance. Standing at attention for a long time seems like an invitation to lower blood pressure. So why don't the guards at Buckingham Palace keel over?

Maybe it's because they don't lock their knees. Dr. Mader suggests keeping your knees slightly flexed rather than locked. "If you flex your knees slightly, you maintain muscle tension in your leg muscles to help pump blood back up to your heart."

Take time to cool down. When you've been exercising vigorously and you suddenly stop, there may be a dizzying drop in blood pressure. "For the next ten minutes or so following exercising, continue your activity at a slowed-down pace," suggests John Duncan, Ph.D., associate director of the Exercise

When to See the Doctor

Since low blood pressure can contribute to falls, you should see the doctor if you have any blackouts or if you repeatedly feel faint and light-headed during the day. You should also see the doctor if you are taking any medication, since many drugs—especially those for *high* blood pressure—can affect the contraction and dilation of blood vessels. Usually you can be switched to a different medication that can still treat your condition without causing problems.

In some cases, low blood pressure may be one symptom of diabetes or nervous system diseases, according to Scott L. Mader, M.D., assistant professor of medicine at Case Western Reserve University in Cleveland.

Low blood pressure after standing can be treated. Often a change in diet or activity level will be enough. However, there are more potent therapies available if needed.

Physiology Department at the Cooper Institute for Aerobics Research in Dallas. That gives your breathing a chance to return to normal and your heart a chance to resume its regular pace.

Stick with nonalcoholic drinks. Alcohol temporarily dilates blood vessels, causing a pleasantly warm flush. But those dilated vessels don't sustain their shape as well as normal, undilated vessels. So when your blood vessels dilate, your blood pressure can hit some dizzying new lows.

Don't restrict salt unless you need to. "I tell a lot of my patients with low blood pressure after standing up to lightly salt their food at each meal," suggests Dr. Mader. This is only for some people, however. If you've been put on a low-salt diet by your doctor, you shouldn't go off it without his permission.

Lie head-high. Sleeping with your head slightly elevated may help your body better adjust to an upright position, Dr. Rosenthal says. Try four-inch blocks under the legs at the head of the bed.

Rise and shine . . . slowly. Take lessons from a cat. Stretch before getting up, contracting and relaxing the muscles in your legs, abdomen and arms. When you sit up, dangle your feet over the side of the bed and flex your calves and arms. "Squeeze your fists and pump your stomach in and out a few times," suggests Dr. Mader. "Arm exercises are particularly effective at raising blood pressure."

Of course, if dizziness is a problem, it's a good idea to keep a chair or handrail by the bed to grasp as you stand.

Eat like a bird, not a boa constrictor. If you feel woozy after a big meal, try eating smaller, more frequent meals, experts recommend. After a big meal, blood rushes to your digestive area, and as a result, there's less blood getting to your brain. By eating smaller, more frequent meals, you're more likely to maintain more constant blood flow.

Walk it off. In one study of older people with low blood pressure after meals, walking afterward restored their blood pressure to normal. "These findings support an old German proverb—'After meals, you should rest or walk a thousand steps,'" says researcher Lewis A. Lipsitz, M.D., director of medical research at the Hebrew Rehabilitation Center for the Aged and assistant professor of medicine at Harvard Medical School, both in Boston.

Marine Bites, Stings and Cuts

About the only thing smaller than the amount of flesh covered by a thong bikini is your risk of an up-close-and-too-personal encounter with some sort of sea critter.

"Sunburn is still the most common and probably the most serious problem a beach-goer faces," says Glenn G. Soppe, M.D., a San Diego physician who lectures on aquatic bites and stings. Still, those murky depths hold more surprises than the contents of Davy Jones's locker.

Minor fish bites should be handled with the usual first-aid treatment like any other wound, and they don't present any extra risk of infection. (There's no such thing as a rabid barracuda!) But what about stings from jellyfish and

When to See the Doctor

Most marine bites, stings and cuts suffered by the average beach-goer are minor, but you should seek emergency medical care if you experience nausea, vomiting or intense swelling or if you have trouble breathing following your mishap, says Glenn G. Soppe, M.D., a San Diego physician who lectures on aquatic bites and stings. Fish-hook injuries should also be treated by a doctor or other trained personnel.

stingrays or cuts from coral, sponge and common seashells? These nautical nuisances may initially seem as frightening as losing your car keys in the sand, but they're usually remedied a lot faster. And here's how.

Take charge with a charge card. You can remove jellyfish tentacles with a credit card, and it won't even show up on your monthly bill. Jellyfish tentacles that get embedded in the skin deliver an attention-grabbing venom. Though painful, the venom is usually harmless (unless you swim in the South Pacific, where box jellyfish stings can be fatal).

"You have to scrape them out, just as you would remove a bee stinger," says Dr. Soppe. "If you try to pull them out with your fingers, you'll inject more venom into your skin. If you have trouble scraping out the tentacles, put some baking soda or shaving cream on your skin to make it easier."

Apply some tenderizing treatment. It may sound as hard to swallow as a cut of gristly beef, but meat tenderizers help neutralize the venom of jellyfish and other sea life. "Most of these stings are protein in nature, and meat tenderizer is meant to degrade protein," explains Arthur Jacknowitz, Pharm.D., professor and chairman of clinical pharmacy at West Virginia University School of Pharmacy in Morgantown.

If you're swimming in an area where there are jellyfish, take along Adolph's or McCormick tenderizer (you can use it for that beachside barbecue, too). "Make a thick paste of meat tenderizer and salt water, and pat it on the skin in the first few minutes after being stung to get substantial relief," suggests Dr. Jacknowitz. When buying meat tenderizer, look for brands that contain either papain or bromelain, the active ingredients that dissolve jellyfish venom. (Bromelain can cause dermatitis in some people, however, so don't apply any more if the skin area begins to look red and inflamed.)

Revitalize with vinegar. Kitchen vinegar is also effective on jellyfish stings. "Just make a 50-50 mixture of vinegar and salt water and apply it to the sting site," says Dr. Soppe. In a pinch, applying some diluted lime juice or ammonia to the site may also work.

Purify with peroxide. "Of course, the best remedy is a good defense. If you don't know what it is, don't touch it, and wear shoes while walking in tide pools," says Dr. Soppe. "But if you happen to cut yourself or get an abrasion from a piece of coral or a sea urchin, give the wound a thorough washing with hydrogen peroxide, followed by a good soaking in diluted vinegar."

Tape provides a sticky solution. You can remove the fine, hard-to-get-to spicules of a sponge or coral by applying a piece of adhesive tape to the abrasion site and then removing it. When you pull off the tape, you pull up the tiny spicules. Then bathe the area with vinegar, suggests Constance L. Rosson, M.D., who practices general medicine at Good Samaritan Hospital in Portland, Oregon.

Get into hot water. "Stingray venom is heat-liable, meaning that heat degrades the protein that causes the pain. Your best bet is to simply soak the area for at least an hour in water that's as hot as you can stand without scalding yourself," says Dr. Soppe. Hot water from the tap is usually around 120°F, which is hot enough for this treatment.

Since the fins of catfish and spines of starfish produce a similar type of venom, adds Dr. Rosson, the hot-water treatment is equally effective after an encounter with either of these sea creatures.

Menstrual Cramps

People who think "What's the big deal?" when it comes to menstrual cramps obviously haven't experienced a full-blown case of these gut-grabbing spasms.

The pain can feel like an abdominal charley horse, and worse yet, this time of month may bring on diarrhea and nausea. Admittedly, menstrual cramps do tend to ease off within a day or two, but who wants 48 hours of misery if it can possibly be avoided?

When pain is that intense, doctors recommend a checkup to make sure your menstrual cramps aren't being caused by something that may require medical treatment, such as endometriosis or a pelvic infection, says Penny Wise Budoff, M.D., director of the Women's Health Services affiliated with the North Shore University Hospital in Bethpage, New York, and author of *No More Menstrual Cramps and Other Good News.*

But once you've ruled out other causes, here are some techniques to maximize comfort and minimize monthly pain.

Say yes to drugs. Nonsteroidal anti-inflammatory drugs such as ibuprofen (Advil) work best to relieve menstrual cramps, and they may also take the edge off the breast pain and the diarrhea that sometimes go along with cramps. That's because these drugs inhibit the formation of prostaglandins, chemicals that cause muscle cramps and pain.

"The trick to easing your pain is to take medication at the very onset of pain or discomfort and repeat every six hours until the pain subsides," says Andrea Rapkin, M.D., associate professor of obstetrics and gynecology at the University of California, Los Angeles, School of Medicine. "Don't save the medication for times of severe pain."

Walk it off. Exercise is a muscle tension reducer and a mood elevator. And it may reduce menstrual cramps by improving circulation in the pelvic organs, experts say. "If you're walking, strike a relaxed pose that lets you swing your hips and arms freely and lets you breathe rhythmically," suggests Robert Thayer, Ph.D., professor of psychology at California State University, Long Beach. If your normally brisk pace wears you out during this time, do yourself a favor and slow down, he adds.

Seek heat. A warm bath or a heating pad on your belly or the small of your back can relax muscle spasms and ease cramping pain, according to doctors. When you're walking outdoors in cold weather, wear a warm jacket that reaches below your hips. That will help keep pelvic muscles warm and relaxed.

Stretch your iliopsoas. No, it's not some sort of strange tropical vine. The iliopsoas are three muscles (major, minor and iliacus) on both sides of your pelvis, stretching from your lower spine to your femur—the upper thigh bone. Tight 'psoas have been implicated in a variety of pelvic organ disorders, including painful menstrual cramps, says Robert King, co-director of the Chicago School of Massage Therapy and a nationally certified massage therapist. To make it easier to stand up straight and to open the area between your ribs and hipbone, you need to stretch these muscles, King says. Here's how.

In a partial side lunge, spread your feet apart and turn your body over the trailing leg, partially bending the knees, then lunge to the other side and repeat. This stretches the musculature of the pelvic area and the 'psoas.

Strike a diamond pose. Yoga can provide exceptional pain relief for menstrual cramps, says Patricia Hammond, a yoga instructor and director of the Sarasota Center of the American Yoga Association in Sarasota, Florida. "We recommend a light routine that stretches and limbers the hips and other joints but doesn't vigorously compress or stretch the abdomen," she says.

Try this pose: Sit on the floor with your back erect. Bend your knees, keeping them as close to the floor as possible. Bring your feet together, sole to sole, making a diamond shape with your legs. Keeping your back straight, breathe in, then slowly bend forward as you exhale. Breathe in and straighten. Bend forward again as you exhale. Repeat several times—feel yourself sink lower with each exhalation.

Curl up in a ball. Here's another yoga pose that's a sure-bet cramp reliever. Kneel, then sit back so that your buttocks rest on your heels and bend forward to rest your chest on your thighs. Place your forehead on the floor, with your arms stretched in back of you so that your hands are by your feet. If your head doesn't touch the floor comfortably, rest it on your folded arms. Breathe normally, and as you exhale, imagine your whole body becoming more limp and relaxed.

If this pose is uncomfortable, you can do a modified version of this pose in a chair, Hammond says. "Sit way back in the chair, with your feet flat on the floor, and lean forward, wrapping your arms around your knees or lower legs." If this pose is uncomfortable, simply rest your arms on top of your knees.

Try drinking some herbal tea. Gingerroot tea can help relieve menstrual cramps. To make it, slice a handful of gingerroot and simmer it in water for 15 minutes.

Add calcium. "Calcium helps maintain normal muscle tone and helps prevent cramps and pain," says Susan Lark, M.D., medical director of the PMS and Menopause Self-Help Center in Los Altos, California. Aim for about 800 milligrams a day, the amount contained in about three cups of milk.

Increase your magnesium. This mineral optimizes your body's calcium absorption and helps decrease menstrual cramps, Dr. Lark says. Good food sources include beans, whole grains such as buckwheat and whole wheat flour, salmon, shrimp, tofu, vegetables and nuts.

Migraines

Referring to a migraine as a headache is like saying the Grand Canyon is a large hole. While a run-of-the-mill headache can make your head spin, migraines can make you feel like Linda Blair in *The Exorcist*. Besides intense head pain, there's often nausea and vomiting as well.

The onset of a migraine is not like the creeping-in head pain of the "classic" tension headache. About 20 minutes before the war between your ears, a migraine can cause flashes of light, blind spots, dazzling zigzag lines, dizziness and numbness on one side of the body. You may feel thirsty or crave sweets, feel elated and energetic or drowsy and depressed. There's also hypersentivity to light and sound.

Heredity plays a role, and women are twice as likely as men to suffer migraines. These mega-headaches usually start around puberty and tend to dwindle after age 45. (But for some reason, they rarely occur during pregnancy.) Although the exact cause of migraines is unknown, evidence suggests that these one-sided headaches (they don't affect the *entire* skull) have something to do with the blood vessels in your head. Triggers also include certain foods, stress, light and even perfumes or other odors.

Your doctor may prescribe ergotamine for these hard-to-handle headaches, but that drug can produce distressing symptoms of its own. Luckily, the experts say, there are other ways to control migraines.

Sleep it off. "Generally, the best treatment for a migraine is to sleep," says Glen Solomon, M.D., a headache specialist at the Cleveland Clinic Foundation in Cleveland and associate professor of medicine at Ohio State University in Columbus. "Relief comes from falling asleep—even if it's for a short time." Dr. Solomon warns, however, that napping can trigger other types of headaches. So if you're susceptible to other headaches *besides* migraines, the best policy is to get on a regular sleeping schedule rather than taking catnaps.

Say no to NutraSweet. The popular artificial sweetener isn't so sweet to migraineurs: Aspartame (sold commercially as NutraSweet) can trigger migraines or make them worse. "Various studies have implicated NutraSweet but *not* other artificial sweeteners," says Fred Sheftell, M.D., director of the New England Center for Headache in Stamford, Connecticut, and coauthor of *Headache Relief.* "There's no question, medically, that many people prone to migraines or headaches will do better if they eliminate NutraSweet."

Take time to relax—literally. "Most migraines occur on weekends or while people are on vacation, and I think it may have to do with a *reduction* of stress," says Dr. Solomon. "When the body's stressed, it produces adrenaline—and adrenaline protects blood vessels against migraines. When you relax and don't have this adrenaline protection, you're more prone to an attack. You need to ease into relaxation, make it more of a gradual transition than just going full blast until 5:00 P.M. Friday and then suddenly stopping everything. I suggest practicing some sort of relaxation technique to slowly unwind—exercise, listening to music, whatever helps you relax—rather than just leaving work Friday afternoon and hitting the bar."

Munch on magnesium. Research by K. Michael Welch, M.D., a neurologist at Henry Ford Health Sciences Center in Detroit, suggests that most migraine sufferers may have a shortage of magnesium in their brains. "Magnesium is a muscle relaxer, and it can help those with migraines," explains Allan

When to See the Doctor

A headache hurts. A migraine can feel even worse. But for either ache, it's unlikely you'll need emergency medical care. However, you *should* call the doctor immediately if your headache is accompanied by convulsions, fever, severe mental confusion or a drop in alertness.

Other signals that you should see the doctor include a sharp pain in the ear or an acute pain in any point around your face or head. And if you have a headache following a severe head injury, don't hesitate to call the doctor or emergency room. You should also see a doctor if regular headaches become much more severe.

Finally, if you have a child who frequently complains of a recurring headache, be sure to consult a pediatrician.

Magaziner, D.O., a Cherry Hill, New Jersey, family practitioner who specializes in nutritional therapy and preventive medicine. Good sources of this mineral include dark green, leafy vegetables, fruits and nuts.

Watch what you eat. About 10 to 15 percent of people plagued by migraines are food-sensitive, which means that consuming some foods or drinks can trigger a severe migraine, says Dr. Solomon. "There are certain foods that we know are triggers—chocolate, red wine and other items containing the animo acid tyramine. Also, foods cooked with MSG (monosodium glutamate) can trigger attacks. I tell my patients to eat what they want but to note if they get headaches after eating certain foods. If they do, stay away from those foods." (For a complete list of tyramine-rich foods, see "Foods That Bring Pain" on the opposite page.)

Take an aspirin every other day. A landmark Physician's Health Study found that aspirin reduced the risk of heart attack. Less publicized was the finding that aspirin is also very beneficial for alleviating migraines. In the 22,000-person study, migraine-prone participants who took a 325-milligram aspirin tablet every other day cut their attacks by 20 percent. "Even a *daily* dose of aspirin seems to help prevent migraines," says Seymour Diamond, M.D., executive director of the National Headache Foundation and director of the Diamond Headache Clinic in Chicago. But check with your doctor before you start an aspirin-a-day program, and never give aspirin to children because of the risk of Reye's syndrome.

Ice your head. You have a 50-50 chance of getting some pain relief *within three minutes* of applying a soft, cold ice pack wrapped in a towel to your head, says Lawrence Robbins, M.D., an assistant professor of neurology at Rush Medical College and the University of Illinois College of Medicine, both in Chicago, who also has his own headache clinic in Northbrook, Illinois. That's because ice constricts blood vessels, returning them to normal size.

Be aerobically inclined. Doctors have long known that exercise is a great way to reduce the stress that often triggers migraines in some people. But now there's research suggesting that cardiovascular fitness may also help lessen migraines—no matter what the cause. Research psychologists at Carleton University in Ottawa, Ontario, report that the severity of migraines decreases as cardiovascular fitness increases. "Regular exercise is a great idea for anyone who has migraines," agrees Dr. Diamond. But he warns: Exercise *during* an attack can make it worse.

Foods That Bring Pain

Certain foods are known to trigger migraines in some people. Leading culprits include:

- Alcohol (especially red and fortified wines).
- Foods containing tyramine (an amino acid)—chocolate, aged cheeses, organ meats, vinegar, ketchup, salad dressings, sour cream, yogurt and yeast extracts.
- Foods containing MSG (monosodium glutamate).
- Other offenders—citrus fruits, onions, dairy products, pickled herring, deli meats, hot dogs, lima/fava beans and seafood.

Relax—as often as possible. Whether you just "imagine" yourself on a beach or actually go to one, practicing a *regular* activity that helps you unwind, relax and manage stress is *essential* for preventing migraines, say *all* our experts. Try to find some time every day for activities such as listening to music, reading or practicing yoga.

Don't pop the Pill. If you're a migraine-prone woman who takes birth control pills, you might want to consider discontinuing them. One in three women with migraines has increased attacks when she takes oral contraceptives.

Try feverfew. Fevers are fewer after taking this white-flowered plant, and so are migraine headaches. Research conducted at University Hospital in Nottingham, England, has shown that people who take feverfew get fewer and less intense migraines. You can grow feverfew, a common herb, or check your local health food store for supplements or powders. *Note:* Don't take feverfew if you're pregnant. And if you experience swollen lips, dulled taste buds or a sore mouth and tongue after trying the herb, be sure to stop taking it.

Morning Sickness

No one likes to hop out of bed at the crack of dawn. But in the earliest stages of pregnancy, some women get acquainted with the *pre*dawn hours. Weeks 6 to 13 can turn into a time of too-early rising, all because of morning sickness. Knowing this, too, shall pass may be comforting, but for those who beeline straight from bed to the bathroom during those 7-plus weeks of intestinal upset, this introduction to motherhood can be distinctly annoying.

Although morning sickness *usually* occurs immediately or soon after waking up, it doesn't have to. During pregnancy, your sense of smell becomes *very* sensitive, and certain odors can trigger the nausea at *any* hour of the day or night, according to doctors. Stress or fatigue is also a trigger. Even though you may not stop morning sickness, avoiding some of the triggers can help a lot.

So here's how to calm the queasiness.

Start your day with saltines. "The best thing is to eat some dry crackers or biscuits first thing in the morning," says John Willems, M.D., associate clinical professor of obstetrics/gynecology at the University of California, San Diego, and a researcher at the Scripps Clinic and Research Foundation in La Jolla. "You'll actually feel better if you have something in your stomach—and the best thing is some sort of dry carbohydrate." Other good foods to choose, besides crackers, include a plain, unbuttered bagel, a piece of matzo or dry toast.

Eat a little a lot. If you're prone to morning sickness, you can lessen its impact by eating five or six "small" meals a day rather than a traditional breakfast, lunch and dinner, says Jack Galloway, M.D., clinical professor of obstetrics and gynecology at the University of Southern California School of Medicine in Los Angeles.

"Morning sickness is caused by high levels of estrogen," says Dr. Galloway. "And excessive estrogen makes your stomach churn. But by constantly keeping something in your stomach, you eliminate this churning, which is caused

When to See the Doctor

Morning sickness is usually a normal part of pregnancy that doesn't cause concern. But obstetricians say you should see a doctor if:
- You are losing weight. Normally, weight gain during pregnancy continues even if you aren't keeping all your meals down.
- You feel dehydrated or you are not urinating.
- You can't keep *anything* down—including water and/or juice—over a period of four to six hours.

by increased stomach acids." Eating a big meal may immediately soothe your stomach, but the churning returns several hours later when food leaves the stomach for the intestines.

Go nuts over almonds. They are high in B vitamins and contain fat and protein—what you and your baby need right now. And they help fulfill the requirement of small meals, says Deborah Gowen, a certified nurse-midwife with the Harvard Community Health Plan in Wellesley, Massachusetts.

Walk away from your problems. Stress makes morning sickness worse, which is one reason why so many working women suffer from morning sickness. "The boss is yelling at them, people calling in are yelling, and when they go home, their husbands yell at them, too," says Dr. Galloway. "You can bet they'll feel nauseated." But whether or not you have to report to a boss at the office or a grump-prone spouse at home, lots of walking is recommended as a stress reliever.

Many experts recommend walking for morning sickness and throughout pregnancy—especially if you've previously been sedentary. "Start at 10 minutes, but if your legs hurt, skip a day," says Dr. Galloway. "Work up to 45 minutes a day, five days a week." Light weight lifting also helps stress, but be careful to *not* hold your breath while pumping iron.

Relieve the pressure with acupressure. While a daily all-over body massage might sound ideal, Wataru Ohashi, founder of the Ohashi Institute in New York City, recommends this quick technique that he claims will cure or reduce morning sickness.

Ask for your partner's help with this. Either sit or lie down on your side, with your partner behind you. He should press his thumb down your back,

What Causes Morning Sickness?

Why does morning sickness afflict so many pregnant women?

Doctors know that it's caused by a hormone called estrogen that is rushed into peak production during your eighth or ninth week of pregnancy. It may be hard to believe while you're camped at the toilet, but morning sickness is actually a *good* sign. Studies show that women with morning sickness are less likely to miscarry or deliver prematurely. But even though it may be a good sign for your pregnancy, the nausea certainly doesn't feel good to you.

first following the groove between your left shoulder blade and your spine, then keeping up the thumb pressure around the perimeter of your shoulder blade, moving out toward your side. Keep the pressure on for five to seven seconds at intervals along this path. The pressure should be comfortable. If you feel a sore spot, ask your partner to keep his thumb there, giving that spot extra attention. Do the massage three times. Repeat the procedure down the right side. "If you stimulate the external, you can eliminate the internal discomfort," says Ohashi, who believes the trigger points you use in this exercise affect the stomach and the hormonal system.

Lift an hourly glass. Getting extra liquids is important if you've been vomiting, so drink several ounces of clear broth, water, fruit juice or flat ginger ale or cola every hour or so. When you feel queasy, a cup of raspberry leaf, chamomile or lemon balm herbal tea can help soothe your stomach.

"At the drugstore you can buy a high-carbohydrate nonprescription drink that helps: It's called Emetrol. It helps calm the emetic center, the portion of your brain that controls nausea," says Dr. Galloway. And sports drinks like Gatorade are also recommended, because they replace electrolytes—substances that regulate the body's electrochemical balance—that are lost when you vomit.

Trust your body's wisdom. "Eat whatever appeals to you, as long as you're not eating junk," says Gowen. "If all you crave is pasta, then eat it. It really does work when women listen to their bodies." The exceptions include sweets and other foods with "empty" calories, which can upset your stomach and trigger nausea. And doctors strongly recommend that you avoid caffeine, artificial sweeteners and fried foods.

Motion Sickness

Whatever the mode of transportation—car, boat, plane or even roller coaster—if you suffer from motion sickness, all roads lead to misery. Nausea. Headache. Dizziness. Cold sweats. Sometimes your lunch is moving faster than the vehicle you're traveling in. You feel like you just want to crawl under a rock and die—but you sure as heck don't want to be driven there.

"Motion sickness is caused by a conflict between what your eyes tell your brain and what your other senses tell your brain," says Robert M. Stern, Ph.D., professor of psychology at Pennsylvania State University in University Park and a researcher on motion sickness and nausea for the National Aeronautics and Space Administration (NASA). For instance, if you're sitting in the back seat of a car and your eyes are focused on the front seat, your eyes are telling your brain that you're not moving. But there is a part of your inner ear that tells your brain differently. And you feel the bumps on the road; you hear the sounds of passing traffic; you may even smell the fumes. In other words, your senses signal your brain that you *are* moving. It's this mixed message that mixes up your insides. But here's how to remedy the problem.

Don't worry. "Nobody ever died from motion sickness, even though they've felt like they wanted to," says Dr. Stern. "That's important to mention: Anxiety is just going to make you feel worse, because it provokes some of the same undesirable body changes as motion sickness. If you relax and realize this is just a passing thing, you'll fare much better."

Face it on a full stomach. "The biggest mistake people make is *not* eating, mostly out of fear that if they eat, they will vomit," adds Dr. Stern. "But avoiding food is the worst thing you can do. When you don't eat, the electrical activity of the stomach becomes very unstable, and it's very easy for anything—a bad smell, the sight of another passenger getting sick, whatever—to push you over the boundary and make you vomit. You should eat a small, low-fat meal before

353

traveling, because the stomach is slower to empty fatty foods into the intestines, and you want a meal that will pass through the stomach quickly. And then, while you're traveling, I recommend going no more than two hours without eating something, even if it's just crackers."

Look where you're going. "Being able to look out the window and follow the movement helps a great deal," adds Dr. Stern. "One reason that kids get sick in the back seat of cars so often is that they can't follow the movement of travel. They see only the back of the front seat. Of course, it's easier to watch things go by when you're in a car or boat than in an airplane. But wherever you are, if you're feeling sick, it usually helps just to 'see' where you're going."

Hold your head still. "Minimizing head movements as much as possible can prevent or lessen the effects of motion sickness," suggests Millard Reschke, Ph.D., senior scientist for sensory function and director of the Neurosensory Lab at NASA in Houston.

Cruise Control

They warned you about sailing. All that movement—churning, bobbing and tossing about. But, silly you, you thought they were talking about the *waves*, not your insides. And now, you're as green as the ocean . . . and feeling lower than Davy Jones's locker.

To keep yourself shipshape during your next cruise, here are some exercises that may relieve dizziness and other symptoms of seasickness. "If you practice them before a cruise, you may help train your body and your brain not to become dizzy," says Christopher Linstrom, M.D., chief of otology and neurotology and director of residency training at the New York Eye and Ear Infirmary in New York City. "If you do these exercises during or after the cruise, they may help reestablish your sense of balance."

And according to the doctor, since the nausea of seasickness oftentimes is closely related to dizziness, preventing the dizziness may help prevent the churning stomach for many people.

You can do these exercises anytime, except when you're actually dizzy or seasick. (But they are not a replacement for any medication your doctor has prescribed).

Don't read. "Reading is one of the worst things you can do if you suffer from motion sickness—in any mode of transportation, including an airplane," says Dr. Reschke, an expert on motion sickness. (Gee, maybe it's more than coincidence that airlines place those cute little air sickness bags right next to magazines in the seat pocket in front of you.)

The reason? Focusing your eyes on the page, rather than the movement, is one way to worsen your condition.

But keep your mind busy. Listening to music, doing problems in your head or other diversionary tactics take the punch out of motion sickness. "That includes doing the driving yourself," says Dr. Stern. "People who usually get motion sickness rarely get it when they drive."

Consider nonprescription medications. Two popular over-the-counter drugs, Dramamine and Bonine, are both effective at preventing motion sickness, but they can cause drowsiness. They're most effective when taken an hour or two

Nod your head. Slowly, then quickly, bend your head forward, then backward, with your eyes open, 20 times. Turn your head from one side to the other slowly, then quickly, 20 times. As dizziness subsides, repeat with your eyes closed.

Shrug it off. While sitting, shrug your shoulders 20 times. Turn both shoulders to the right, then to the left, 20 times. Now bend forward and pick up an object from the ground; then sit back. Again, repeat this exercise up to 20 times.

Stand up, sit down. Change position from sitting to standing and back to sitting again 20 times. First do this routine with your eyes open, then repeat with your eyes closed. (It's okay to open your eyes if you feel yourself losing balance.) Now throw a small ball from hand to hand above eye level.

Keep on moving. Walk across the room with your eyes open, then closed, 10 times. Walk up and down a slope with your eyes open, then closed, 20 times. Repeat on a flight of stairs. (Hold on to a railing for the portion of this exercise that's done with your eyes closed.)

before traveling. They can, however, have side effects, so check with your doctor first.

Try ginger for a queasy stomach. For generations, travelers on sailing ships and in bumpy carriages took gingerroot as a cure for nausea. Today, the same motion sickness cure comes in capsules containing the powdered root, and some modern-day travelers find it effective. How much should you take? That depends on how nauseated you are, but "you will know you've had enough when you burp and taste ginger," says Daniel B. Mowrey, Ph.D., a psychologist and psychopharmacologist in Lehi, Utah.

Take the interstate instead. When traveling by car, many people avoid or minimize motion sickness by taking a route *without* a lot of stop-and-go movement.

Mumps

Thanks to immunization, which is recommended at 15 months of age, few children under regular medical care ever get the mumps. If they do, there's usually little to be concerned about. But because mumps can occasionally lead to more severe problems, it's important to have your child vaccinated as recommended.

The virus may cause moderate fever, pain in the neck muscles and headache. There is usually pain and swelling in the salivary glands, which causes the cheeks to puff out. Your child should be seen by a doctor to confirm or exclude mumps. (In adults, however, mumps may be more serious and require medical care.)

Should your child be one of the unlucky few to come down with mumps, here's how to reduce the discomfort and nurse your tyke back to better health.

Avoid acidic drinks. "Lemonade, orange juice and other acidic drinks increase saliva flow," says Henry M. Feder, Jr., M.D., professor of family medicine and pediatrics at the University of Connecticut Health Center in Farmington.

When to See the Doctor

Roughly 15 percent of children who come down with mumps may develop meningitis, which may require hospitalization and additional diagnostic or treatment measures. Meningitis can lead to impaired hearing or other serious problems.

Any child should be taken to the doctor when there's fever, swelling, drowsiness, severe headache, vomiting or signs of delirium. Even if you think you recognize the cheek swelling that is typical of mumps, it's important to find out whether your child actually has mumps or whether it's some other kind of childhood illness, such as strep throat or meningitis, according to Edgar O. Ledbetter, M.D., former chairman of the Department of Pediatrics at Texas Tech University in Lubbock.

But what if *you* have signs of fever, headache, muscle pain in the neck and swollen cheeks? See your doctor, suggests Dr. Ledbetter. When adults get mumps, it can lead to complications. Men may get an inflammation of the testes that in rare cases leads to infertility. In young women, mumps may produce some abdominal pain, which indicates inflammation of the ovaries. It may also provoke spontaneous miscarriage.

"The more saliva flows, the more it's going to hurt." It's better if the child drinks just nonacidic fluids such as water or milk.

Go bland on food, too. "Spicy foods provoke contractions of the salivary glands and increase discomfort, so your child will appreciate a bland diet," says Edgar O. Ledbetter, M.D., former chairman of the Department of Pediatrics at Texas Tech University in Lubbock. "Of course, most children realize this as soon as they eat something spicy," since the spiciness almost instantly leads to greater pain.

Apply some warmth. You may help your child find relief by applying localized heat to his swollen salivary glands, says Dr. Ledbetter. A warm heating pad or even a warm cloth can be used.

Muscle Soreness

Tree fact: The guy who first used the phrase "No pain, no gain" was *not* talking about oral surgery, auto repair bills, bosses, barking dogs, traffic jams or those hidden objects you smash your bare feet on when you're walking to the bathroom in the dark. He was talking about the kind of pain you get when demanding exercise such as weight lifting, running and gymnastics creates tiny tears in your muscle. It's called muscle soreness. And even though this soreness lies in muscle matter, you can ease it—and still make training gains—if you just use your head before, during and after your workouts.

Be hot and cold. A hot-and-cold shower remedy for muscle soreness takes some courage—but Patrice Morency, a sports injury management specialist in Portland, Oregon, who works with Olympic hopefuls, swears by it. Take a hot shower for two minutes. Then turn on the cold and let it run full throttle for 30 seconds. Repeat the process five to ten times. As you switch from hot water to cold, your blood vessels actually open and close, flushing lactic acid—which causes muscle soreness—out of the muscles, says Morency.

Massage away the pain. At the University of Colorado in Boulder, the Buffaloes football team has its own secret weapon for combating muscle soreness: massage. Following games and after the Buffaloes' toughest workouts, key players are given body massages to help move along waste products that are caused by exercise, such as lactic acid. Massage helps push the acid out of the muscle. "That helps recovery time a lot," says Steve Willard, a trainer for the team.

Have a tablet. Over-the-counter anti-inflammatories such as Nuprin, Advil, Tylenol and Anacin-3—medications containing ibuprofen or acetaminophen— can help calm inflammation and soreness, says Jennifer Stone, head athletic trainer at the U.S. Olympic Training Center in Colorado Springs, Colorado. The only caveat: "You've got to know whether you're dealing with just soreness or something more serious before you start taking them," says Stone.

Head for a hot tub. When muscles are tight and stiff the day *after* a workout, nothing beats a hot bath, according to Stone. "You don't want to take a bath right after you train, but I'd recommend it several hours afterward," she says. The reason: Heat increases circulation, promoting inflammation. But if you wait a while before taking your bath, you'll get a more soothing effect and less inflammatory action.

Take the ice plunge. After a tough workout, use this well-tested method from the University of Miami football team in Coral Gables, Florida. Fill a plastic garbage can with ice and water to create a cold bath that's a nippy 55°F (test it with a thermometer to make sure). Then step inside for instant relief, suggests Andy Clary, head trainer for the team.

Although Clary calls it "the best thing we've done for muscle soreness," he recommends that you go slowly the first time you test these icy waters. First fill the can just calf-high and step in. If you don't have problems with that, fill the can higher and sit so that the water comes up to your waist—but for no more than five minutes. "It's a pretty quick in and out that shocks the system and helps with any inflammation and soreness," he says.

Warm up before working out. Want to *avoid* muscle soreness? A warm-up not only helps you avoid unnecessary injury, it also helps get you ready for one of the best next-day soreness busters: stretching. "Our philosophy is that you need to warm up before you do anything else," says Clary. "Get some circulation to your peripheral muscles and increase that circulation to warm up the muscles and tendons. Once you increase circulation and the muscles are warm, then you can stretch them properly."

Stretch right for your sport. When you're getting ready to play hard and tough, don't settle for just a few hastily performed side bends or trunk twists. Instead, make your stretches sport-specific, says sports injuries specialist Craig Hersh, M.D., of the Sports Medicine Center in Fort Lee, New Jersey. "If you're a runner, you want to concentrate on the legs and back. If you're a pitcher, you want to concentrate on the shoulders, neck and upper back."

For other sports, think about which muscles you use most, and get them limber and warm first. The best way to stretch is with no bouncing. "Bring the stretch out to its extreme and hold it for 15 to 20 seconds," says Dr. Hersh.

Do some postgame stretching, too. "Stretching is even more important *after* the activity, because it helps prevent soreness the next day," says Clary. Stretching after exercise is also easier: Your muscles are more elastic after they've been warmed up.

Follow the 10 percent rule. Training with abandon seems macho—until your muscles refuse to help you out of bed in the morning. Instead of suffering, try this simple rule: Never increase the difficulty of your activity more than 10 percent from week to week.

If you're a runner who's logging 3 miles every day, continue to do that for a week, then try 3.3 miles daily during the next week. Or if you're running 20 minutes a day, you can up the time to 22 minutes the following week. This 10 percent rule ensures that you increase the level of difficulty in manageable increments.

Wear down pain. Elastic nylon shorts actually help prevent muscle soreness by providing support, says Clary. They also gently massage sore muscles, he adds.

Swap your sports. Instead of sticking strictly with your favorite sport, you can keep from surprising your muscles by cross-training, suggests Clary. If you're a tennis player, that means taking frequent bike rides. Into running? Try racquetball.

Have a carbo drink. One of the University of Miami football team's best-kept secrets for fighting muscle soreness is probably carried by your nearest supermarket: electrolyte/carbohydrate replacement drinks like Gatorade. It all started one season when each player was asked to down a glass of sports drink after practice, after each game and at dinner. (Sports drinks are high in carbohydrates, which the body quickly turns into glycogen to be used as fuel for the muscles.) By the end of the season, Clary noticed something startling: Far fewer players complained of muscle soreness than the year before. "I'm not kidding—we are believers in fluid replacement," he says.

Start half as fast. In your haste to get back into your training groove—or simply start—be careful not to go too fast. "If someone is just starting or coming back from an injury, I tell him to figure out what he *thinks* he can do and then cut that in half," says Stone. "People grossly overestimate their capacities. You're better off making a mistake by going a little too slow than going too fast. If you go too fast and get too sore, you'll be tempted to skip exercising the next day."

Muscle Spasms

A human muscle can knot up quicker than an overzealous Boy Scout can tie a figure eight.

Knots occur when your muscle suddenly contracts, or "shortens"—producing immediate and intense pain. Often muscle spasms result when you have overused the muscle while exercising or have injured it in some way.

But muscle spasms are sometimes caused by inactivity, such as sitting in the same position for too long. And you can also get spasms from a pinched nerve. They may even signal a mineral deficiency.

"Most people call these muscle *cramps,* but technically, it's a muscle spasm if the pain is sustained and you can actually feel a lump of muscle tissue under your skin," says sports medicine specialist Charles Norelli, M.D., staff physiatrist at Good Shepherd Rehabilitation Hospital in Allentown, Pennsylvania. But no matter what you call it, here's how to ease a muscle that goes into spasms and prevent the same painful thing from happening again.

S-t-r-e-t-c-h. Logic tells you that *pulling* on that shortened muscle is the simplest way to get relief. When you get a muscle spasm, treat it with "gentle, gradual stretching of the affected area," suggests Robert Stephens, Ph.D., chairman of the Department of Anatomy and director of sports medicine at the University of Health Sciences–College of Osteopathic Medicine in Kansas City, Missouri. "Besides pulling on the muscles, stretching helps improve blood flow to the area, which may reduce spasm pain."

If you're in one position too long, muscles tend to shorten. The movement of stretching can prevent this type of spasm.

"A woman who wears high heels all day might get muscle spasms in her feet after she takes off her shoes," says Dr. Norelli. That's because her feet have been "locked" in the same uncomfortable position all day. "One way to prevent muscle spasms is to stretch your legs and feet after you take off your shoes. Walking around barefoot for a while is usually the best remedy."

When to See the Doctor

Muscle spasms are usually not serious, and occasional occurrences shouldn't cause you concern. But if you *frequently* get intense leg cramping, it could be a sign that you have restricted blood flow or blood clotting in your legs—both of which can be extremely serious.

Cramping may also signal a nerve injury, says Allan Levy, M.D., director of the Department of Sports Medicine at Pascack Valley Hospital in Westwood, New Jersey, and team physician for the New York Giants professional football team and the New Jersey Nets professional basketball team. The bottom line: If your pain is very severe or if it occurs several times in one week, consult your doctor.

Apply moist heat. A hot bath or shower is another way to end muscle spasms. "Like stretching, heat improves blood circulation," says Dr. Stephens. "Heat also helps the connective tissue around the muscles: The warmer that tissue is, the more liquid it is. The colder, the stiffer." In fact, he recommends that you hit the showers *before* your workout to *prevent* muscle spasms. "I think you'll get your muscles ready for exercise better if you take a hot bath *before* exercise," he says.

Consume more calcium. "Sometimes muscle spasms are the result of a calcium deficiency," says A. J. Hahn, D.C., a chiropractor in Napoleon, Ohio, who specializes in natural remedies. He recommends getting calcium in your diet "if you suffer recurrent muscle spasms that don't result from overactivity." Good sources of calcium include low-fat dairy products such as yogurt, skim milk and ricotta cheese. Always check with your doctor before adding a calcium supplement.

Say no to acidic foods. Try to limit your intake of acidic foods such as tomatoes and vinegar if you suffer from recurrent muscle spasms, according to Dr. Hahn. That's because these acids can interfere with the body's ability to absorb calcium.

Pump up your potassium. Another nutritional deficiency that's been linked to muscle spasms is inadequate potassium. "Particularly if you're very active— like a long-distance runner or a soccer player—it's very important to make sure you eat plenty of potatoes, bananas and other foods high in potassium," says Dr. Stephens. Other good sources of potassium include dried peaches, prune juice and beet greens.

Take it easy. Since most muscle spasms come from overusing muscles, try to give yourself a break every now and then when doing anything physical. "Most people try to work through the pain—and the next morning, they'll pay for it with stiff muscles and intense soreness," says Dr. Hahn. "If you're spading your garden or painting your house (when you get a muscle spasm), take a break at the first sign of pain. Rest for 15 minutes or so and *then* resume your work. I think that giving your body a break when it needs it goes a long way toward preventing muscle spasms."

Nail Biting

T *a-dum.* Yes, it often begins with boredom. Or impatience. Or fidgeting. Then a nibble. And the next thing you know, your fingernails look like the Mad Nail Nibbler went on a binge.

If you are among the millions who regularly bite their nails, you know the Mad Nail Nibbler all too well. And you've probably said to yourself (how many times?) "I *wish* I'd stop biting my nails!"

Anyone can be a nail biter—and it often begins in childhood. Forty to 50 percent of all children regularly pick and chew their nails and cuticles, though many of them manage to kick the habit by the time they get to be adults. But nail biting can also get *started* in adulthood—sometimes out of the blue.

"While nail biting in some people may be a nervous reaction to stress, those who engage in it generally are not nervous individuals," according to R. Gregory Nunn, Ph.D., a clinical psychologist and president of R. G. Nunn and Associates, a private clinic in San Diego. "Nail biting is a learned behavior that usually results from factors that have nothing to do with stress. Ironically, one of the most common causes is the physical condition of the nails."

"If the nails become irregular or damaged, it promotes attempts to try to smooth them, and biting is one such means," says Nathan H. Azrin, Ph.D., professor in the Department of Psychology at Nova University in Fort Lauderdale, Florida. "But biting just worsens the condition of the nails and encourages further biting."

How, then, do you resist this urge to indulge in a five-finger feeding frenzy? Just sink your teeth into these proven tips.

First, pretend to bite your nails. That's right. And do it in slow motion in front of a mirror, so you can actually see all the movements that are involved.

"Most nail biters begin by running their thumb along the nails' edges, feeling for irregularities, before bringing the hand to the mouth," explains Dr. Azrin. "We want them to identify the *initial* parts of the movement. It's much easier to interrupt it at the initial stage than to wait until the finger is nearly in the mouth." Other signals: rubbing your face or cupping your hands just before you bite.

Keep a daily record. Build up your awareness by noting when nail biting occurs—that is, how often, when, where and with whom. Your goal is to identify all the situations in which you are more likely to engage in the habit, then consciously remind yourself *not* to bite your nails in those situations as you enter them.

Grip, grab and clench. You can't bite your nails if your hands are involved in other activities. So if you realize you're getting the urge to bite, immediately do something else with your hands. If you're sitting on a sofa, for instance, grab the armrest. If you're reading, hold the book firmly. And if you're in a meeting, gently grab your knee. Just hold on for a couple of minutes and the urge will pass.

File your nails daily. "Keep your nails well trimmed and short, especially for the first few weeks," says Trisha Webster, a hand model with the Wilhelmina Modeling Agency in New York City. "Use an emery board instead of a metal file or scissors—it is gentler and won't weaken your nails."

She recommends filing your nails into a rounded or oval shape. "If you file your nails straight across," she warns, "they will have two sharp points that are tempting to bite."

Baby them. "Soak or massage your nails with baby oil, olive oil, vitamin E oil or a gentle dish detergent at least twice a day to replenish lost moisture, stimulate growth and prevent cracking and chipping," says New York City skin care specialist Lia Schorr, author of *Lia Schorr's Seasonal Skin Care.* "Also, use a moisturizing hand lotion several times a day to keep the skin around the nails healthy and attractive."

Make your nails less tasty. Schorr and Webster both suggest coating your fingers with hot pepper or lemon juice: Any nontoxic, bitter substance will make you think twice about putting your fingers near your mouth. But make sure you also keep your hands away from your eyes.

Go undercover. When you're at home, suggests Schorr, try wearing some light cotton gloves. They're surefire protection against nail biting.

Dress up your digits. Once the appearance of your nails has improved, don't hide them—show them off! Dr. Azrin and Dr. Nunn both suggest wearing rings and jewelry and putting your hands on top of a desk or table rather than hiding them underneath. After you've given up nail biting, you should begin to feel comfortable extending the fingers rather than cupping them. If you draw attention to your fingers and receive compliments, that's a wonderful incentive to keep up the good work.

Nail Fungus

It doesn't hurt. It won't threaten your health. And the odds are that no one else will even notice that you have nail fungus—at least in its early stages. A long-term condition, however, can be marked by thick, yellow, raggedy-looking nails on your fingers and toes.

This isn't a condition you want to ignore. "The fungus starts at the free edge of the nail and works its way to the root. Once the fungus infects the root of the nail, there is virtually nothing you can do other than take the nail out and destroy it," says Houston podiatrist William Van Pelt, D.P.M., former president of the American Academy of Podiatric Sports Medicine.

Nail fungus is usually caused by an immune system deficiency, but it's aggravated by moisture, so keeping hands and feet clean and dry is the best way to prevent or control it. And here are the best ways of doing that before this bothersome blight gains a toehold.

Aim a cool hair dryer. Your feet spend all day in a warm, damp environment—namely, your shoes. To get your toenails dry before you put on your shoes and socks, use a hair dryer set on the cool setting. Then blow-dry under, around and between your toes after bathing, suggests podiatrist James Graham, D.P.M., of the Mayo Clinic in Rochester, Minnesota.

Apply antiperspirant. Sweating makes matters worse, since it creates a warm, moist environment—perfect for spreading nail fungus. "One of the best ways to stop sweating before it starts is to apply an unscented antiperspirant to your feet," says Dr. Van Pelt. "You can use either a roll-on or a spray, but the key is to use an *unscented* brand, because the perfumes in scented kinds are too harsh for many people."

Snip nails short. Long nails act like levers. When you catch the end of a long nail on something, it lifts the nail from its bed, and that invites fungus inside. Clip back your nails so that none protrudes beyond the nail bed, suggests Lowell Goldsmith, M.D., professor and chairman of the Department of Dermatology at the University of Rochester School of Medicine and Dentistry in Rochester, New York.

But don't clip your cuticles, advises Dr. Graham." When cuticles are damaged, that removes your nail's protective barrier and allows easy entry for the fungus and bacteria," he says. And use an orange stick rather than a nail file to clean under your nail tip. "Digging debris from under your nail tip too vigorously may create space that allows the fungus to grow," says Dr. Graham.

Smooth away dead skin. Fungus often attaches itself to dead, dry skin, then moves on to other areas. "Soap and water and a gentle scrub brush will remove dead skin buildup," says Richard L. Dobson, M.D., professor of dermatology at the Medical University of South Carolina in Charleston.

Wash your hands. Fungal infection can spread from your feet to your hands. So wash your hands after inspecting your feet, advises Dr. Graham.

Wear breathable footwear. "Man-made materials such as vinyl and patent leather (which isn't actually leather) don't breathe, so I advise wearing shoes made of natural materials such as leather or canvas," says Dr. Van Pelt. It's also a good idea to *not* wear the same shoes two days in a row, adds Dr. Graham. That way, each pair will be thoroughly dry before you put it on again.

Socks should also be made from a blend of fabrics—preferably acrylic and wool—that wicks away moisture and retains its softness. If your socks feel

NAUSEA

moist throughout the day, change them frequently. And for extra drying power, sprinkle a medicated antifungal powder into your socks. But avoid using cornstarch. Besides caking, "it could prompt bacteria to breed and compound your problem," says Dr. Graham.

Nausea

Nausea is a universal malady—*everyone* gets it at one time or another. And depending on the sensitivity of your stomach, it can be caused by just about *anything*—from the smell of a skunk to (very rarely) appendicitis.

The usual way to end nausea, of course, is to vomit. Fortunately, there are other remedies that aren't so drastic.

Drink a Maalox cocktail. "Put a few drops of spirits of peppermint into Maalox and mix it with one quart of distilled water," says Christa Farnon, M.D., associate director of Occupational Medical Services for SmithKline Beecham, a pharmaceuticals company in King of Prussia, Pennsylvania. Take a few sips of this to soothe your upset stomach and use the rest later, as needed.

Eat crackers. "In general, when people are slightly nauseated, if they can make themselves eat some very plain food they will feel better," says Robert M. Stern, Ph.D., professor of psychology at Pennsylvania State University in University Park and a researcher on motion sickness and nausea for the National Aeronautics and Space Administration. "I recommend low-fat foods, such as crackers." Don't overdo it, though. A few crackers will ease your nausea, but too much of any food may make you feel even worse.

Exercise your mind. "Sometimes keeping busy can help people," suggests Dr. Stern. "Before they know it, the nausea passes." Play a mental game, read a book or strike up a conversation with someone to keep the nausea out of your mind.

Rest your body. Astronauts on the first space flights had few complaints about motion-induced nausea. The reason may have been that they were

367

When to See the Doctor

Repeated or prolonged nausea can be a symptom of a wide range of conditions, from flu and food poisoning to intestinal disorder and tumors.

"If you're nauseated and there's not an obvious reason, you should see a doctor," says Robert M. Stern, Ph.D., professor of psychology at Pennsylvania State University in University Park and a researcher on motion sickness and nausea for the National Aeronautics and Space Administration. And even if you do know the reason for it—such as car sickness or seasickness—you should see a doctor if the nausea doesn't go away after a day or two.

You should also see a doctor if your nausea is accompanied by fever, especially if you are elderly, according to Dr. Stern.

forced to remain still, because the area inside the capsule was so confined. Try not to move around too much, even when your stomach is doing somersaults, recommends Dr. Stern. Most important of all: Try to keep your head still.

Say "I'll pass" on the milk. "Milk and milk products are much more difficult to digest than other foods," says Dr. Farnon. "They contain proteins and fats and create mucus. This means that they are harsher on the stomach." She advises clear liquids such as tea or juices served at room temperature, never cold, when you are trying to recover from nausea.

Try acupressure. Some people find relief from nausea—especially the kind that comes from motion sickness—by applying pressure to the inside of the wrist near the center. Those who practice acupressure believe this is the point that controls things such as nausea and vomiting, says William Grant, Ed.D., vice chairman of the Department of Family Medicine and research associate professor at the State University of New York Health Science Center at Syracuse.

Wrist-wrap with a Sea Band. Sea Bands, special wristbands that put pressure on the inside wrist area, were created for seasickness but are now used for other types of nausea. They can be found at boat dealers, in some sporting goods stores and in most local American Automobile Association offices.

Seek relief in nonprescription drugs. Some over-the-counter medications such as Pepto-Bismol, Maalox and Mylanta are known to help calm nauseated stomachs. It depends on the cause of nausea, doctors agree, but an irritated stomach may feel better after a couple of spoonfuls.

Don't forget Dramamine. "Some nauseated people might be helped by the anti–motion sickness drugs such as Dramamine," says Dr. Stern. Although he acknowledges that little is known about how Dramamine works to ease nausea, he suggests that you give it a try and keep this over-the-counter medication on hand if it works.

Drink flat soda. "Just open up a carbonated soft drink and let it go flat," says Dr. Grant. He recommends ginger ale, but other soft drinks work just as well. Dr. Farnon suggests the flat syrup of Coca-Cola, available in most drugstores, sipped over cracked ice when your tummy becomes queasy.

Nicotine Dependency

The good news is that each year, a few thousand Americans manage to quit smoking. The bad news is, that's a mere fraction of the 50 million Americans who can't. Blame it on nicotine, the active ingredient in cigarette smoke (as well as in snuff and chewing tobacco) that's as addictive as heroin. Seconds after you light up a cigarette, nicotine rushes to the brain, bringing a quiet fix of pleasure and satisfaction—especially to those who have been without a cigarette for an hour or more and may be experiencing withdrawal cravings. But nicotine also quickens the heart rate and constricts blood vessels, impairing normal blood flow, making your heart work harder and putting you at risk for heart disease.

The pleasure brought on by nicotine quickly convinces the brain to require more, and the smoker soon develops a tolerance for these effects—needing greater "doses" to feel satisfied. Habitual smokers who fail to get a dose of nicotine every 30 minutes or so may show irritability, inability to concentrate, anxiety, confusion and insomnia.

Quitting is never easy, but the worst part usually comes up front. The physical withdrawal symptoms last a week or two, so getting through that period is usually toughest. Here are some ways to make the rough road a little easier, once you crush out your last butt and retire your habit for good.

Drink orange juice. If you're quitting cold turkey, you'll get over withdrawal symptoms faster if you drink a lot of orange juice. "By making your urine more acidic, you'll clear your body of nicotine faster," says Thomas Cooper, D.D.S., professor of oral health sciences at the University of Kentucky in Lexington and a nicotine dependency researcher. "However, if you're using the nicotine patch or gum (which need a doctor's prescription), then *don't* drink orange juice, because you want to keep nicotine in your body."

Write a letter to a loved one. When the craving to pick up a cigarette hits, pick up a pen instead—and write a letter to loved ones explaining why smoking is more important than they are. "Explain to your son or daughter why cigarettes are so important to you that you would choose to die early rather than live to see them go to their prom or graduate from college, or see them married and have their own children," according to Robert Van de Castle, Ph.D., professor of behavioral medicine at the University of Virginia Health Sciences Center in Charlottesville.

The letter is realistic, he says, "because that's what is going to happen if you continue to smoke. Certainly heart disease or stroke or lung cancer will get you before you'll be able to share important moments in the lives of your family or loved ones."

When Dr. Van de Castle's patients attempt these letters, they usually don't finish writing. "After a while, you begin to feel so foolish, so selfish and so out of control that you're putting these white sticks ahead of the people who mean most to you that it's often enough to convince you to quit smoking—withdrawal symptoms and all," he explains.

Soak yourself. Another way to distract yourself from the urge to smoke is with a nice hot shower or relaxing bath. And that soothing hot water carries another bonus for the nicotine-dependent: "One of the best ways to deal with pain is to do something relaxing," says Jack E. Henningfield, Ph.D., chief of the Clinical Pharmacology Branch of the Addiction Research Center at the National Institute on Drug Abuse in Baltimore.

Get a lot of exercise. Taking a walk is one of the best ways to walk a mile *away* from a Camel. "Exercise is an excellent method of distraction for people trying to quit," says psychologist Gary DeNelsky, Ph.D., director of the Smoking Cessation Program at the Cleveland Clinic Foundation in Cleveland.

The Only Way to Quit

Many smokers mistakenly think that switching to a low-tar and low-nicotine brand will ease their nicotine addiction, making it easier for them to quit smoking. "Actually, the tobacco is the same in all cigarettes," says Thomas Cooper, D.D.S., professor of oral health sciences at the University of Kentucky in Lexington and a nicotine dependency researcher. "The only difference is that the 'low' brands have more holes punched into their paper or filters, so you don't get as good a draw when inhaling. But to compensate, people smoking low brands tend to inhale more deeply and take more puffs, so they wind up getting the same amount of nicotine."

Same goes for cutting down the number of cigarettes you smoke. If you smoke fewer every day, "you'll just take longer and more frequent puffs, so you'll still be getting the same amount of nicotine," according to Dr. Cooper. "In studies, I found that the average smoker has 30 cigarettes a day (1½ packs), taking ten three-second puffs on each butt. When he cuts down to only 10 cigarettes, the number of puffs increases, and each puff becomes longer and more deeply inhaled, up to eight seconds. So cutting down is not an effective way to stop smoking. You have to stop smoking completely."

"When you exercise, you're not as aware of your internal state. So if you're in the middle of a tennis game, you're not going to think of those cravings; you're focused too much on the game. Besides, the longer you exercise, the more healthy you feel, and many people find that a regular workout psychologically turns them off to smoking."

Most experts, including ex-smoker Dr. DeNelsky, suggest daily exercise during the quitting stage. Some even suggest a brief walk or another workout whenever you feel cravings.

Drink a baking soda cocktail. If you're not on a low-sodium diet, researchers at the Mayo Clinic in Rochester, Minnesota, say you may get short-term relief from nicotine withdrawal symptoms by dissolving two tablespoons of baking soda—sodium bicarbonate—in a glass of water. Have this drink with every meal. *Note:* This is *not* recommended if you have peptic ulcers.

Pay yourself. A federally funded, $1.3 million study on smoking habits found that people who are paid $1 for every day they go without a smoke are more successful at staying off nicotine than other quitters.

"I think the key is to reward yourself quickly," says Doreen Salina, Ph.D., a clinical psychologist and research scientist at DePaul University in Chicago who is the project director of the study. "If you simply put money in a kitty, it won't have the same effect."

Actually, Dr. Salina says *any* reward will do; money is just one option. "Some people allow themselves a nice bath, or they watch a certain TV show they normally wouldn't," says Dr. Salina. Try whatever works, she suggests: "The point is to indulge yourself in some way to compensate for the sacrifice you're making."

Go to the library. "In order to be successful at quitting smoking, you have to prepare to leave situations where smoking is permitted. Modify your activities so that you spend more time in places where smoking is *not* permitted," says Dr. DeNelsky. "Go to the library. Go to church. Visit places where you cannot smoke. It's important to understand that these nicotine cravings will pass, but they will pass more easily if you're someplace where you cannot indulge."

Monitor your vices. "Once you get off cigarettes as a source of nicotine, it's essential that you reduce both your caffeine and alcohol consumption," says Dr. Cooper. "That's because your body loses some of its capacity to process both of these substances as you reduce the amount of nicotine in your body.

"Someone who smokes will process caffeine 2½ times faster then someone who doesn't," Dr. Cooper points out. "That means if you quit smoking, you'll need only about a third as much coffee to get the same 'rush' you got from coffee drinking while still smoking. And you'll get drunk faster without nicotine in your body, so don't drink as much as before."

Nightmares and Sleep Terrors

W e may spend one-third of our lives sleeping, but it's not always time well spent. Sometimes our imaginations take us to the wrong side of the railroad tracks in dreamland.

Nightmares are perhaps the most common form of sleep disturbance. "Probably 75 percent of people can remember at least one nightmare from their childhood," says Gary Zammit, Ph.D., director of the Sleep Disorders Institute at St. Luke's–Roosevelt Hospital Center in New York City. "Nightmares are distinctively frightening experiences that may be a reflection of significant psychological stress or may mean absolutely nothing." They tend to occur toward the end of sleep, usually an hour or two before awakening.

Sleep terrors are different from nightmares because technically they aren't bad dreams; rather, they're "scary images" that tend to occur a few hours after going to sleep. Most common in children under age 12, sleep terrors can be associated with stress, sleep deprivation, fever and some medications.

"The child wakes up in sheer terror and can't remember what caused so much fear," says Dr. Zammit. "It's even more frustrating the following morning, when the child remembers waking up scared but does not recall what scared him." A child might say "The bad man was going to get me," but his description is vague.

While both nightmares and sleep terrors may scare you as much as Junior, they're a normal part of childhood—or even maturity. "As long as the nightmares or sleep terrors don't interfere with your or your child's daytime activities, you shouldn't be too concerned," says Peter Hauri, Ph.D., co-director of the Mayo Clinic Sleep Disorders Center in Rochester, Minnesota. "Mostly, the best thing you can do is endure it and be supportive of your child."

Well, maybe. But when kids are in distress, parents naturally want to help out. So here are several ways to take at least some of the fright out of your child's night.

When to See the Doctor

If your nightmares are so frequent and disturbing that they are beginning to interfere with your daytime life, you should visit a sleep disorders center, according to Peter Hauri, Ph.D., co-director of the Mayo Clinic Sleep Disorders Center in Rochester, Minnesota. The experts at the center can determine whether your nightmares are related to psychological causes such as anxiety, agitation or overstress or to physical causes such as epilepsy or sleep apnea. And they can refer you to an appropriate specialist for treatment.

"Play" it out. If your child is unable to express what he's feeling, use creative play to help him "say" what's bothering him. "Having the child draw a picture or play with figures that represent different situations or family members can reveal a lot about how that child is feeling," says Dr. Zammit.

Encourage enough sleep. "Being overtired is one cause of sleep terrors, and putting the child to bed earlier is one way to remedy them," says Marc Weissbluth, M.D., author of *Healthy Sleep Habits, Happy Child* and director of the Children's Memorial Hospital Sleep Disorders Center in Chicago.

Control allergies. Allergies also impair sleep quality and therefore can cause sleep terrors, says Dr. Weissbluth. "It's likely that your child has allergies if he or she snores, sleepwalks, sleeptalks or wets the bed."

Don't be Perry Mason. "When a child wakes up terrified, it's important for parents to be comforting and soothing. They should avoid long and detailed questioning about the dream or telling the child what it may have meant," advises Dr. Zammit. "Whatever discussions are needed should be handled the following day and should be brief."

Secure the area! One way to help children deal with frequent nightmares is to show them that their sleeping environment is a secure one, suggests Dr. Zammit. "You might want to 'check the room' with the light on, looking in the closet and under the bed. Then turn the light *off* and talk about the shadows and what's causing them, to reassure your child."

Provide a bell. Another strategy that has been used to help soothe a frightened child is to give him a "special" small bell to ring to scare away monsters. According to Dr. Zammit, this gives the child some control over his anxiety. Of course, the ringing bell also tells parents how often the child is waking up because of "monsters" or other frightening images.

Nosebleed

Whatever the cause—and there are about a dozen, from allergies to too much nasal spray—a nosebleed can be an alarming experience. In most cases, though, pride is injured more than your nose, since nosebleeds are seldom anything more than a nuisance. In fact, rarely is more than tablespoon of blood ever shed. But here's how to stop the flow fast.

Gently blow your nose. A gentle honking of your honker can help clear out blood clots that could be preventing a blood vessel from sealing, says Louis D. Lowry, M.D., professor of otolaryngology at Thomas Jefferson University Hospital in Philadelphia.

Pretend you're about to jump into a pool. "Pinch your nostrils the same way you would if you were jumping into the water," recommends Leonard Rappaport, M.D., assistant professor of pediatrics at Harvard Medical School and a senior associate in medicine at Children's Hospital in Boston. "Then hold it that way for five minutes, breathing through your mouth. When you let go and resume nose breathing, *don't* blow your nose."

Stand tall. Sit up straight, because lying back or putting your head back causes you to swallow blood, says Alvin Katz, M.D., an otolaryngologist and surgeon director at Manhattan Eye, Ear, Nose and Throat Hospital in New York City.

Humidify your surroundings. Being in a heated room can dry out mucous membranes, making you more susceptible to nosebleeds. But humidifying your surroundings, especially in winter months, can keep moisture in your

When to See the Doctor

If, after blowing out the clots and applying pressure, your nosebleed doesn't stop or slow down after ten minutes, or if blood flow is severe, you probably need emergency care to help stop the bleeding, says John A. Henderson, M.D., assistant clinical professor of surgery/otolargyngology at the University of California, San Diego, School of Medicine.

If you feel blood running down the back of your throat after you pinch your nostrils, you need medical attention as soon as possible. It means you're losing blood, even if you stop the nosebleed in front, according to Dr. Henderson.

home—and your membranes, suggests Paul Edelson, M.D., chief of pediatric infectious diseases at The New York Hospital–Cornell Medical Center in New York City.

Take your vitamins. If you're prone to nosebleeds, consider boosting your iron and vitamin C intake. Iron helps your body rapidly replace the blood supply, says Gilbert Levitt, M.D., an otolaryngologist with the Group Health Cooperative of Puget Sound in Redmond, Washington.

Vitamin C, along with the B-complex vitamins, is necessary for the formation of collagen and free-flowing mucus, creating a moist protective lining in your sinuses and nose, adds John A. Henderson, M.D., assistant clinical professor of surgery/otolargyngology at the University of California, San Diego, School of Medicine.

Oily Hair

If you've noticed that your hair is oily and you're wondering how it got that way, there are between 90,000 and 140,000 good reasons. That's how many strands of hair are on a reasonably well-covered head, according to Philip Kingsley, a New York City and London hair care specialist. And each strand has its very own oil gland. Strenuous exercise only increases oil production, as do heat and humidity. Plus there's pollution. And hormones. And sweat. And residue from all those hair products you may have used to control the oiliness.

It goes for anyone: If you've got a full head of hair and live a relatively active life, then some extra oil is almost inevitable. But hair color does make some kind of difference, adds Kingsley. Redheads with thick, coarse hair, for example, rarely have problems with oily hair, while blondes with silky, baby-fine hair have the worst problem. (So much for having more fun!)

But whatever your hair color or the problems with your hair, here's how to ease the oiliness.

Choose the right shampoo. The obvious answer to oily hair is to shampoo often—*daily* is recommended by most of our experts. But if you're using the wrong shampoo, you could be disappointed with the results. "Look for a shampoo that's designated as 'deep cleaning' and for other descriptions on the packaging that indicate the shampoo cleanses well," suggests John Corbett, Ph.D., vice president of technology for Clairol, based in Stamford, Connecticut.

"Clear, see-through shampoos tend to have less goo in them," adds Thomas Goodman, Jr., M.D., assistant professor of dermatology at the University of Tennessee Center for Health Sciences in Memphis. "They clean away oil more effectively and don't leave a residue."

And use it the right way. Most often recommended is a double shampoo, leaving the suds on your head for *at least* five minutes each time, says Lowell Goldsmith, M.D., professor and chairman of the Department of Dermatology at the University of Rochester School of Medicine and Dentistry in Rochester, New York. (If your head isn't especially oily, a single shampoo is enough, as long as you leave the shampoo on for the full five minutes.)

Rinse your hair with vinegar. One teaspoon of apple cider kitchen vinegar added to a pint of water makes an excellent finishing rinse that adds shine and luster to your hair while removing soap residue that can weigh down oily hair. A thorough rinsing with plain water will remove the smell.

Or freshen it with lemon. Squeezing the juice of two lemons into a pint of distilled water makes another excellent rinse that helps cut oiliness, adds David Daines, owner of David Daines Salon in New York City.

Take a powder. "If your hair is oily after a difficult, tense day, I suggest you do a temporary 'dry' shampoo by sprinkling a tiny amount of talcum powder

(I recommend Zeasorb-AF) onto your hair one section at a time. Rub the powder first onto the scalp, then through the hair with your fingers," says Karen E. Burke, M.D., Ph.D., a dermatologist and dermatologic surgeon in New York City. "The powder very effectively absorbs some of the oil." But be careful not to use too much powder or your hair will look white and dull, and you may even have difficulty with static electricity, making your hair difficult to style.

Oily Skin

Maybe your forehead shines a little. Okay, so maybe it shines *a lot*. There are many reasons for a facial gloss that resembles 10W-40 motor oil: hormones (particularly when you're pregnant), stress, the cosmetics you use and *especially* heredity.

But before you start chopping down your family tree, know there's some good news. Just as it protected your ancestors against the harsh weather, that excess oil can protect your skin from Father Time, helping you age more gracefully and wrinkle less than those with dry or normal skin.

Still, promises of future youth may not convince you to accept the oil of today. So if you want to change things a bit oil-wise, here's how.

Give your face a "tea" steam bath. "A good treatment for oily skin is to steam the face using some Swiss Kriss herbal laxative. Make a 'tea' by boiling about two tablespoons of Swiss Kriss in a big spaghetti pot filled with about two to three quarts of water," says Karen E. Burke, M.D., Ph.D., a dermatologist and dermatologic surgeon in New York City. "After you take the pot off the stove, place your head over the steam for about one to three minutes, then rinse your face with cold water." Doing this about once or twice each week opens pores and removes excess oils, says Dr. Burke. Swiss Kriss is sold in many health food stores.

Go synthetic. Oily skin should be cleansed at least twice daily, but use your fingertips, *not* stiff washcloths or polyester scrubs, advises Nelson Lee Novick, M.D., associate clinical professor of dermatology at Mount Sinai

School of Medicine in New York City. Use sensitive-skin cleansers labeled "synthetic," he suggests. The synthetic cleansers won't leave scummy deposits on your skin, as regular soap can. (The deposits can further clog your pores and contribute to oiliness.)

Mask yourself in mud. Clay or mud masks—available at most stores where beauty products are sold—offer temporary relief, adds Howard Donsky, M.D., associate professor of medicine at the University of Toronto and author of *Beauty Is Skin Deep.* Generally, the darker the color of the mud, the more oil it will absorb. White or rose-colored clays are best suited for sensitive skin.

Wipe yourself clean. If you have exceptionally oily skin, you can remove oil from your skin by gently blotting your face with soft tissues, advises Michael Ramsey, M.D., clinical instructor of dermatology at Baylor College of Medicine in Houston.

Cast the witch hazel spell. For extra punch, dab a little witch hazel on the tissues—it's one of the most effective oil absorbers for the money, according to Dr. Burke. But don't use rubbing alcohol, because it's too harsh.

Wash with hot water. Using hot water when you wash your face dissolves skin oil more effectively than using cool or tepid water, says Hillard H. Pearlstein, M.D., assistant clinical professor of dermatology at Mount Sinai School of Medicine.

Take a lesson from your child. The same products that teenagers use to clean their faces during those traumatic "acne years" are effective on your oily skin. (After all, acne is caused by clogged oil glands, among other factors.) When shopping, look for benzoyl peroxide gel, preferably in a low-strength (2.5 percent) formulation to minimize potential irritation.

Osteoporosis

As you age, your bones erode a bit. That's normal. But some people lose so much bone that their skeletons become riddled with weak spots. That's osteoporosis, and it causes a lot of hip, spine and forearm fractures. At its worst, bones become so frail that they crack under the body's own weight!

Anyone can get osteoporosis, but women are more likely to get it than men. They have lighter bones than men, and they lose bone rapidly after menopause, because their bodies are producing less estrogen. But men aren't immune, especially if they drink heavily, smoke or have taken steroid drugs.

But your bones don't have to crack under the strain of this disease. You can slow, stop or even reverse bone loss. For women, medical treatment with estrogen replacement therapy (ERT) is the most effective way to accomplish this. But even if you choose ERT, there are natural methods to help it along. (And not surprisingly, they're the same tips and techniques that can help *prevent* osteoporosis in the first place.)

If you want to step lively and stall bone loss, here are the tactics doctors recommend.

Build those bones. "We suggest, as a minimum, that people follow the American College of Sports Medicine recommendations to exercise aerobically for 20 minutes a day at least three days a week," says Miriam Nelson, Ph.D., an exercise physiologist and research scientist at the U.S. Department of Agriculture (USDA) Human Nutrition Research Center on Aging at Tufts University in Boston. Exercise actually stimulates bones to lay down new tissue, she explains.

What's the best aerobic exercise for strong bones? "It's one you will continue doing, because if you don't do it *for life,* the bone-building benefits fade," explains Dr. Nelson. In her studies, walking won top ratings—20 minutes a day three or four times a week—but you may prefer running, biking, swimming or aerobic dance classes.

Stop Training for the Olympics

An intense exercise training schedule that leaves a woman so lean that she stops having menstrual periods also robs her bones of necessary calcium. "This usually happens only with elite female athletes, but it can also happen with women who are obsessed with staying thin and who exercise several hours a day," says Christine Wells, Ph.D., professor of exercise science at Arizona State University in Tempe.

The solution: "Aim for quality, not quantity, when you exercise. Train hard, eat well, and maintain a weight that normalizes your menstrual periods," Dr. Wells recommends.

Walk in water. If you've already had a fracture or two, your best choice of exercise may be walking in chest-deep water, working up to 30 minutes at least three times a week, suggests Sydney Lou Bonnick, M.D., director of Osteoporosis Services at the Cooper Clinic in Dallas. The water will help support your body weight and take stress off bones and joints.

Make your "exercise equipment" a chair and the floor. To complement water walking, do some easy muscle-strengthening exercises in a chair or on the floor, suggests Mehrsheed Sinaki, M.D., a physiatrist in the Department of Physical Medicine and Rehabilitation at the Mayo Clinic in Rochester, Minnesota. Such exercises can include abdominal curls, shoulder blade squeezes and back extensions.

To do back extensions, lie on the floor on your stomach, with a pillow under your hips and your arms at your sides. Using only your back muscles, not your arms, raise your upper body a few inches off the floor. Hold for as long as comfortable, then relax downward. Work up to doing this six to ten times a day.

Chow down on calcium. Doctors agree that you should try to get 1,000 milligrams a day of calcium, even if you haven't reached menopause. And they suggest 1,200 to 1,500 milligrams a day for postmenopausal women who are not getting ERT.

Most women consume far less than those amounts. Reaching 1,000 milligrams through diet alone means drinking a quart of skim milk a day or eating two cups of low-fat yogurt or four cups of low-fat cottage cheese.

"Figure out, realistically, how much calcium you can get through your diet, then make up the rest with supplements," says Bess Dawson-Hughes, M.D., chief of the Calcium and Bone Metabolism Laboratory at the USDA Human Nutrition Research Center on Aging at Tufts.

Aim for maximum absorption. Spread your calcium supplements out over the day rather than taking them all at once, and take each one with a meal, Dr. Dawson-Hughes suggests. Most doctors recommend calcium carbonate, a relatively inexpensive source of calcium that's fairly well absorbed if taken in divided dosages and with meals.

Get enough vitamin D. For maximum protection, aim for 400 international units of vitamin D per day (twice the Recommended Dietary Allowance), especially if you don't get much sun, suggests Dr. Dawson-Hughes. "Here in Boston, we tell people they need a more reliable source of vitamin D than the sun, especially during the winter months."

A cup of milk contains about 100 international units of vitamin D, so four cups a day is ideal. But don't count on other dairy products, such as cheese, yogurt or ice cream, to fulfill your vitamin D needs. Unlike milk, these foods are *not* fortified with vitamin D.

Do not exceed the recommended dosage of 400 international units, however. Vitamin D is toxic in high amounts.

Graze far and wide. Bones are not made from calcium alone. They're an amalgam that includes zinc, boron and copper, among other minerals. "These trace elements are best gotten through a varied and broad-based diet that includes mostly unprocessed foods, such as whole grains, beans, fresh fruits and vegetables, fish and shellfish and lean meats," Dr. Dawson-Hughes says.

If you smoke, stop. "Smoking accelerates bone loss," Dr. Dawson-Hughes says. It speeds the rate at which the body metabolizes estrogen, virtually canceling out the bone-beneficial effects of ERT. "And smoking must have other bone-rattling effects, too, because it causes bone loss in postmenopausal women not taking estrogen and in men," she adds.

Monitor your medications. Some drugs can hasten bone loss, says B. Lawrence Riggs, M.D., president of the National Osteoporosis Foundation and professor of medical research at the Mayo Clinic.

Those most likely to cause problems: corticosteroids, which are prescribed for a variety of conditions such as rheumatic disorders, allergic conditions and respiratory disease; L-thyroxine, a thyroid medication; and furosemide, a diuretic often used against fluid retention associated with high blood pressure and kidney problems.

"Talk with your doctor about this possible side effect," Dr. Riggs suggests. "If you have other risk factors as well, your doctor may want to check your bone density and, if it's low, alter the dosage or stop the drug entirely."

Pass on the pop. Colas and some other carbonated soft drinks get their sharp taste from phosphoric acid, which contains phosphorus, a mineral that in excess amounts causes your body to excrete calcium.

Salt lightly. As with phosphorus, too much salt causes your body to excrete calcium. So go easy on the shaker, and check food labels. Avoid products with more than 300 milligrams of salt per serving.

Overweight

At this very moment, as many as half of *all* American adults are on a diet. Millions more are eagerly burning up calories with aerobics classes, clocking record mileage with walking or running or wearing out rowing machines and stair-climbers. All very serious enterprises when those extra pounds seem as though they're here to stay.

If you're among the more than one in three Americans who are overweight, you probably already know the keys to a slimmer body: a low-fat diet and regular exercise. But even with rice cakes and daily trips to the gym, those stubborn pounds may seem to stay around as long as deadbeat relatives on a long holiday. How come those pounds don't take a hint and *leave*?

Just wishing won't do the trick. But other methods will. Here's how you can speed up weight loss and make the most of your weight-control efforts.

Eat beans several times a week. "If you keep beans in your diet, you'll lose more weight, and you'll lose it faster," says Maria Simonson, Ph.D., Sc.D., professor emeritus and director of the Health, Weight and Stress Program at Johns Hopkins Medical Institutions in Baltimore. "That's because beans,

Beware of This Dieters' Trap

Dieters may actually *gain* weight while consuming "lite" foods and no-calorie sweeteners. How? When you think you're "saving" calories by choosing this diet fare, you may overeat other foods, according to Richard Mattes, Ph.D., of the Monell Chemical Senses Center in Philadelphia. An example: allowing yourself to have extra cookies because you "save calories" by using a sugar substitute in your coffee.

The trick to effective weight loss is to cut *total* calories and exercise regularly, says Dr. Mattes.

which are very low in fat and calories, give you a feeling of fullness that can last up to *four hours longer* than meals without beans." Naturally, the more full you feel, the less likely you are to eat.

Drink more water. It's no secret that water is an effective weight-loss tool, and the more water you drink, the more weight you lose. Drinking a glass of water whenever you feel hungry helps take the edge off "food cravings," which often are actually cravings for fluid, says George Blackburn, M.D., Ph.D., chief of the Nutrition/Metabolism Laboratory at New England Deaconess Hosptial in Boston. A glass before dining also helps you eat less.

Plan exercise around your meals. You probably know that aerobic exercise is essential to weight loss—even more important than diet, in fact, if you're over age 35. Still, many people don't know *when* to exercise to reap maximum benefits. The answer: light exercise after you eat.

Why? "A moderate workout after you eat uses just-consumed calories instead of storing them," says Bryant Stamford, Ph.D., director of the Health Promotion Center and professor of allied health at the University of Louisville School of Medicine in Louisville, Kentucky. He points out that when you avoid storing calories, you also avoid turning them into fat.

Dr. Stamford recommends an easy walk or other mild exercise *after* eating. You burn calories while digesting food, of course—but you'll *double* the calories burned if you get some exercise after the meal.

Lift weights to lower your weight. Although weight lifting has long been maligned as a second-rate fat burner (*aerobic* exercise takes the prize), new research indicates that the more muscle you have, the higher your metabolism rate. In fact, extra muscle makes your metabolism go up even when you're at rest.

Over the course of an 8- to 12-week weight-training program, you typically gain about three pounds of muscle. That extra muscle makes you burn an additional 250 calories a day, even when you're just sitting still, says Wayne Wescott, Ph.D., national strength-training consultant for the YMCA.

Make breakfast your biggest meal. Breakfast should *always* be your biggest and most caloric meal of the day. "You burn calories faster and more completely one hour after you wake up than at any other time of the day," says Dr. Simonson. She suggests that the single best dieting strategy is to eat a big meal before 9:00 A.M. every day, even if you aren't accustomed to eating a sizable breakfast.

Don't eat too *little.* Although many commercial diets call for 1,000 calories a day or less, experts say normal-weight women need *at least* 1,200 calories for long-term dieting success, and normal-weight men need about 1,500. Those calories are critical for good health.

A Secret of Dieting Success: Get a New Tablecloth

*P*ssst, dieters, pay attention to the colors in your dining room: Choosing the right hues may help weight loss.

"Color influences the process of eating much more in the overweight than the underweight," says Maria Simonson, Ph.D., Sc.D., a professor emeritus and director of the Health, Weight and Stress Program at Johns Hopkins Medical Institutions in Baltimore who *halved* her weight of 300-plus pounds before becoming a leading weight-loss researcher.

Her advice: "If you're overweight, get a tablecloth that's dark green, dark blue or coffee-colored brown, because it will help suppress your appetite." Painting your kitchen shades of dark blue, violet or green may also help.

And what has the opposite effect? Shades of orange, yellow and red tend to stimulate appetite and make us overeat—one reason why these are popular color choices in restaurants and most fast-food chains.

"Ultra-low-calorie diets very rarely work over the long term," says Wayne Callaway, M.D., associate clinical professor at George Washington University Medical Center in Washington, D.C., and a member of the U.S. Dietary Guidelines Advisory Committee. "From a biological point of view, people on ultra-low-calorie diets are 'starving.' " When your body is that deprived, he says, your metabolism slows down—so you're really undermining the success of your weight-loss plan. It's also very difficult for your body to get all the nutrients it needs.

Dine to Dvořák. Listening to classical or other "soft" music during meals results in more chews per minute, according to studies at Johns Hopkins Medical Institutions. "People who eat fast often get hungry again soon after eating," says Dr. Simonson. If you take longer to complete a meal, you'll feel fuller and *stay* feeling full for a longer time. "It's also easier to digest your food when you take longer to eat," she notes.

But stick to soft music: Hard-driving heavy metal and rock and roll can actually make you eat *faster!*

Seek out other pleasures. "A lot of people who think they want food really want pleasure, solace, comfort and relief from boredom," explains Howard Flaks, M.D., an obesity specialist in Beverly Hills and chairman of public relations for the American Society of Bariatric Physicians. "Food is only one of an infinite number of pleasures."

Dr. Flaks gives his clients a list of 150 pleasures to try instead, such as taking a hot bath, calling a friend, getting a pedicure or planning a fantasy vacation. His advice: Instead of reaching for food, give yourself another pleasure.

Panic Attacks

An upset stomach or chest pain could be this afternoon's lunch acting up. A racing heartbeat or shortness of breath could indicate you've exercised too much. Feeling "tingly" all over could suggest you're lucky at love.

The fact is, *any* of these symptoms could mean any number of things. But put them together—along with an almost uncontrollable feeling of impending doom—and it usually spells panic attack. Panic attacks are the primary symptom of panic disorder, which is one of the most common and more terrifying of all psychological disorders. These intense, unpredictable feelings of overwhelming anxiety and fear are so common that they affect an estimated 1 in 20 people.

Panic attacks vary in intensity and frequency, but they usually last from 5 minutes to an hour—averaging about 20 minutes. The typical sufferer gets them two to four times a week, but some people can get several in one day. "There are a lot of theories about what causes panic attacks: Some say it's genetic, others say it stems from childhood insecurity," says Christopher McCullough, Ph.D., a psychotherapist in Raleigh, North Carolina, and former director of the San Francisco Anxiety and Phobia Recovery Center. "But when you're having an attack, forget about insight and take care of the symptoms." Here's how.

Take a whiff of your childhood. Your nose knows—which is exactly why researchers urge you to sniff aromas that remind you of happy childhood memories. A sniff or two can almost *instantly* help curb fears and induce a more relaxed state—the first step in stopping a panic attack. "One odor that seems to work for just about everybody is baby powder," according to Alan R. Hirsch, M.D., a psychiatrist and neurologist who heads the Smell and Taste Treatment and Research Foundation in Chicago. "Other odors have similar impact, depending on where you were born. Research shows us that for people from the East Coast, it's the smell of flowers. For those from the South, it's fresh air; in the Midwest, farm animals; and in the West, the smell of barbecuing meat." Other anxiety-easing smells include salt air, fresh-baked chocolate chip cookies and Mom's home cooking.

Stay active. "Probably the *worst* thing you can do is what most people tell you to do when you're in a state of panic—sit down and relax," according to Dr. McCullough. "No matter what theory you have about the cause of panic attacks, at the point of the actual *attack,* it's a physiological event. It's all related to the sudden release of adrenaline—the fight-or-flight syndrome. So what you need to do is burn that adrenaline by exercising—taking a walk or moving around in some way."

Note: Studies show that people who practice a *daily* exercise program—rather than *just* when anxiety hits—bounce back faster in anxious situations.

Slow down your breathing. During a panic attack, you often hyperventilate—and that short and shallow gasping only adds to your state of fear. "You have to

Phobias: When Anxiety Goes Awry

Let anxiety go out of control and it can result in a panic attack. Let the fear of having a panic attack get out of hand and you're likely to develop a phobia.

"A phobia is an involuntary fear reaction that usually revolves around a particular place or situation and is so intense that a person will do almost anything to get out of it," says Jerilyn Ross, director of the Ross Center for Anxiety and Related Disorders in Washington, D.C., and president of the Anxiety Disorders Association of America. "The important thing to understand about phobias is that the anticipating anxiety is usually worse than actually being in the 'scary' place or situation. The way to treat phobias is to gradually approach the situation you're afraid of and stay there long enough that the frightening feeling will pass. At the same time, refocus your thinking to positive thoughts. Each time you do this, you reinforce the fact that although the feelings are frightening, they are not dangerous. And that gives you courage to face the situation the next time."

make a conscious effort to take long, deep diaphragmatic breaths," explains Dr. McCullough. To practice deep diaphragmatic breathing, try to keep your chest and shoulders in position while you slowly expand and contract your stomach area.

Count backward from 100. "The purpose is to focus on *something* specific such as counting or touching, but not on your anxiety," says Jerilyn Ross, director of the Ross Center for Anxiety and Related Disorders in Washington, D.C., and president of the Anxiety Disorders Association of America. "Counting backward, counting the stripes on the wall, snapping a rubber band—doing anything that takes your mind off your panic attack helps, because it refocuses your thinking. You pay attention to things around you, rather than trying to fight the anxiety."

Get a massage. Particularly on the back of your neck, around your throat and in your diaphragm area, advises Dr. McCullough. "Those are the three areas where you can tense up because of anxiety. Rubbing your neck helps relieve tension, which can soothe or possibly prevent a panic attack, while breathing deeply relaxes the diaphragm area." When massaging the neck, massage only one side at a time. (If you rub both sides too enthusiastically, there's a risk you may cut off your blood supply and become unconscious.)

Remember, it's just a passing phase. No matter how scary a panic attack is, it helps to remember that it's only a passing phase. "You need to remind yourself that what you're feeling are normal bodily functions that are happening at the wrong time, and they're not going to hurt you," says Ross. "You're not going to die from it. You're not going crazy. And it will be over soon."

Don't leave your situation. It's not advised to run to get *away* from your fears, says Fred Wright, Ed.D., director of education for the University of Pennsylvania Hospital's Center for Cognitive Therapy in Philadelphia. "Escaping" your environment during a panic attack encourages the development of phobia—an irrational fear reaction to the place or situation you were in when the panic attack hit. Many of the people who have panic attacks eventually develop phobias, such as fear of driving, because they associate the attacks with a particular object or situation, rather than trying to remedy the anxiety itself.

Switch to decaf. People who get panic attacks are often highly sensitive to caffeine, says Alexander Bystritsky, M.D., assistant clinical professor of psychiatry and director of the Anxiety Disorders Program at the University of California, Los Angeles. So if you're prone to panic attacks, try to limit your intake of coffee, tea, chocolate and colas that contain caffeine.

Paper Cuts

The pen is mightier than the sword"—at least according to playwright Baron Edward Bulwer-Lytton. But slice your finger on the edge of an innocent-looking piece of paper and . . . *yowwwwwww!* You'll learn firsthand of the awesome power of office supplies.

But here's what you can do about this skin-deep slice of life.

Use glue to renew. It's not exactly the kind of stuff they teach in medical school, but Krazy Glue, Super Glue or any other clear, super-strength bonder offers the fastest relief known to modern medicine. "It's really the best thing there is," says Rodney Basler, M.D., a dermatologist and assistant professor of internal medicine at the University of Nebraska Medical Center in Omaha. "It eliminates pain in about three seconds, because it immediately stops the air from hitting nerve endings—and air touching the nerves is what causes the pain. Just place a drop on the cut and repeat it the following day."

Although it "seals" instantly, a drop of this glue wears off in a day or so. Just be sure you don't touch something in the instant or so before it dries, because it does bond very quickly to whatever you touch.

Adds Nelson Lee Novick, M.D., associate clinical professor of dermatology at Mount Sinai School of Medicine in New York City: "These glues plasticize so quickly that they act as a sealant, so healing can take place while the finger is protected from air and germs. And they're completely safe, because a paper cut is so minor that they never enter the bloodstream." However, Elmer's and other white and yellow glues don't work this way.

Apply New-Skin. "A product called New-Skin, also available at your drugstore, stings a little but acts as a liquid dressing and is excellent for paper cuts," says Dr. Novick.

Feel serene with Vaseline. If you have no super-strength bonder or antibiotic ointment, apply some petroleum jelly (Vaseline) to the cut. "It acts as a coating that prevents air from getting to sensitive, exposed tissue," explains Dr. Basler. "It also provides a moist base, so new skin tissues can grow more easily than if you apply nothing."

Nail that pain with nail polish. In a pinch, dabbing some clear nail polish *after* cleaning the wound will also seal it against air and germs, adds Dr. Novick. However, it doesn't promote faster healing.

Paroxysmal Atrial Tachycardia

H^{uh?}

H That's right, *paroxysmal atrial tachycardia.* The name may escape you, but it's a condition that's estimated to affect as much as 40 percent of the U.S. population. And if you're among them, it's an experience you'll never forget: Your heart rate suddenly shoots upward to 220 beats a minute, and it feels like it won't slow down. You feel flushed and have body chills. You may also feel nauseated and dizzy and be almost overwhelmed by a sense of panic and doom.

Heart attack? It sure seems like it. But with paroxysmal atrial tachycardia, or PAT, there's no severe, viselike physical pain in the chest. And another important difference: PAT is *not* fatal.

It's basically a temporary internal "electrical malfunction" that throws the heart's pacemaking system out of sync, causing instantaneous rapid heartbeat and the sudden release of adrenaline. Your heart goes into "high gear" for up to 30 minutes. (If an episode lasts longer, seek *immediate* medical treatment.) "It's the same sort of fight-or-flight reaction you experience if someone sneaks up behind you and yells 'Boo!' " says James Frackelton, M.D., president of the American Institute for Medical Preventics in Cleveland and a PAT researcher.

And it can be scarier than a Freddy Krueger movie. But this is no nightmare on Elm Street, health-wise. PAT causes no significant tissue damage to the heart—despite a heart rate *three times* that of a normal resting pulse.

Still, the fear of recurrent bouts can be emotionally devastating and may be an early sign that heart-healthy people are stressing their bodies. If you've been diagnosed with PAT, here's what you can do to keep it under control.

Take it easy. "If you can control the stress and anxiety in your life, you're drastically cutting your risk of suffering an attack," according to Michael Crawford, M.D., chief of cardiology at the University of New Mexico School

When to See the Doctor

Although heart attack and paroxysmal atrial tachycardia (PAT) have similar symptoms, *any time* you feel chest pain you should take it seriously—particularly if you haven't already been told by your doctor that you have PAT. If you have any of these symptoms, seek emergency care.

- Intense chest pain that lasts 15 minutes or longer (this pain is often described as a feeling of heavy pressure)
- Pain that could, but doesn't necessarily, extend to the *left* shoulder and arm, back and/or jaw
- Prolonged pain in the upper abdomen
- Shortness of breath
- Feeling faint or fainting
- Nausea, vomiting and intense sweating along with the pain

of Medicine in Albuquerque and former chairman of the American Heart Association's council on clinical cardiology. Not surprisingly, studies show that PAT strikes hard-driving, Type A personalities who are easily touched off. So if that's your style, try taking things a bit slower.

Kill that killer instinct. Even during R and R, PAT can strike—especially if you take your playing too seriously and are up against stiff competition. "People notice attacks during competitive exercise, like during a game of tennis, whereas they wouldn't be as likely to get one when running by themselves," says Dr. Crawford. "It's that added factor of psychological stress that makes the difference."

Pass on that second cup of joe. Caffeine can trigger an irregular heartbeat, so some experts suggest that those with PAT limit their daily caffeine intake to about two cups of coffee or tea, says Dr. Frackelton.

Limit the booze, too. "If you drink, even if it's an *occasional* binge, you may experience symptoms," says Dr. Crawford. "I recommend no more than two glasses of beer, wine or mixed drink at a time."

Take a cold shower. Cold water helps slow down the heartbeat when you're feeling stressed or having an attack.

Cut down on calcium. PAT, like some other forms of arrhythmia such as irregular heartbeat, is sometimes treated with calcium-blocking drugs. "The theory among preventive medicine specialists like myself is that PAT can be triggered by excess calcium," adds Dr. Frackelton. "Eat less calcium and more magnesium and manganese, found in soy products, leafy vegetables and nuts. I advise eating more fruits and vegetables, but eat *twice* as many vegetables as fruits."

Go easy on flour and sugar. "Both can spark the release of adrenaline, triggering an attack," says Dr. Frackelton.

Stock up on potassium. Potassium helps "flush" excess sodium and other harmful substances from the body. It's abundant in fruit juices, raisins and sardines as well as in bananas and potatoes.

Passive Smoking

It's a hot topic: Smoking is now known to cause or contribute to scores of health problems, ranging from asthma and wrinkles to cancer and heart disease. And what really gets people burned up is *other* people's smoke, since research shows that you don't have to be a smoker to suffer harm from smoke inhalation.

In fact, breathing someone else's cigarette fumes—so-called passive smoking—often produces health hazards as bad as or even *worse* than the effects of puffing your own cigarette. That's because when you're standing or sitting next to a smoker, you inhale smoke from the burning tip of the cigarette, which contains *higher* concentrations of many toxic and cancer-causing chemicals than what the smoker gets inhaling through a filter. The National Academy of Sciences and the U.S. Surgeon General have concluded that nonsmokers are also at risk for lung cancer, heart disease and other problems caused by cigarettes, resulting in smoking restrictions or bans in many public buildings and workplaces.

But what can you do about it? According to Jack E. Henningfield, Ph.D., chief of the Clinical Pharmacology Branch of the Addiction Research Center at the National Institute on Drug Abuse in Baltimore, "There's only one answer: Get away and stay away from anyone who smokes."

Sometimes that's easier said than done. True, passive smokers have become more active in their stance against smokers, but you may still find yourself too close for comfort to a smoke-filled room. If so, here's how to limit your exposure when you're near smokers.

Designate a "smoking room" at home. If you live with a smoker, establish a designated area outdoors or set aside *one* room in your house for smoking. The preferable area is the best ventilated, and it's not a central meeting place such as the kitchen or family room, suggests Joan Belson, R.N., a smoking cessation specialist in Newton, Massachusetts. If the smoker keeps the door closed and windows open while smoking, it will eliminate some of the indoor air pollution that you and other family members would normally inhale. (Better yet, make your home smoke-free: Ask smokers to step outside.)

Speak up. Frankly but politely, ask the smoker to stop. This is a much more direct and appropriate response than waving your hands or grumbling—sending signals that smoking annoys you. Hand waving and grumbling usually cause the smoker to dig in his heels and continue puffing away. "People

What to Say When Someone Lights Up

Politely butting in and *asking* people around you to abstain from smoking in public places is the best way to get them to put out their butts and prevent them from lighting up again. Here are some lines suggested by Barry Lubetkin, Ph.D., a psychologist and director of the Institute for Behavior Therapy in New York City.
- "I would really appreciate it if you blew your smoke in another direction."
- "I know that you want to smoke, and that's fine, but could you please hold your cigarette in your other hand?"
- "We'll be leaving in a few minutes. If you can hold off smoking until then, I'd really appreciate it."

If you have no luck with those polite requests, bring in the heavy artillery: "Excuse me, I have trouble breathing, so I must ask you to put out your cigarette."

have the most resistance to change when others aren't completely frank around them," says psychologist Barry Lubetkin, Ph.D., director of the Institute for Behavior Therapy in New York City. "If someone just waves away the smoke but doesn't say anything, it gives the smoker a chance to disengage himself from responsibility for his act." But if you confront the smoker politely, he must take responsibility for what he's doing—and is more likely to stop smoking in your presence.

Or let your money do your talking. Give your business to restaurants and other public places where smoking is controlled or eliminated entirely. Your local chapter of GASP (Group against Smoking Pollution) and other non-smokers' groups usually have lists of these places. Or you can simply call a restaurant before going there, explain that you don't want to be exposed to cigarette smoke and ask for a table far from smokers. If the manager says there are no separate accommodations, it's fine to say you'll refrain from spending your money there until the policy changes.

And if you find yourself at a restaurant where you are bothered by smoke, do mention it to the waiter or manager. "If patrons don't say anything, restaurateurs think there's no demand for nonsmoking sections," says Regina Carlson, executive director of GASP in Summit, New Jersey.

Phlebitis

It's a pain in the leg—or both legs. That's how it begins, anyway. And when the pain doesn't go away, you probably want to pick up the phone and call the doctor.

Well, that's exactly the right thing to do, because anyone with the warning signs of phlebitis needs to find out as soon as possible which *kind* of phlebitis he has. And only a doctor can tell you that.

Phlebitis (the full name is *thrombophlebitis*) is an inflammation or blood clot in a vein, usually in the legs. There are two kinds. Deep-vein thrombophlebitis is the risky variety. It affects the veins that are deep beneath the skin (that explains the name), and it can be fatal if a blood clot dislodges from the vein

When to See the Doctor

If you have been diagnosed with superficial phlebitis, be sure to call your doctor if there's a sudden increase in pain or swelling, if you notice any lumps or if you develop a fever, suggests Robert Ginsburg, M.D., director of the Unit for Cardiovascular Intervention at the University Hospital in Denver and professor of medicine at the University of Colorado in Boulder.

Increased pain or swelling could be an indication of deep-vein thrombophlebitis, which requires immediate attention. Though it rarely happens, a blood clot could break loose and travel to the lungs. Prompt treatment may include hospitalization and medication with anticoagulants, prescribed drugs that prevent blood clots from forming.

Since fever may be a sign of infection, also see the doctor if you develop a higher-than-normal temperature. Infection can usually be cleared up promptly with antibiotics, but you'll need a physician's diagnosis and prescription.

and travels to the lungs. So doctors recommend immediate action if an exam turns up any warning signs of deep-vein phlebitis.

More often the problem is superficial thrombophlebitis, which means that you have some blockage in the superficial veins near the surface of the legs. Painful, yes—but not dangerous. Be ready to call the doctor again if you see any sign that it's getting worse. But in the meantime, there are many things you can do to ease the pain and reduce the worry associated with this problem.

The tips here should be used only by people who have been diagnosed with superficial phlebitis and are under a doctor's care. If that means you, here's what you can do to reduce your chances of another bout with pain, redness, tenderness and itching in your legs.

Take a load off. "Superficial phlebitis can be treated by elevating the leg and applying warm, moist heat," suggests Michael D. Dake, M.D., chief of cardiovascular and interventional radiology at Stanford University Hospital in Stanford, California. Keep legs elevated 6 to 12 inches above the level of the heart, and apply a heating pad to the affected area. In fact, it may help to keep your feet up all night long. You can elevate the foot of your bed several inches with wooden blocks.

Put the pressure on. Any kind of exercise, but especially walking, allows you to stay one step ahead of phlebitis. Muscular activity puts pressure on the veins, which helps empty them. Essentially, the walking motion helps prevent pooling of blood in the veins, says Robert Ginsburg, M.D., director of the Unit for Cardiovascular Intervention at the University Hospital in Denver and professor of medicine at the University of Colorado in Boulder.

Pop some aspirin. Besides reducing pain and easing inflammation, aspirin has blood-thinning properties, so it may reduce phlebitis by preventing rapid clot formation. For best results, take aspirin before prolonged periods of bed rest or travel, which are the times when your circulation is most sluggish. And if you're phlebitis-prone, your doctor may recommend aspirin before you have any kind of surgery.

But don't down the Pill. "If you've had a history of phlebitis or blood clots, you definitely shouldn't use oral contraceptives," says Jess R. Young, M.D., chairman of the Department of Vascular Medicine at the Cleveland Clinic Foundation in Cleveland. (The incidence of *deep-vein* thrombophlebitis in oral contraceptive users is estimated to be three to four times higher than in nonusers.)

And don't smoke. Another no-no is cigarettes, which can also cause recurring phlebitis in a more complicated circulatory condition called Buerger's disease.

Massage Can Be Dangerous

If you have phlebitis, you might be tempted to "massage away" the pain when you have a flare-up. But that's not advisable *unless* you have explicit permission from your doctor, according to Robert Ginsburg, M.D., director of the Unit for Cardiovascular Intervention at the University Hospital in Denver and professor of medicine at the University of Colorado in Boulder.

Massage can be dangerous for people who have superficial *or* deep-vein phlebitis, because you could dislodge a blood clot and cause a stroke or heart attack. So don't try hands-on healing without your doctor's blessing.

Think of zinc. If itching is a problem, a dab of zinc oxide in the bothersome areas can bring relief, according to Dr. Young. Zinc oxide is sold in most drugstores and doesn't require a prescription.

Sock it to yourself. Many phlebitis sufferers find that it helps to wear support stockings (the same kind used to treat varicose veins). The rule of thumb: If the stockings ease the discomfort, wear them. However, wearing support hose won't *prevent* a recurrence of phlebitis if you've had it before.

Ease your air travel. "On airplanes you tend to be confined to your seat a lot more than when traveling by car. So if you've had phlebitis, this is a case where you ought to put on your elastic stockings before boarding, then get out of your seat and walk up and down the aisle every half-hour or so after taking off," advises Dr. Young.

Pinkeye

If your overall health is in the pink, your eyeballs shouldn't be. But when you have an allergic reaction to something—pollen, cosmetics, chlorine in a swimming pool or even substances in the air—or when you come in contact with someone who has an eye infection, the white portion of your eyes can suddenly turn (*ugh!*) the color of Malibu Barbie's Corvette. As if that weren't bad enough, your eyes can be itchy and irritated; in some cases, there may also be a discharge of pus or fluid around the eyes.

All because of conjunctivitis, or pinkeye, a highly bothersome but usually relatively harmless inflammation of the surface of the eye. Aside from your own allergic reaction, you can get pinkeye from irritants in your environment, such as chemicals, or as the result of casual contact with someone who's infected. So you can get pinkeye by using the same towel as someone who's infected or even by touching the person's hands and then rubbing your eyes. That's one reason why conjunctivitis is especially common in children. Usually the inflammation will disappear on its own within 48 hours. But here's how to quicken your recovery and ease your discomfort.

When to See the Doctor

If you *still* can't see the whites of your eyes after two or three days of self-care, then shoot right over to your eye specialist. When caused by a virus, pinkeye is rarely serious. But when caused by bacteria, pinkeye can damage the eye if not treated quickly with antibiotics.

If for some reason you can't get to the doctor immediately, it's a good precaution to use an over-the-counter antibiotic ointment such as Polysporin (but still see a doctor as soon as possible).

If your symptoms include blurred vision, pain or "halos" around lights, see an ophthalmologist promptly, says Merrill M. Knopf, M.D., an ophthalmologist in Long Beach, California, and an officer of the California Association of Ophthalmology. These are not symptoms of pinkeye and could be something much more serious.

Don't cover your eye. Covering your sore eye is perhaps the *worst* thing you can do when you have pinkeye. "Putting a covering or patch over the eye—which, believe it or not, is actually a fairly common practice—raises the temperature of the eye, and those little buggers causing conjunctivitis grow faster in a warm environment," says Merrill M. Knopf, M.D., an ophthalmologist in Long Beach, California, and an officer of the California Association of Ophthalmology. "Besides that, a patch interferes with the flushing mechanism of tears, which removes the waste products. It's much better to leave the eye exposed."

Try two minutes of shut-eye. If you use over-the-counter eyedrops to soothe the itch, keep your eyes shut for at least two minutes after applying the drops, suggests Major William White, M.D., oculoplastic surgeon at Brook Army Medical Center at Fort Sam Houston in San Antonio, Texas. That's because when your eyes remain open, you blink—and blinking can wash away medication. But use eyedrops sparingly: Using them for more than three days can be counterproductive and can actually *induce* redness.

Apply a compress. Place a warm compress over your eye for ten minutes three or four times a day to soothe your inflamed peeper, suggests Robert Petersen, M.D., director of the Eye Clinic at Children's Hospital in Boston. Covering the eye briefly does *not* mean leaving on the compress. But if your

Remove Contact Lenses
at the First Sign of Pinkeye

People who wear contact lenses are, in general, more susceptible to eye problems than people who don't. But besides being more likely to get conjunctivitis, they also face more serious problems because of it.

"If you wear contact lenses, remove them at the very first sign of conjunctivitis," warns Merrill M. Knopf, M.D., an ophthalmologist in Long Beach, California, and an officer of the California Association of Ophthalmology. "People who wear contacts can get serious cornea infections from pinkeye. In some rare cases, it can lead to blindness."

His advice: "Think of your eyes like the warning light on your car: When you first notice they're red, get your lenses out as soon as possible."

eye itches and a warm compress doesn't work, Dr. Knopf suggests trying a cool compress.

Wash your hands—again and again. "Soap kills bacteria and viruses that cause pinkeye," notes Dr. Knopf. "Wash your hands as often as you can to prevent aggravating your own case and prevent spreading it to others." Frequent washing is important, because people touch their eyes more often than they might suspect.

Get grown-up help with baby shampoo. Although *not* advised for children, here's a solution for adults with a lot of discharge: Make a solution of one part baby shampoo to ten parts warm water. Dip a sterile cotton ball in the solution, and while keeping the eye closed, use it to clean off crusty eyelashes, advises Peter Hersh, M.D., chairman of ophthalmology at the Bronx-Lebanon Hospital Center in New York City. Another alternative for adults is an over-the-counter product called Eye-Scrub that works the same way.

Pizza Burn

B ite into a slice of steaming hot pizza and . . . *yow!* That nasty burn you get on the roof of your mouth could make you consider take-out Chinese next time.

It's an agonizing encounter: Searing hot cheese meets the tender parts of your upper palate. What you can expect are a blistering lesion, moderate pain that lasts for about a week and sometimes a loosened piece of flesh that hangs down from the roof of your mouth. The symptoms are so typical that this condition has made it into the pages of authorative medical journals as—what else?—"pizza burn."

But actually, pizza is only one of the hot foods that can burn. The tissue on the roof of your mouth is only millimeters thick. Just about any food or drink that retains heat well—any melted cheese dish, many soups and sauces, beverages like tea and hot chocolate, even *hot* hot fudge topping—can damage that tissue and cause swelling. Until recently, these other culprits have been bit players in this oral drama. Pizza was the main villain. But now, in the age of the microwave, any hot food can produce a sneak attack.

So here's what to do if you singe your mouth.

Ice it. "Put an ice cube in your mouth immediately to neutralize some of the tissue reaction," suggests Fred Magaziner, D.D.S., a spokesdentist for the Academy of General Dentistry and host of "Open Wide—A Look at Dentistry," a Baltimore TV talk show about dental care. "Besides lessening some of the pain, it will reduce the chance of any additional swelling and irritation. That's why it's also a good idea to never bite into pizza without a cold drink handy."

Gargle with salt water. "I recommend frequent saltwater rinses—every hour or so if you can manage," says Bernard Dishler, D.D.S., a dentist in Elkins Park, Pennsylvania. "Make your own rinse of ½ teaspoon of salt mixed with eight ounces of warm water to promote the healing process."

When to See the Doctor

Do nothing and pizza burn will heal on its own in a week to ten days. But if you have an ache or pain on the roof of your mouth that doesn't go away, see your dentist. It could be a problem that's unrelated to hot food.

"The lesion caused by pizza burn can mimic the early stages of cancer of the mouth," says Allen R. Crawford, Jr., D.M.D., a dentist in Macungie, Pennsylvania. A dentist who is trying to tell the difference will probably ask you how long you've had the pain, according to Dr. Crawford. "Pizza burn usually doesn't last beyond ten days and rarely lasts past two weeks."

Avoid "sharp" foods. That means sharp in taste and in edges. "Spicy foods, particularly Italian, will increase the pain from an existing pizza burn and may trigger infection," says Allen R. Crawford, Jr., D.M.D., a dentist in Macungie, Pennsylvania. "You'll also want to avoid potato chips and other foods with sharp edges, which will aggravate the lesion."

Head for the drugstore. "A product called Orabase, which is available over the counter, is a pectin ointment that sticks to wet tissue to protect the lesion from the heat you eat—particulary spicy foods," says Dr. Magaziner. Apply Orabase directly on the burn to protect as well as heal.

Drink plenty of milk. "Milk provides a mild coating that protects the lesion slightly," adds Dr. Crawford.

Let microwaved foods "sit." Foods prepared in microwaves cook unevenly, so the outside and inside may be different temperatures, says Dr. Magaziner. "Most people get burned because they don't do what you're supposed to do with microwaved food."

And what should you do? "Let the food sit in the microwave for two minutes after the buzzer rings before you eat it," advises Dr. Magaziner.

Plantar Warts

They're small, usually less than ¼ inch, but they can be larger. They're slow, often taking months to spread—or even be *noticed*. But plantar warts pack a painful punch.

Plantar warts are caused by a virus that invades the skin through a microscopic cut or abrasion on the sole of the foot. And then they grow inward—*under* the skin. The pressure of your weight flattens them until they are covered by a callus that sometimes has tiny black dots on the surface. As you walk around, the callus hardens under pressure, and the harder it gets, the worse it feels. When a plantar wart reaches maximum foot-torture stage, it feels as though you're stepping on a tack.

More bad news: Plantar warts are very difficult to treat, because the virus often lies dormant for several months before it reappears. Your podiatrist may wind up having to burn it off with a laser, freeze it off with liquid nitrogen or cut it off with his trusty scalpel. But first . . . try these do-it-yourself treatments when trouble's afoot.

When to See the Doctor

Before you treat a wart, make sure that it *is* a wart—not a corn, callus, mole or cancerous lesion. "Normally you'd think it would be pretty easy to identify a wart, but it's amazing how many people end up treating skin cancers or other growths as warts," observes Alvin Zelickson, M.D., clinical professor of dermatology at the University of Minnesota Medical School in Minneapolis.

So if you have the slightest doubt about what you're dealing with, see a doctor.

Give it the corn treatment. "You can use commercial corn remover preparations," says Stephen Weinberg, D.P.M., a podiatrist who specializes in sports medicine at Columbus Hospital in Chicago. The acid in the corn remover irritates the wart and causes it to go into remission. Look for a product, such as Duofilm, that contains salicylic acid.

Avoid them with cleanliness. "Practicing good hygiene is probably the best way to avoid getting plantar warts in the first place," says Robert Diamond, D.P.M., a Pennsylvania podiatrist affiliated with Muhlenberg Hospital Center in Bethlehem and Allentown Osteopathic Hospital. "Since they're caused by a virus, they are passed by contact. So if you're using public showers or walking barefoot in any public area, wash your feet afterward and wear thongs."

Poison Plants

Who else but prolific Mother Nature could provide us with itches in triplet form—poison ivy, oak and sumac? These three plants are annoying as all outdoors to an estimated 50 million people each year. At least half of the U.S. population has some allergic reaction to this trio. In fact, this is the most common allergy known to humans.

The wicked itch and bothersome rash of these "poisons" are caused by urushiol oil, a light, colorless or slightly yellow oil, one of the world's most potent toxins. A mere one-billionth of a gram is enough to cause sensitive folks to scratch themselves silly. And far more than one-billionth is released whenever the plant is "bruised," which happens *any* time there is direct contact with the leaves, stems or roots.

The potency of urushiol oil lasts about five years, so you can get a reaction from handling unwashed garden tools that were used to dig up poison ivy years earlier. But the oil does wash away. So if you wash yourself and your garden tools with soap and water within 15 minutes after contact, you can help avoid a later rash. Applying calamine lotion and taking oatmeal baths are probably the best-known cures once you've been exposed, but here are some other ways to rush the rash and nix Mother Nature's mother of all itches.

Know Your Poison Plants

Poison ivy usually grows east of the Rocky Mountains as either a vine or a shrub. Its leaves are in clusters of three, and it has white berries.

Poison sumac grows in southern swamps and northern wetlands. It's a tall shrub with 7 to 13 small leaves per branch and cream-colored berries.

Poison oak grows west of the Rockies, usually as a shrub or small tree but sometimes as a vine. It has yellow, "hairy" berries as well as hair on the leaves and trunk.

Have a milk soak. "A compress with ice-cold milk helps dry the rash and soothe the itch," says John F. Romano, M.D., a dermatologist and clinical assistant professor of medicine at The New York Hospital–Cornell Medical Center in New York City. "Just soak milk in gauze and apply it to your skin." *Note:* Whole milk seems to work; skim milk doesn't have the same effect, though doctors aren't sure why. Also, since milk can leave skin smelling "sour," be sure to rinse yourself off with cool water after each application.

Rub on baking soda. "If your rash is blistering or weeping, make a paste of water and baking soda and apply it to the skin," advises dermatologist Rodney Basler, M.D., assistant professor of internal medicine at the University of Nebraska Medical Center in Omaha. "This helps dry up the oozing blisters." If the area itches without blistering, however, the baking soda paste won't have much effect.

Enlist help from M.O.M. "Although it's not made for this purpose, milk of magnesia can relieve poison ivy itch as well as calamine lotion," according to Dr. Romano. That's because anything alkaline usually helps relieve itch, and milk of magnesia is alkaline. And since it's a thinner solution than calamine, it's easier to apply, Dr. Romano points out.

Try a dose of deodorant. The U.S. Forestry Service asked William Epstein, M.D., professor of dermatology at the University of California, San Francisco, School of Medicine, to come up with an inexpensive way to protect forest rangers from poison ivy. He found an unusual answer: spray deodorant. Aluminum chlorohydrate and other agents in spray deodorants prevent oils in

---

A Rash of Rumors

Misconceptions about poison ivy, oak and sumac are almost as widespread as the plants. Let's set the record straight.

- Myth: Poison ivy is contagious. Fact: Rubbing the rashes won't spread poison ivy to other parts of your body (or to another person). You spread the rash only if urushiol oil—the sticky, resinlike substance that causes the rash—has been left on your hands.
- Myth: You can get poison ivy simply by being near the plants. Fact: Direct contact is needed to release urushiol oil.
- Myth: Leaves of three, let them be. Fact: Poison sumac has 7 to 13 leaves on a branch, although poison ivy and oak have 3 leaves per cluster.
- Myth: Don't worry about dead plants. Fact: Urushiol oil stays active on any surface, including dead plants, for up to five years.

---

poison ivy from irritating the skin. So in a pinch, spraying arms and legs with a deodorant can help protect you. But Dr. Epstein notes that there are commercial products that work better.

Stop the itch with ice. "By far the cheapest effective remedy once you have contracted poison ivy is to apply an ice cube to the affected area for about one minute," says Dr. Romano. "The ice cools the itch." If you don't have any ice cubes, it helps to run cold water over the areas.

Zap it with zinc. Although it's not the most effective choice, zinc oxide, according to some experts, helps soothe itching and may help dry the rash. An inexpensive, over-the-counter skin ointment best known as the stuff lifeguards wear on their noses, zinc oxide is one of the active ingredients in calamine lotion.

Learn not to burn. Don't try to rid your backyard of poison ivy by burning it. That releases droplets of urushiol oil, which can be inhaled and cause serious damage to your lungs. Instead, dig it up—roots and all—and dispose of it in a sealed container. Then wash yourself, your clothes and your tools thoroughly.

Go commercial. To help prevent another attack, there are several over-the-counter poison ivy repellents such as Ivy Shield, which is sold in most drugstores.

Poor Posture

Sure, some kids act like know-it-alls, but who would suspect them of knowing about good posture? Even toddlers display perfect posture—naturally, according to Bill Connington, board chairman and president of the American Center for the Alexander Technique in New York City, where people are taught to develop greater ease, grace, flexibility and freedom from strain in their daily physical activities.

"Children use their joints well, and there's a wonderful sense of flow and freedom that lasts until the age of four or five," observes Connington. "Then they begin to imitate whoever is around them."

And that's not such a great thing, says Connington. Their movements become more restricted, and they pick up habits such as hunching over a desk or a dinner table. These habits can last for life and can lead to back problems.

But like any habit, bad posture can be broken. Connington recommends that you simply study and imitate small children in your daily routine. With this in mind, try the following tips for better body alignment.

Stand tall, but not straight. "Once people realize that they have problems with their posture, they tend to think 'Oh, I have to stand up straight.' They pull themselves up, pushing their shoulders and head back," says Connington. "Because this position is so uncomfortable, within a few minutes they fall back to their old habits." So relax: Good posture should be natural, not ramrod stiff.

Get motivated. "Good posture is really a matter of motivation," says Christa Farnon, M.D., associate director of Occupational Medical Services for SmithKline Beecham, a pharmaceuticals company in King of Prussia, Pennsylvania. "For instance, if an adolescent wants to stand tall, she will." When you find yourself slouching, remind yourself that better posture will make you appear more attractive, and self-confidence will naturally follow.

Exercise for Better Posture

Sometimes improving your posture is simply a matter of gaining flexibility and relaxing your muscles. To improve your balance and to limber your shoulders, neck and back and relieve back and neck strain, try these exercises recommended by Patricia Hammond, a yoga instructor and director of the Sarasota Center of the American Yoga Association in Sarasota, Florida.

Do a balancing act. Try this simple technique for improving your balance and posture. Starting on your hands and knees, breathe in and slowly raise your right arm and left leg until they are in line with your back and directly parallel with the floor. Look forward as you hold your position and breathe in, then lower your arm and leg, breathing out. Repeat with your left arm and right leg. Do three repetitions, alternating sides.

Stretch for better posture. Start by lying on your back with both arms resting on the floor over your head. First reach upward with your right hand, as if you were stretching to grasp something overhead. At the same time, push down with your right foot, keeping the foot flexed. Repeat with the left side. Then stretch your left hand and right foot; next stretch your right hand and left foot. Remember to keep your foot flexed during the sequence of exercises.

Try a sun pose. Once you have mastered the other exercises and are reasonably limber, try this more challenging one, called the sun pose. Stand straight, with your hands clasped behind your back. Straighten your arms and pull them away from your body. Breathe in deeply, then exhale slowly, bending at the hips and flexing your arms up and away from your back. Exhale as you are bending forward. Hold the bent position for a second or two, then breathe in slowly as you come up. Repeat this exercise three times.

Tune up your upper muscles. Strong upper body muscles are an essential part of lifelong good posture. Dr. Farnon suggests a planned program of weight-bearing exercises to build muscles in your upper body and give you more strength and better back protection. Those exercises also ensure better posture in the future: With more exercise, you deposit more calcium in your bones, which helps prevent osteoporosis.

Toss the heels. High heels are a major cause of swayback in women, according to Dr. Farnon. "Heels really throw off your balance, because they prevent your pelvis from staying where it should, which is in line with your shoulders." Save your back by opting for low-heeled shoes.

Rest one leg. "When you have to stand for long periods of time, it is important to get one foot up," says Margaret Fankhauser, D.O., associate professor in the Department of Physical Medicine and Rehabilitation at Michigan State University in East Lansing and medical director of a rehabilitation unit at Lansing General Hospital. When you stand completely straight, you get some curve in your lower back, she says. By raising one foot, you tend to straighten that curve. Rest one foot on the edge of the bathtub while you are brushing your teeth or on the floor of an open cupboard while you are cooking. If you are waiting in line, put one foot up on a curb or step if one is available. These simple techniques will help take the pressure off your back.

Choose your chair carefully. "It is important to find a chair that supports your lower back," says Deborah Caplan, a physical therapist and a founding member of the American Center for the Alexander Technique. "If you sit all the way in the back of the chair, you should have support for the normal curves of your back." Look for chairs and pillows that offer lumbar support, available at drugstores, surgical supply stores and some department stores.

Postnasal Drip

Some mucus is always gliding effortlessly down the back of your throat, but what happens when that normal trickle turns into Chinese mucus torture—the steady drip you know (and dread) as *postnasal*?
You hack. You ahem. You swallow. You snort.
In short, you suffer.

Some causes of postnasal drip are well known, such as colds and allergies. A less recognized cause is aging, when mucus turns a bit thicker and more obtrusive. So much for the causes. How about the cures?

Water down your woes. "You want to keep that mucus as thin as possible," says Alexander C. Chester, M.D., clinical professor of medicine at Georgetown University Medical Center in Washington, D.C. Steaming your nose in a hot shower or sauna, drinking a lot of water and humidifying the air will lighten the load on your nose and throat, he says.

Squirt in some salt and soda. Saline sprays or drops will help flush away excess nasal secretions, says Gailen D. Marshall, Jr., M.D., Ph.D., assistant

Postnasal Drip: A Gut Reaction?

We've all seen a faucet that drips down the drain, but how do you visualize a drip that goes up? What we sometimes think is that postnasal drip actually is bubbling up from the belly.

"I've seen many people undergo numerous surgeries for postnasal discharge, and they still have the problem," says Mark Loury, M.D., assistant professor in the Department of Otolaryngology/Head and Neck Surgery at Johns Hopkins University Hospital in Baltimore. "That's because the secretions are usually coming not from above the mouth but from below."

Thanks to a leaky valve separating your esophagus from your stomach, saliva, food and digestive enzymes may gurgle up your throat into the back of your mouth, a condition called gastroesophageal reflux. You may vomit a little or at least have a sour taste in your mouth when it is severe.

But more often a patient will complain of a dry, nonproductive cough, throat clearing, occasional hoarseness and a drip sensation in the throat area. "Because they may have the feeling it's coming from the nose," explains Dr. Loury, "many people think it's postnasal drip."

Fatty foods, alcohol and caffeine all encourage reflux, as does a large meal. When you do overindulge or feel that reflux feeling, reach for a Tums, Dr. Loury advises. Taking an antacid about 30 minutes after eating and then again before going to bed eases the symptoms.

professor and director of the Allergy and Clinical Immunology Division at the University of Texas Medical School at Houston. In eight ounces of water, dissolve ¼ teaspoon of table salt and ¼ teaspoon of baking soda. Use a nosedropper to squirt about half of the solution up your nose, he advises.

Give your throat a saline swish. Once you've rinsed out your nostrils, gargle with the remainder of the saline solution. "That will soothe a scratchy throat and help eliminate the drainage sensation," Dr. Marshall says.

Get a rise out of lying down. If you notice the sensation of secretions in your throat at night, try raising the head of the bed by putting a few books under the legs of the headboard. (Be sure the bed will remain steady.) The drip won't pool in the back of your throat, and any stomach contents that might be creeping up your throat will drain back to where they belong, says Mark Loury, M.D., assistant professor in the Department of Otolaryngology/Head and Neck Surgery at Johns Hopkins University Hospital in Baltimore.

Don't scoff at a cough cure. Over-the-counter anticough preparations such as Robitussin and Vicks Formula 44 also thin the mucus, explains Horst R. Konrad, M.D., chairman of the Division of Otolaryngology/Head and Neck Surgery at Southern Illinois University School of Medicine in Springfield. These preparations will at least allow your mucus to take a smoother ride down your throat.

Premature Ejaculation

For men who experience premature ejaculation, lovemaking can be bad news. The good news, though, is that premature ejaculation—the most common sexual problem among men—is also the easiest to cure.

"With the right treatment, the cure rate for premature ejaculation is near 100 percent," says Sheldon Burman, M.D., founder and director of the Male Sexual Dysfunction Institute in Chicago, the country's largest treatment center for male sexual problems. More good news: The right treatment is usually painless, inexpensive and relatively easy.

Premature ejaculation is usually easy to identify: It means that a man reaches orgasm too soon. "If you *and* your wife think you're too fast, then you're a premature ejaculator," says Dr. Burman. Here's how to delay ejaculation for more satisfying lovemaking.

Practice makes perfect. "The simplest thing to do if you're a premature ejaculator is to have sex more often," says J. Francois Eid, M.D., director of the Erectile Dysfunction Unit at The New York Hospital–Cornell Medical Center in New York City. "For one thing, you're more likely to ejaculate prematurely if there's a long gap between sexual sessions. Besides, most men find they perform better with practice. You learn more about your body and your limitations."

Try the "stop-start" approach. This technique involves stimulating the penis almost to the point of ejaculation, then stopping; stimulating it again, then stopping; and repeating this until you learn to control your ejaculations, says Oakland, California, psychologist Bernie Zilbergeld, Ph.D., author of *The New Male Sexuality*.

Do Kegel exercises. The same pelvic muscle strengthening that women practice to hold their urine after childbirth can help men delay ejaculation, reports Dr. Zilbergeld. To perform Kegel exercises, simply contract your buttocks for one second as though you were trying to delay a bowel movement. Do this 15 times in a row, working up to 60 to 75 contractions twice a day. The purpose of Kegels is to strengthen your pelvic muscles so that you can contract or relax as you near orgasm, delaying ejaculation. (Some men last longer when squeezing the muscles, and others, when relaxing them.)

Do your bodybuilding later. While exercise is part of a total healthy lifestyle that can prevent or reverse premature ejaculation, it's unwise to exercise just before sex, according to Dr. Burman. "Whenever you exercise, the body directs blood to that group of muscles. For instance, if you do bicep curls, blood will be directed to your arm muscles—and away from your penis. So save your exercise for another time."

Reverse position. "Men are most easily aroused when they are on top in the missionary position, so it might be best for her to be on top," says Dr. Burman. "When a woman is on top, you can control her motion by guiding her hips. That way, if you become too aroused, you can guide her to slow down or stop her movements."

Diet for better sex. Premature ejaculation is often due to physical changes in the body. Men over age 30 may begin to have problems with premature ejaculation even though their sex lives were fine when they were younger.

"The problem is often an inadequate blood supply in the penis," according to Dr. Burman. When the arteries in the penis become partially clogged with fat and cholesterol, maintaining an erection becomes more difficult. "When this occurs, your brain tells your body that you'd better ejaculate before you lose your erection, and a pattern for premature ejaculation is developed," says Dr. Burman.

His recommendation: Live a healthy lifestyle in order to maintain good arterial health. "Your potency will be prolonged if you eat a low-fat, low-cholesterol diet, exercise regularly, don't smoke and keep your stress managed," says Dr. Burman.

Premenstrual Syndrome

S ugar and spice and *everything* nice? What about breast pain, bloating, weight gain and acne? Or cramping, headaches, food cravings and mood swings? When it comes to describing that aspect of womanhood known as premenstrual syndrome (PMS), *nice* isn't exactly the first word that pops to mind.

Common might be the word that better describes this complex of problems brought on by fluctuating hormone levels. About half of all American women between the ages of 20 and 50 have PMS, and upward of nine in ten women may experience at least some of its symptoms. But even though PMS brings on many kinds of discomfort, luckily there are also plenty of treatments.

Finding the best ones for you, however, may take some experimenting. PMS seems to be affected by stress, doctors say, and they agree that diet may be a large factor. So if the up-and-down symptoms of PMS are all too familiar, you might begin by looking at what's on your menu.

Get the saturated fat off your plate. Eating a lot of fatty foods will increase PMS symptoms and pain, according to Guy Abraham, M.D., a PMS researcher in Torrance, California, and former professor of obstetrics and gynecologic endocrinology at the University of California, Los Angeles. It helps to avoid fatty cuts of beef, lamb and pork. Better yet, substitute poultry and fish. And replace butter (which is high in saturated fat) with polyunsaturated oils such as flaxseed, corn and safflower, suggests Dr. Abraham.

Go without salt. "People don't realize that foods with a high salt content can contribute to water retention," says Susan Lark, M.D., medical director of the PMS and Menopause Self-Help Center in Los Altos, California.

Most snack foods and other processed foods are high in salt—and some fast-food meals can be extremely high. So stay away from these foods if you're going on a low-salt diet, suggests Dr. Lark. Also, some boxed cereals and many condiments are higher in salt than many people realize. So read labels on

The Vitamin Cure

Some experts suggest eating certain foods high in key vitamins and minerals to avoid symptoms of premenstrual syndrome (PMS).

Here's an overview.

Do your skin a favor with vitamins A and D. This dynamic duo may play a part in suppressing premenstrual acne and oily skin, says Susan Lark, M.D., medical director of the PMS and Menopause Self-Help Center in Los Altos, California. Among the best food sources for vitamin A are raw carrots, cooked spinach, cooked sweet potatoes and fresh cantaloupe. Sunshine provides vitamin D, but you can also get this nutrient from fortified milk—and cereal.

Feel better with vitamin B₆. Increasing your intake of this B vitamin can help alleviate symptoms such as mood swings, fluid retention, breast tenderness, bloating, sugar craving and fatigue, says Dr. Lark. Supplements of 25 to 100 milligrams per day are well tolerated by most women. And be sure to eat foods that are high in vitamin B₆, including many kinds of fish and the white meat of chicken and turkey, in your diet. Potatoes and bananas also are good sources of vitamin B₆.

Try vitamin C to reduce stress and allergies. Vitamin C may help relieve the stress felt during PMS, says Dr. Lark. And since it's also a natural antihistamine, it can be helpful for women whose allergies worsen be-

packaged and processed foods, and whenever possible, choose fresh fruits and vegetables.

Counter the cravings with carbohydrates. Food cravings are common during PMS, and often those cravings focus on sweets and snacks such as ice cream, chocolate and potato chips. But you'll do yourself a favor if you can switch to other kinds of fare when you get the cravings.

"Eating complex carbohydrates such as whole grains, pasta, cereal and bagels is probably the best way to ward off food cravings experienced during PMS," says Dr. Lark. These foods also are a good source of fiber, which helps clear excess estrogen from your body, according to Dr. Lark. (High levels of the hormone estrogen have been shown to contribute to PMS.)

fore a period. You get good doses of vitamin C from vegetables such as broccoli, brussels sprouts and raw peppers. And many kinds of fruit and fruit juices are excellent sources, including cantaloupe, grapefruit, oranges, cranberry juice and citrus fruit drinks.

Relieve symptoms with vitamin E. This vitamin may have a powerful effect on the hormonal system, helping to relieve painful breast symptoms, anxiety and depression, says Guy Abraham, M.D., a PMS researcher in Torrance, California, and former professor of obstetrics and gynecologic endocrinology at the University of California, Los Angeles. Among the food sources of vitamin E are many of the oils used in cooking and in salad dressings, such as olive oil, safflower oil and corn oil, as well as a few fruits such as blackberries and apples.

Take calcium and magnesium to fight PMS. These two minerals work together, says Dr. Lark. Calcium helps prevent premenstrual cramps and pain, while magnesium helps the body absorb the calcium. Magnesium also helps control premenstrual food cravings and stabilize moods.

Skim milk is a good source of calcium if you are not lactose-intolerant. Other good food sources include green leafy vegetables, beans, peas and tofu as well as canned salmon. Good food sources of magnesium include spinach, tofu, rice bran and certain fish such as halibut and mackerel.

Eating high-carbohydrate, low-sugar foods provides another benefit as well, according to Judith Wurtman, Ph.D., a researcher at the Massachusetts Institute of Technology in Cambridge. She has found that cereal and other high-carbohydrate foods actually relieve the psychological symptoms of tension, anxiety and mood swings that accompany PMS.

Dr. Wurtman suggests having a heaping bowl of unsweetened cereal when you get hungry. (Reminder: Read the package label first, and choose a low-salt variety.) "It works like Valium," says Dr. Wurtman. In general, she has found, women who have PMS are more alert and happier when they eat high-carbohydrate foods rather than high-protein, low-carbohydrate foods.

Go for locomotion. When your mood takes a walk on the wild side, take a walk. "Exercising has been found to significantly reduce many physical and psychological PMS symptoms," says Ellen Yankauskas, M.D., director of the Women's Center for Family Health in Atascadero, California. That's because exercise releases endorphins, brain chemicals that ease pain and produce a sense of well-being. And in PMS sufferers, that means less crying and anxiety. Exercise has also been shown to help reduce breast tenderness, food cravings, fluid retention and depression.

"It's best to exercise at least three times a week, even when you don't have PMS," she says. "Walking is the exercise I recommend, because weight-bearing exercises help keep bones strong." She suggests going out for at least 12 minutes, though 30 minutes or more is even better.

Screen out foods with caffeine. If you happen to be caffeine-sensitive (and some people are more so than others), then you should avoid coffee, tea, colas and chocolate, according to Annette MacKay Rossignol, Sc.D., professor and chairman of the Department of Public Health at Oregon State University in Corvallis. Studies have suggested that the risk of PMS is between two and seven times greater in women who consume two or more cups of coffee or tea each day, according to Dr. Rossignol. Caffeine is a stimulant and can contribute to anxiety and irritability. Caffeine may also contribute to painful breast tenderness.

Read labels on pain relievers. Since caffeine can worsen PMS symptoms, you should make sure any pain relievers you take are caffeine-free. "You have to be a label reader," says Dr. Yankauskas. An over-the-counter pain reliever that contains caffeine can actually make your PMS symptoms worse.

Stay on the wagon. Alcohol is a depressant and diuretic that can worsen PMS headaches and fatigue and can accentuate depression, adds Dr. Yankauskas.

For this reason, it's advisable to avoid drinking any alcoholic beverages, including wine or beer, when you've been having trouble with PMS, according to Dr. Yankauskas.

Prostate Problems

Forget about those yearnings for red convertibles and shapely young blondes. The *real* midlife crisis occurs in a man's prostate, the gland that adds fluid to semen so that he can ejaculate. Four of every five men over age 50 develop an enlarged prostate—or, more specifically, a condition called benign prostatic hyperplasia (BPH). One-fourth to one-third of them will experience BPH's uncomfortable and potentially dangerous symptoms.

"BPH causes no pain, but it does make urination more difficult," says Stephen Rous, M.D., professor of surgery at Dartmouth Medical School and a urologist at Dartmouth-Hitchcock Medical Center in Lebanon, New Hampshire. Because the prostate surrounds the urethra, the tube that carries urine from the bladder, when it enlarges it restricts urine flow. This results in a need to urinate more frequently, often with increased difficulty getting started.

With prostate problems, you may also experience dribbling, because the prostate isn't as strong as it used to be and you can't urinate with the same force. Some men with this problem are unable to sleep through the night without waking to urinate, while others are completely unable to urinate—an emergency condition.

Surgery to remove the prostate is one alternative, and there are several medications—some of which take months to work—that can reduce an enlarged prostate and improve urination. But for tried-and-true *home* treatments, here's what the experts recommend.

Cut the caffeine. "Caffeine in any form—coffee, tea, chocolate or soft drinks—tends to tighten the bladder neck and make it more difficult to pass urine," says urologist Durwood Neal, Jr., M.D., associate professor of surgery, urology, microbiology and internal medicine at the University of Texas Medical Branch at Galveston. "Some of the prostate is made up of smooth muscle, and any-

417

When to See the Doctor

An enlarged prostate may cause difficulty urinating, but you shouldn't experience pain. "The only prostate condition that leads to pain or discomfort is prostatitis, a bacterial infection that is treated with antibiotics," says Stephen Rous, M.D., professor of surgery at Dartmouth Medical School and a urologist at Dartmouth-Hitchcock Medical Center in Lebanon, New Hampshire. If you experience painful urination, coupled with lower back pain, fever and pelvic pain, you may have a prostate or bladder infection. See your doctor.

Of course, it's wise for *all* men over age 50 to see their doctors to be tested for prostate cancer, a leading cancer among middle-aged and older men. And if you can't urinate at all, head straight to the emergency room: Urinary retention is extremely uncomfortable and can be life-threatening if left untreated.

thing that causes that muscle to constrict will make urination more difficult. Caffeine does this quite a bit."

Don't serve yourself. Alcohol also tightens the bladder neck to hamper urination. And since it's a diuretic, it increases the amount of urine that builds up inside the bladder, adds Dr. Neal. "Drinking alcohol also makes the bladder operate a lot less efficiently. And the more you drink, the more problems you'll likely have."

Give a cold shoulder to cold medicines. Antihistamines and decongestants can cause even more harm to some men. In fact, taking large doses of cold medications occasionally leads to urinary retention—a potentially life-threatening condition in which you completely stop urinating. "Decongestants cause the muscle at the bladder neck to constrict, restricting the flow of urine," says Peter Nieh, M.D., a urologist at the Lahey Clinic Medical Center in Burlington, Massachusetts. "And antihistamines simply paralyze the bladder."

If you have allergies as well as prostate problems, Dr. Nieh suggests you speak to your doctor about prescribing astemizole (Hismanal) or terfenadine (Seldane), two medications that have no antihistamines. If you must buy over-the-counter medication, take half of the suggested dose. If no problem ensues, move to the full recommended dosage.

Be wary of spicy foods. Spicy and acidic foods bother some men with enlarged prostates, says Dr. Neal. "If you notice more problems after eating salsa, chili or other spicy or acidic foods, then you're among those men—and you should avoid that cuisine."

Manage your stress. Perhaps the most underrated trigger is unmanaged stress. "Stress plays a major role in prostate-related discomfort, because the bladder neck and prostate are both very rich with nerves that respond to adrenal hormones," says Dr. Neal. "When you're under stress, there are more of those hormones floating around—causing more difficulty in urinating."

Stress also triggers the release of adrenaline in your body, prompting a fight-or-flight response. "Just as it's impossible to get an erection during the fight-or-flight response, it can make urination difficult, too," Dr. Neal adds.

Get more amour. One way urologists help ease urination problems is to massage the prostate. For men with mild to moderate voiding difficulties, an alternative may simply be to have more sex. "Many men notice that the more they ejaculate, the easier it is to urinate," says Dr. Rous. That's because ejaculation helps empty the prostate of secretions that may hamper urination.

Empty your bladder before you go to bed. "Many men get the urge to urinate in the middle of the night, and it can be a real problem," says Dr. Neal. "But if you limit your intake of beverages after 6:00 P.M. and make sure you urinate before going to sleep, you can eliminate much of this problem."

Flee south in the winter. If at all possible, spend winters somewhere in the Sunbelt. "In the urology trade, we usually say that summer is the season to pass kidney stones and winter is the time for urinary problems. I'm not exactly sure why, but people have more trouble urinating and are most likely to go into urinary retention during cold weather. Perhaps this is due to an increase in upper respiratory infections, which many men treat with over-the-counter antihistamines and decongestants. These further aggravate BPH," says Harold Fuselier, M.D., chairman of urology at Ochsner Medical Institutions in New Orleans. "Since an enlarged prostate already makes urinating more difficult, you'll do much better in a warm climate during cold weather."

Psoriasis

I f there ever was a medical condition that could convince Sherlock Holmes to get out of the business, it's psoriasis. The clues are obvious—after all, it's hard *not* to notice that maddening itch, the inflammation and those bothersome silvery scales that usually occur on the elbows, knees, trunk and scalp. But when it comes to finding its cause or cure, that's even more of a mystery than Watson's first name.

What *is* known about psoriasis is that it causes skin cells to go hyper. A normal skin cell takes about a month to mature, but in those with psoriasis, this process takes only three or four days. These skin cells are poorly developed, and they can't shed fast enough. Instead, they pile up—forming raised, scaly "plaques" that itch and leave skin below red and inflamed.

Psoriasis *isn't* contagious, but beyond that, researchers can't speak about the condition's causes with any degree of certainty. There may be a genetic link, however: In one in three cases, the disorder can be traced through the family, although it sometimes skips a generation. Also, doctors have observed that stress can spark new outbreaks (or make existing cases worse). Other suspected triggers include damage to the skin from injury, dryness or chafing and reaction to certain drugs and infections (such as strep throat).

But instead of the proverbial heartbreak, there is reason to take heart. While there's no cure as yet, you can *control* psoriasis and lessen its impact on your life. Your doctor has probably told you about tar shampoos and ultraviolet light treatments, but here are some other ways to keep those plaques from giving you flak.

Look for lactic. All our experts agree that the most important step in controlling psoriasis is to keep skin well moisturized. "A big problem with psoriasis is scale buildup, and moisturizers are extremely effective at preventing this," says Nicholas J. Lowe, M.D., clinical professor of dermatology at the University of California, Los Angeles, School of Medicine and director of the Skin Research Foundation of California in Santa Monica. "Plain petroleum jelly is a very effective moisturizer. But if you're buying a commercial moisturizer, those that contain lactic acid, such as LactiCare, seem to work better. Also, Eucerin cream works well as a moisturizer for those with psoriasis."

Moisturize after bathing. To get the most from your moisturizer, "apply it within three minutes after leaving the shower or bathtub," advises Glennis McNeal, public information director at the National Psoriasis Foundation headquarters in Portland, Oregon. "We recommend that you pat yourself dry and apply the moisturizer liberally all over your body—*not* just on plaques. That's because even 'clear' skin in people with psoriasis is drier than in people who don't have psoriasis. It's thought that little cracks on dry skin might encourage more psoriasis."

Soak up the sun. Many psoriasis patients are prescribed a specific regimen of ultraviolet light treatments. Getting artificial sunlight from a special lamp or tanning booth can help. An easier and less expensive method is simply to hit the Great Outdoors. "We know that exposure to sunlight is extremely helpful for treating psoriasis," says David Kalin, M.D., a family practitioner in Largo, Florida. A moderate amount of sunlight enhances the production of vitamin D, which may be effective in controlling psoriasis.

But don't soak up the booze. Doctors are still trying to find out for sure why alcohol exacerbates psoriasis. They suspect that alcohol increases activity of a certain kind of white blood cell that's found in psoriasis patients but not in other people. (But it's also possible that drinkers are just more highly stressed— and therefore more prone to psoriasis.)

"Alcohol is a definite problem," according to Stephen M. Purcell, D.O., chairman of the Department of Dermatology at Philadelphia College of Osteo-pathic Medicine and assistant clinical professor at Hahnemann University School of Medicine in Philadelphia. "It's best to *not* drink at all if you have psoriasis."

Spice up your bath. Bathing is often a catch-22 for those with psoriasis. That's because soaking in warm water helps soften psoriasis plaques, but it sometimes dries skin and worsens itching. "One way to get the benefits of a bath without the dryness is to add a couple of capfuls of vegetable oil to your bath," says McNeal. "The best way to do it is to get in the tub first, so your body soaks up the water, and *then* add the oil." Another alternative suggested by McNeal: Mix two teaspoons of olive oil in a large glass of milk and add that to your bath.

Be extra careful stepping out of the tub, since oils can make surfaces very slippery. (Be sure to scrub the tub afterward.)

Head to the kitchen to soothe that itchin'. To soothe itching caused by dry skin and psoriasis, dissolve ⅓ cup of baking soda in a gallon of water. Soak a washcloth in the solution, wring it out, and then it apply to the itchy area. Or add a cup of apple cider kitchen vinegar to the water and apply that to the skin.

Cover the cracks with cow cream. If your skin is cracked because of psoriasis—which can cause itching and more plaques—do what dairymen do. "They found that Bag Balm, a product originally used to relieve cracking in cow udders, worked just as well on their cracked hands," says McNeal. "Then people with psoriasis found it worked *great* on their dry or cracked skin." Bag Balm is available at most feed stores; some drugstores may be able to order it.

Take care of mind and body. Stress is a known trigger of psoriasis, so managing your mental state—through exercise, relaxation techniques or whatever mellows you out—is one way to keep your condition under control.

Guard against infection and injury. "Infection may lead to an outbreak or worsen your condition, so it's important to try to avoid infectious disease," says Dr. Kalin. New lesions may also appear on injured skin, so try to avoid cuts and scrapes.

Watch what you eat. "Although there are no specific links that have been proven, it appears a diet high in oily fish—such as tuna, mackerel, sardines and salmon—helps reduce the itching and inflammation of psoriasis," says Dr. Lowe.

Avoid certain foods. "Some anecdotal reports suggest patients do better when they reduce or eliminate tomatoes and tomato-based dishes—possibly because of high acidity levels," says Dr. Kalin. "Also, some of my patients with psoriasis have noticed a decrease in plaques by avoiding or limiting their intake of pork products and other fatty meats as well as caffeine."

Go electric. If you have plaques on your face, neck, legs or other areas that require shaving, use an electric razor instead of a blade. "An electric razor won't cut skin as easily, and every time you cut yourself, you risk new lesions," says dermatologist John F. Romano, M.D., clinical assistant professor of medicine at The New York Hospital–Cornell Medical Center in New York City.

Pulled Teeth

E ver wonder why those often-yanked molars are called "wisdom teeth"? Have them pulled and you'll soon question the wisdom of that decision. Actually, get *any* of your teeth pulled and you'll note the healing process has plenty of hurt—as well as its share of physical foolishness. Just look in the mirror and you may see cheeks as swollen as those of a Type A squirrel prepping for the winter. Here's how to pull the plug on the pain of pulled teeth.

Try hands-on healing. According to some doctors, there are "pressure points" on the body, and pressing on or massaging those areas can help relieve pain. "Massage either your earlobe or the area of your hand between your forefinger and thumb on the same side as your pain to bring relief," says Wistar Paist, D.M.D., a dentist in Allentown, Pennsylvania. "Gently massage that spot with your other hand for about 10 minutes. You should get relief in 15 or 20 minutes. If the pulled tooth is on the right side, rub your right earlobe or right hand; if the pain is on the left side, rub the left side." (You can also numb the area with a piece of ice instead of rubbing; the procedure is the same.)

Take vitamin C. Taking 1,500 milligrams of vitamin C daily (500 milligrams with each meal) can take a lot of the punch out of extractions, according to researcher Robert Halberstein, Ph.D., associate professor in the Department of Epidemiology and Public Health at the University of Miami in Coral Gables, Florida. He recommends those doses both *before* and *after* dental work.

"We found that people who take 1,500 milligrams of vitamin C daily—that's one 500-milligram tablet with each meal—for a couple of days *prior* to the extraction and then for a week afterward have a significantly faster healing process than those who don't take the supplements," says Dr. Halberstein. "Vitamin C speeds the healing process because it plays a major role in the

Curb Extraction Bleeding with a Tea Bag

A cool tea bag of any variety of tea containing tannic acid, such as green, black or oolong, can stop bleeding problems that often follow a tooth extraction.

"Just take a tea bag, soak it, and squeeze out most of the water," says dentist Wistar Paist, D.M.D., of Allentown, Pennsylvania. "Place the cool tea bag over the spot where your tooth was pulled, then bite gently. The tannic acid in the tea helps promote clotting, which will help stop your bleeding."

manufacture of collagen in the body, which is a protein material that's instrumental in forming scar tissue."

Bonus: Following this 1,500-milligram formula can reduce by *sevenfold* your chances of developing the painful inflammation of "dry-socket," which occurs in 1 of every 20 extractions.

Chill out . . . and then warm up. "Timing is very important in order to relieve the pain of a pulled tooth. For the first 24 hours after the extraction, place an ice pack (wrapped in a towel) on the area outside the mouth where the tooth was pulled in order to prevent swelling—20 minutes on and 20 minutes off in order to minimize the swelling and pain," says Nabil Abaza, D.M.D., Ph.D., professor of dental medicine and oral and maxillofacial surgery at the Medical College of Pennsylvania Hospitals, Main Clinical Campus, in Philadelphia. "But after the first 24 hours, switch to gargling gently with warm salt water. The heat soothes, and the salt water helps prevent infection and remove any food particles."

Swallow that pain reliever. Forget about placing aspirin directly on the socket to bring quick relief. "It's okay to swallow aspirin for the pain, but placing it directly on the gums causes a terrible irritation on the tissues," says Dr. Paist. If you're sensitive to aspirin, try swallowing ibuprofen (Advil) or acetaminophen (Tylenol). Also, don't give aspirin to children because of the risk of Reye's syndrome.

Don't wait too long to get help. The longer you wait before getting a painful tooth pulled, the longer your pain will continue *after* it's pulled. "Don't wait until you can no longer stand it before you see your dentist, because you will pay for it with more pain and infection," says Dr. Abaza. "The quicker a damaged tooth is removed, the easier it is to extract—and the less pain you will have in recovery."

Puncture Wounds

Nothing feels better than being footloose and fancy-free, but when one of those loose feet meets a very sharp object, your carefree thoughts may phase out quickly. One tiny hole in the skin can often produce a lot of major concern, not to mention some pain.

A big-league wound calls for emergency care, or at least a call to the doctor. But if your wound is minor enough to be treated at home, here's how.

Irrigate immediately. Even if there's some bleeding, the first thing you should do is wash the puncture thoroughly with soap and water. "Your biggest

When to See the Doctor

While minor cuts and scrapes can usually be treated at home, some wounds need a doctor's attention as soon as possible, according to Birt Harvey, M.D., professor of pediatrics at Stanford University School of Medicine in Stanford, California.

If any cut is bleeding bright red and spurting, that's a sign that you may have punctured an artery. Apply pressure to control bleeding and be sure to call the emergency room or see your doctor.

You'll also need a doctor's help cleaning the wound if you can see there's dirt or grime in it but you can't wash it out. And a cut may require stitches if the ends of the wound don't come together.

Also be sure to visit the doctor if you notice any red streaks, pus or redness around the cut as it begins to heal. These may be signs of infection, says Dr. Harvey.

concern isn't the blood but the risk of infection, so it's essential that you clean the wound as quickly as you can," says Arthur Jacknowitz, Pharm.D., professor and chairman of clinical pharmacy at West Virginia University School of Pharmacy in Morgantown. "If you don't have soap, then just use water. But the sooner you dilute the punctured area with water, the more likely you are to remove all debris and reduce risk of infection later on."

Rub-a-dub with a washcloth. Birt Harvey, M.D., professor of pediatrics at Stanford University School of Medicine in Stanford, California, has found that scrubbing with a clean washcloth is especially effective. "Forget all the advertisements about special cleansing agents," he says. "The best way to clean a puncture wound is with a soapy, clean washcloth. The scrubbing of the washcloth seems to get more of the bacteria or debris."

Let it bleed (for a few minutes, anyway). If there's no water around, let your blood wash away the bacteria. "People get all upset when they see blood and think the most important thing they should do is control the bleeding. But actually, you *want* to see a puncture wound bleed a little," says Dr. Harvey. "It's blood that washes away the bacteria." After a few minutes, of course, bleeding should be controlled by pressing on the puncture site. (Reminder: If there's spurting blood, or if the bleeding won't stop, call a doctor at once and apply firm pressure while waiting.)

Is Your Tetanus Booster Up-to-Date?

Tetanus has a fearful reputation, and it's true that this bacteria can cause lockjaw and death. If you've had a tetanus booster within the past five years, there's no need to worry, according to Birt Harvey, M.D., professor of pediatrics at Stanford University School of Medicine in Stanford, California. But what about the story that you'll get tetanus if you step on a rusty nail?

"People worry about rust, but the real problem is that the nail has been on the ground outdoors," says Dr. Harvey. Any nail that's been lying on the ground has been exposed to bacteria and may be carrying tetanus.

If you do get a scratch or puncture wound from a nail and you can't remember whether you've had a tetanus booster in the last five years, doctors advise that you get one within 24 hours.

Heal it with warmth. "If you notice redness around the puncture site, a hot-water soak can help by increasing blood flow," says Dr. Harvey. The increased blood flow from heat brings in white blood cells that kill bacteria, he notes. "Soak the area for 15 minutes four times a day in hot water."

Keep the puncture uncovered if possible. "If you don't have to cover the wound with a bandage, don't," advises Dr. Harvey. "It's always better to let it dry in the air, so it gets a 'crust.' That crust acts as a natural bandage. But if the area will get rubbed, then cover it with a bandage."

Rashes

Anyone who's ever had athlete's foot, eczema, chafing, hives, food allergies, razor burn, poison ivy or any of umpteen other dermatological dilemmas knows what a rash looks like. Redness, itching, spots, blisters—whatever the type of outbreak, it can turn your skin into a hair shirt of prickles and pain.

Most annoying of all, there are probably times when you just don't know why you get a rash, since they can be caused by just about anything. Of course, there are *other* times when it's easy to determine the cause: If your skin turns red after applying a new brand of blusher, then it's a good bet that the makeup is to blame. Drive back from a camp-out with a wealth of itchy welts around your arms and legs and you can probably point an itchy accusing finger at poison ivy. And it doesn't take Sherlock Holmes to figure out the cause of heat rash or diaper rash.

But other rashes can leave you scratching your head as well as your skin as you try to determine the cause. Well, scratch no more. When you've got a rash and you don't know why, investigate these lesser-known causes and cures.

Take time-outs on toothbrushing. If you get a mysterious rash around your mouth, it could be caused by your toothpaste: Tartar control toothpastes (but not other types) contain compounds that leave skin cracked and cause redness and itching around the corners of your mouth.

The cure? "For some reason, if you reduce your use of tartar control toothpastes to only once a day, the rash doesn't occur," according to Bruce E. Beacham, M.D., associate professor of dermatology at the University of Maryland School of Medicine in Baltimore. "It seems to occur most frequently in those who use the toothpastes three times daily as well as in people who have asthma or hay fever."

Stop tartar rash with cream. Besides limiting use of the toothpastes, you can remedy "tartar rash" by applying a 1 percent hydrocortisone cream such as maximum-strength Cortaid on affected areas, adds Dr. Beacham. Cortaid and similar creams are available over the counter at most pharmacies.

Relax before you react. If you get a rash that's not related to a specific condition such as poison ivy, eczema or athlete's foot, some R and R may be the best Rx for curing it. Most doctors agree that stress and anxiety can cause or aggravate rashes. When you're under stress, your body releases chemicals that force white blood cells to clog blood vessel walls beneath the skin. That reaction causes redness and irritation on the skin surface, says George F. Murphy, M.D., a dermatology professor at the University of Pennsylvania in Philadelphia.

Dr. Murphy says a regular stress management program—even something as simple as discussing your problems or feelings with a friend or family member—can potentially help remedy some forms of skin redness and blotching. And those kinds of stress reducers could even help *prevent* rashes such as hives and rosacea.

Get a crush on vitamin C. Applying a lotion of crushed vitamin C tablets and water directly on skin may cure many rashes because of the vitamin's antioxidant qualities, says Douglas Darr, Ph.D., assistant medical research professor at Duke University Medical Center in Durham, North Carolina. "In fact, some cosmetic moisturizers brag that they have vitamin C in them, but the concentrations are usually so low that it's probably degraded even before the consumer buys it," says Dr. Darr.

Razor Burn

Though it's not certain, it seems likely that men invented profanity as an explicit response to the pain and injustice of razor burn.

After all, anyone who has to draw a sharp blade across raw skin every morning to dispense with an overnight growth of stubble *needs* a grab bag of colorful expletives. How else to endure the cuts, nicks and scrapes that occur all too often?

Of course, there's always Styptic—that mysteriously named drugstore item that you can apply to a nick or scratch to stanch the telltale red droplets that say "I goofed" more clearly than words. And if that morning meeting is an urgent one that will be attended by lots of honchos, Styptic may be your best bet for instant damage repair.

But here are some other tactics recommended by razor researchers and dermatologists for getting through your morning shave without getting burned in the first place.

Delay your morning shave. If you reach for your razor the minute you wake up, you're probably walking around with an irritated face. When you sleep, body fluids tend to puff up the surface of your skin and hide the hairs, says Fred Wexler, director of shaving research for Schick, a division of Warner-Lambert Company in Milford, Connecticut. "If you shave right after you jump out of bed, the razor can't get as close to the hair follicle (the place where the hair comes out of the skin). It takes at least 20 minutes after you get out of bed for those fluids to disperse and for your skin to become taut again."

If you're a morning exerciser, shave *after* your workout and shower, suggests Wexler. Your sweat is acidic and can irritate freshly shaved skin, so that burn will feel worse if you shave before you run or exercise.

Soften your bristles. "About 25 percent of men experience razor burn or other forms of shaving discomfort," says John McShefferty, Ph.D., president of the Gillette Research Institute in Gaithersburg, Maryland, one of the corporate research laboratories of the Gillette Company. The reason? "Most of them

For Women: Ways around Razor Burn

Shaving legs and underarms can result in razor burn, too. But here are some ways around it.

If you get underarm pain, it might be from antiperspirant applied *after* shaving. "An antiperspirant is *very* irritating—especially when you consider that the underarm skin is highly sensitive," according to John McShefferty, Ph.D., president of the Gillette Research Institute in Gaithersburg, Maryland, one of the corporate research laboratories of the Gillette Company. "It might be better to shave underarms at night, so you don't have to apply antiperspirant right away.

"For legs *or* underarms, you can cut down on some of the irritation by using shaving creams, gels or foams," suggests Dr. McShefferty.

don't take the time to properly soften their beards before shaving. You need about two to three minutes of soaking before you actually start shaving."

The key, according to Dr. McShefferty, is to *not* dry your face after you wash or take a shower. "While your skin is still wet, apply a shaving gel or foam. Wait for a minute or two and then shave."

Shave the way your hair grows. Most men shave against the grain, thinking they get a closer shave. "Maybe they do, but they also get more razor burn that way," says dermatologist John F. Romano, M.D., clinical assistant professor of medicine at The New York Hospital–Cornell Medical Center in New York City. "You should always shave in the same direction as the way your hair grows. That means shaving on an angle, perhaps, or shaving from the chin to the throat—not the other way around, as most men do."

Use short strokes. "When you use long strokes, you tend to press down harder and cause more friction—and friction causes razor burn," according to Dr. Romano. "It's always better to use short strokes. You'll get just as good a shave, with a lot less irritation."

Make your mug moister. "Don't use colognes or commercial after-shave lotions, because they contain alcohol, which is drying and irritating to a freshly shaved face," says Dr. Romano. "You don't need an antiseptic on your face if you wash it regularly."

Dr. McShefferty recommends applying an over-the-counter moisturizer, after shaving, to soften your skin. "Women tend to do this after shaving their legs, but most men don't, because they think the fragrances of their wife's brand may be too feminine." But there are several products that have more masculine fragrances.

Beware of hydrocortisone creams. These over-the-counter medications for skin irritations are okay for occasional use and quick healing of nicks, cuts and other abrasions caused by shaving. But according to Dr. Romano, you should use them no more than twice a week. "Use them only when your skin is really bad," he says, "because eventually they can cause thinning of the skin."

Rectal Itching

Okay, so it doesn't warrant the same awe-inspiring stories as that knee injury you got when you made the winning touchdown in the Big Game or that shrapnel you took while saving everyone in your platoon during the war: "So, Bob, there I was on this important job interview when, all of a sudden, I got the most uncontrollable, embarrassing itch . . . "

While rectal itching may be the butt of many locker room jokes (particularly in junior high school gymnasiums), it isn't at all funny. In fact, it takes real endurance to put up with the aggravation. But here's how you can reduce the discomfort—or banish it.

De-yeast it with yogurt. "Many times, rectal itching is caused by a yeast infection, and when that's the case, applying plain, unflavored yogurt will do the trick," says Jerome Z. Litt, M.D., assistant clinical professor of dermatology at Case Western Reserve University School of Medicine in Cleveland. "Yogurt with active cultures has bacteria that compete with the growth of yeast; the bacteria literally kill the yeast. The best way to apply it is to sit in a tray of yogurt for about an hour, but you can also apply it with a handkerchief. It's very soothing."

Sit in sitz. "People with hemorrhoids often have rectal itch because they can't clean the area as effectively, and that soil is what causes the itch," says

D'Anne Kleinsmith, M.D., a cosmetic dermatologist at William Beaumont Hospital near Detroit. "Taking sitz baths, or just taking a lot of baths in general, helps stop the itch."

Cast that witch hazel spell. Witch hazel, applied with a cotton ball or hanky, provides cool relief for some. An application also helps dry out the infected area, adds Dr. Kleinsmith. (Medicated pads such as Tucks are also recommended.)

Use a drugstore-bought cleanser. "A product called Balneol, available at your local drugstore, is very good," says Dr. Kleinsmith. "It's very mild and should be used after you go to the bathroom."

Restless Legs Syndrome

Scientists call this condition Ekbom syndrome, RLS or nocturnal jerking movements—and if you're a sufferer, the poor schmoe you sleep with probably has a few choice monikers for it, too. That's because when your restless legs start running at night, you're likely to give your bedmate a swift kick or two as your legs thrash about seeking relief.

But what makes them restless? Maybe your legs seek relief from a cramplike feeling. Or perhaps your thighs feel as though bugs were crawling inside them. Sometimes the pain is deep and throbbing. Other times it feels like pins and needles. The feelings vary but not the scenario: During periods of rest—especially as you're going to sleep—your legs get antsy, and moving them is the action that brings relief. And it's not just legs and feet, either—your hands may go through those nightly motions as well.

One in 20 Americans has restless legs syndrome, which may be inherited. Doctors believe it may be triggered by stress, a nutritional deficiency or some sort of imbalance in brain chemistry. It is not dangerous and doesn't lead to serious neurological disorders. In fact, many doctors think restless legs syndrome is an annoyance rather than a bona fide disease. But here's how to get a leg up on restless legs.

Exercise before bedtime. "People report that if they exercise sometime during the day, they are less likely to be bothered by restless legs at night. For best results, I recommend that you do deep knee bends or other leg exercises as close to bedtime as possible," suggests Arthur S. Walters, M.D., associate professor of neurology at the University of Medicine and Dentistry of New Jersey Robert Wood Johnson Medical School in New Brunswick and a researcher into the causes and cures of restless legs syndrome.

Since leg exercises or taking a walk brings only short-term relief, Dr. Walters stresses that you need to exercise close to the time when you're going to bed. Exercise helps by releasing endorphins, the body's natural painkilling substances that may ease restless legs symptoms.

Take your vitamins. Several studies have shown that iron deficiency can trigger symptoms of restless legs syndrome. Others blame a folate deficiency. To cover all the bases, take a multivitamin/mineral supplement every day to protect yourself against both deficiencies and possibly against restless legs, advises Lawrence Z. Stern, M.D., professor of neurology and director of the Mucio F. Delgado Clinic for Neuromuscular Disorders at the University of Arizona College of Medicine Health Sciences Center in Tucson.

Sip the grape. Douglas K. Ousterhout, M.D., D.D.S., clinical professor of surgery (plastic) at the University of California, San Francisco, and a former restless legs sufferer, says he relieved his symptoms simply by drinking wine. "Ever since I started to drink a glass of wine each night, I've never had a problem," he says. His mother also got over restless legs syndrome by having a glass or two a week. Although Dr. Ousterhout initially thought that red wine did the trick, "I've since learned that white wine works just as well—although I can't think of any scientific explanation and have no idea why it works."

When to See the Doctor

If you have restless legs syndrome, you probably don't have anything to worry about—except the sleep it sometimes causes you to miss. If *nothing* seems to help ease your discomfort, you may need prescription drugs, which have been shown to relieve symptoms.

You should also see your doctor if you're experiencing symptoms for the first time. Although restless legs syndrome usually doesn't occur until middle age, its symptoms could mimic other medical problems, such as lung disease, kidney disease, diabetes and Parkinson's disease.

Stop smoking. "It's certainly worth trying," says Janet A. Mountifield, M.D., a general practitioner in Toronto who noticed that one of her patients was cured of restless legs syndrome after quitting a longtime smoking habit. One possible theory: Smoking impairs blood flow to leg muscles. "I don't know if it was a fluke, but my patient tried everything. Nothing worked for her restless legs—until she quit smoking."

Soak your feet. A cool-water soak just before bedtime is a good way to chill restless leg pain. "Many people soak their feet in cool water, and it seems to help somewhat, so I think it's worth trying," says Ronald F. Pfeiffer, M.D., associate professor of neurology and pharmacology at the University of Nebraska Medical Center in Omaha. Just don't overdo it. Immersing your feet in ice or extremely cold water can cause nerve damage, so be sure to keep the water at least 50°F.

Or massage your legs. "Rubbing your legs briskly, or running a vibrator over them, also brings relief for many people," says Dr. Pfeiffer. Many experts believe it's because massaging can "shut off" the pain impulses caused by restless legs.

Don't eat a big meal late. "It may be the activity of the nervous system involved in digesting a big meal that triggers symptoms," offers Dr. Stern.

And don't drink coffee at all. Some studies show that eliminating caffeine from your diet can bring relief. "In general, stimulants can aggravate restless legs syndrome in some people, and getting rid of stimulants such as coffee can relieve symptoms," adds Dr. Pfeiffer.

Ringworm

We are not alone.

Every day, people around the world, from every walk of life, experience visitations by alien life forms. These silent invaders use our skin as landing sites, burrowing and spreading, as if they were exploring some strange new world. The only evidence of their arrival: a red, scaly, O-shaped lesion, like the rings of Saturn.

Those lesions are the telltale signs of ringworm—which is *not* a worm but a group of fungi identical to the kinds that cause athlete's foot and jock itch. Invading the warm, moist areas of the groin, trunk, extremities and scalp, the fungi multiply to form a pronounced red ring or an itchy, eczema-like patch.

Ringworm is highly contagious. If your skin comes in contact with the fungi *anywhere,* parts of your hide may begin to display the telltale circular design. Bathrooms, gym lockers, theater seats, combs, pets and unwashed clothing have all served as launching pads for a nasty bout with ringworm.

Severe cases, specifically those of the scalp, can be treated only with prescribed oral antibiotics. But with milder cases, you have more down-to-earth weapons at your disposal to fight off this invasion of the body splotchers.

Cream it with an antifungal. "You can stop most ringworm infections of the trunk, groin or extremities with an over-the-counter antifungal cream," says Jack L. Lesher, Jr., M.D., associate professor of dermatology at the Medical College of Georgia in Augusta. "Go with a cream that contains an *-azole* product as its active ingredient. Clotrimazoles (Lotrimin AF, Mycelex) and

When to See the Doctor

There are times when over-the-counter antifungals aren't appropriate or strong enough to stop a bad case of ringworm. That's when you need to see a dermatologist, who is armed with an arsenal of high-strength topical and oral medications. According to Loretta S. Davis, M.D., assistant professor of dermatology at the Medical College of Georgia in Augusta, you should seek medical treatment if any of the following occur.

- The ringworm persists or grows even after you have treated your condition for two full weeks with an over-the-counter antifungal medication.
- It is on your scalp, face or beard.
- You see signs of infection on a baby.
- There are several lesions scattered across the body.
- The ringworm invades the toenails.

miconazoles (Micatin, Monistat) do a great job of controlling ringworm fungi quickly."

"You may also see good results with a product containing a tolnaftate, such as Tinactin or Aftate," says dermatologist Joseph Bark, M.D., past chairman of the Department of Dermatology at St. Joseph's Hospital in Lexington, Kentucky. "These will cool down a ringworm infection, reduce the itching and limit the spread. They're more effective on smaller patches than on large ones."

For directions for application, check the package. You will need to apply any medication twice a day for about two weeks *after* the ring disappears to take care of any stubborn fungi that may be hiding.

Establish a safety zone. "With antifungal creams, it is important to treat both the affected area and the area immediately around it," according to Elizabeth Whitmore, M.D., assistant professor of dermatology at Johns Hopkins University Outpatient Center in Baltimore. "Spread the cream on the area outside the ring, and work your way in toward the center. On a nickel-size patch, try to cover a half-dollar-size area."

Bathe daily. You can't wash away ringworm, but a daily bath or shower may hinder its spread and provide some itch relief. "No astringent, gritty or germ-fighting soaps are needed," says Dr. Bark. "Just use a plain gentle soap to keep the area clean. Avoid harsh scrubbing; it will only aggravate the lesion."

Use a medicated shampoo. Dr. Lesher recommends trying medicated shampoos such as Selsun blue, Denorex or Head & Shoulders for ringworm of the scalp. "It won't cure ringworm, but it will limit its spread, prevent it from looking too scaly and provide itch relief. Don't scrub: Let the shampoo lather well and sit on the scalp for four to five minutes, then rinse."

Blow-dry the cozy crevices. Ringworm fungi thrive in moisture. "They love to make themselves cozy in the warm, moist areas on the body, especially between toes and in the groin area," says Loretta S. Davis, M.D., assistant professor of dermatology at the Medical College of Georgia. "After bathing, thoroughly pat the affected area dry. Then sprinkle on some absorbent powder. (Don't use cornstarch; fungi will use it as food.) You'll also see improvement if you air out problem areas with an electric hair dryer set on cool."

Rotate your shoes. Since shoes often harbor fungi, you need to be careful how you handle them, advises Dr. Davis. "In fact, your medication may not do any good if you step into the same fungus-infested shoes each day," she says.

She recommends that you never wear the same pair of shoes two days in a row. "Give them a chance to air out," she says.

Put on socks before undies. "This will prevent your underwear from coming in contact with fungus-infected feet," says Dr. Davis. "When you pull up your underwear, you won't spread the fungi to your leg, groin or belly."

Wear loose-fitting clothing. "A good way to keep the ringworm area dry is to wear shorts or loose clothing. Tight clothing also generates far too much heat," says Paul Honig, M.D., director of pediatric dermatology at Children's Hospital of Philadelphia. "Cotton fibers are a good choice, because they breathe to keep the area exposed to air and free from perspiration. Change your clothing and bedding daily, so fungi don't have a place to breed."

Machine-wash clothes and linens. "Regular washing in hot water with chlorine bleach as well as detergent is the best way to kill fungi on underwear and linens," says Dr. Whitmore. Washing with detergent alone isn't usually enough. Combs and hats should also be thoroughly cleaned and disinfected.

Go light on the hydrocortisones. You don't want to scratch an itchy ringworm infection. On the other hand, anti-itch hydrocortisone creams alone will only encourage the fungi to grow. "However, a little hydrocortisone applied simultaneously with an antifungal for the first one to two days will diminish severe itching," says Dr. Lesher. "On the third day, continue with the antifungal only."

Take your pet to the vet. Kids love to cuddle dogs and cats. Unfortunately, pets make great homes for ringworm fungi, according to Dr. Whitmore. If you suspect your child's ringworm is coming from a pet, take the animal to a veterinarian for a thorough exam and professional treatment.

Disinfect the trouble spots. Ringworm fungi love to collect in tubs, on bathroom floors and in hampers and dresser drawers. Dr. Whitmore recommends that you destroy these breeding grounds by regularly cleaning them with chlorine bleach.

Runny Nose

When you consider that the average nose produces up to three quarts of mucus each day to keep your upper respiratory tract lubricated, you have to expect a few extra drips now and then. (And if you have allergies, that three-quart average may turn into *six*.) Sometimes a stray ounce or two trickles down the back of your throat in the form of postnasal drip. Other times, that mucus contributes to a classic case of runny nose.

All the blame can't be placed on the mucus-making nasal and sinus cavities, or even on allergies. "Only about half of the people with runny nose are actually allergic," says Hueston C. King, M.D., an otolaryngologist in Venice, Florida, and visiting professor at the University of Texas Southwestern Medical Center at Dallas. "Many other people have nonallergic rhinitis, which can be triggered by the wind blowing, a change in temperature, even eating."

The obvious solution to *any* kind of runny nose is to blow your nose, which brings immediate relief and helps remove any irritants. But here are some other ways to make a nose stop running.

Eat Mexican. It's been well documented that spicy foods—particularly hot peppers, Tabasco sauce and other foods with capsaicin—help relieve congestion. It may seem like a contradiction, because this hot stuff triggers the same reflex that causes a runny nose.

So why eat spicy food? "Blasting yourself with hot and spicy food might be a good way to increase the nasal discharge to the point where it will remove whatever is causing it to run. In addition, this same response releases chemicals in the nose that protect you against infection," says Gordon Raphael, M.D., an allergist and former researcher at the National Institute of Allergy and Infectious Diseases in Bethesda, Maryland. "It certainly won't hurt you and could be very beneficial."

Use antihistamines with care. "If your runny nose is caused by allergies, then taking an over-the-counter (OTC) antihistamine will help," says Dr. King.

What's Causing Your Runny Nose?

Is your runny nose due to allergies or to aging? Many people simply "develop" a tendency toward runny nose as they age, says Hueston C. King, M.D., an otolaryngologist in Venice, Florida, and visiting professor at the University of Texas Southwestern Medical Center at Dallas. Here's how to tell what's causing yours.

You're likely allergic if you get a runny nose only at certain times of the year—usually spring or fall—or when you've been exposed to known allergens such as pet fur, dust or pollen. Also, the "reaction" will come almost instanteously, "occurring within the first few minutes" of being exposed to that substance, according to Dr. King.

But the cause may be attributed to the natural aging process if it happens after you've been out in the wind or after there's been a sharp change in temperature. If your nose runs as soon as you go outdoors, or come inside, or eat a meal, blame it on aging rather than allergies.

"But if you get a runny nose from wind, changes in temperatures or other reasons, don't put much faith in OTCs. You may get some relief from antihistamines, but it won't be *good* relief."

Another reason to exercise caution: "*All* over-the-counter antihistamines cause drowsiness to some degree," adds Dr. King. The only "nondrowsy" antihistamines, terfenadine (Seldane) and astemizole (Hismanal), are available only by prescription.

Soothe with salt water. Another effective way to remove allergens causing a runny nose—and to dry out secretions—is to "irrigate" nostrils with a saltwater solution. It may be uncomfortable at first, says Jerold Principato, M.D., clinical professor of otolaryngology in the Department of Surgery at George Washington University School of Medicine in Washington, D.C., but it gets easier with practice.

Simply dissolve ½ teaspoon of table salt in eight ounces of warm water. Draw the water into a nosedropper (aspirator), and with your head tilted back, put the tip of the nosedropper in your nostril. Then breathe in to "suck" the water into your nostril. You may need to do this a few times before you feel relief. When you're finished, blow your nose to remove the watery discharge.

Nudge out nasal sprays. You can also buy nonprescription saline nasal spray or mist at most drugstores. But these products should be used sparingly, because they can have a "rebound effect" and actually worsen the problem.

"For instance, many people may notice that they get a runny nose when they eat. It's not necessarily the spice but rather the change in temperature of the food that causes a runny nose," says Dr. King. For these situations, according to Dr. King, it's fine to use the nasal spray in advance, just to avoid the awkwardness and discomfort of having a runny nose in a restaurant. "But you should use the nose spray *only* when you dine out," says Dr. King. "When eating at home, you should just endure it."

Scarring

U nless you're a criminal named Mugsy, you probably have little use for scars. Although some wounds will leave you with an eternal etched-in-skin reminder of your misfortune or operation, often you can reduce the chance of scarring simply by treating your skin right during the healing process. Even when a scar can't be completely avoided, there are ways to help it fade faster or more completely.

"C" your way to faster healing. A wound that heals quickly and neatly is less likely to develop a scar than a wound that festers. Foods high in vitamin C, such as broccoli, potatoes and citrus fruits, are thought to promote faster healing by building collagen tissue around blood vessels in the skin, says Las Vegas orthopedic surgeon Michael Rask, M.D., chairman of the American Academy of Neurological and Orthopedic Surgeons and the American Board of Ringside Medicine and Surgery.

Down the zinc. Some experts recommend zinc-rich foods for faster healing. Good sources of zinc include roasted pumpkin and sunflower seeds, Brazil nuts, Swiss and Cheddar cheeses, peanuts, dark-meat turkey and lean beef.

Clean the wound daily. During the healing process, clean the wound daily with hydrogen peroxide or soap and water to help avoid secondary infection—

which may increase permanent scarring. Then sparingly apply an over-the-counter antibiotic ointment, which keeps it moist and prevents infection, says Jeffrey H. Binstock, M.D., assistant clinical professor of dermatologic surgery at the University of California, San Francisco, School of Medicine. And don't pick at scabs.

Massage with moisturizer. "One of the most effective things you can do to eliminate or reduce the size of a scar is to massage the incision or wound site with moisturizer after the skin surface has healed," advises Stephen M. Purcell, D.O., chairman of the Department of Dermatology at Philadelphia

The ABCDs of Mole Detection

Once they were called beauty marks. Now they're often thought of as a mark of skin cancer. Sometimes moles *do* have to be removed, and that can produce some slight scarring. But don't hesitate when it needs to be done: One in three cases of malignant skin cancer starts in moles, says dermatologist Rodney Basler, M.D., assistant professor of internal medicine at the University of Nebraska Medical Center in Omaha.

Although moles aren't necessarily a sign that you'll get skin cancer—after all, the average person has more than 40 moles—the more you have, the greater your skin cancer risk. A change in any mole should warrant an examination by your doctor, who is likely to remove it with a procedure that takes only a few minutes and leaves a tiny scar. But when you observe moles for signs of change, Dr. Basler suggests that you pay special attention to the ABCDs of mole watching.

- *Asymmetry:* "Moles are symmetrical, so one half is the same shape as the other. But cancers are not," says Dr. Basler.
- *Borders:* "Moles have smooth borders. Cancers have an irregular border—notched, ragged or poorly defined," he adds.
- *Color:* Variation in either shade or color from one area of the mole to another is a likely sign that it's cancer. Shades may be tan to brown or varying intensities of black. The presence of red, white or blue in a changing mole is known as a flag sign, usually indicating that cancer is present.
- *Diameter:* Be suspicious of moles larger than six millimeters—roughly the size of a pencil eraser.

College of Osteopathic Medicine and assistant clinical professor at Hahnemann University School of Medicine in Philadelphia. "The massaging improves blood flow to that area and encourages more even distribution of collagen, which results in less of a thickened scar. And the moisturizer is just good for skin."

Sock it with sunscreen. Scars have less pigment than the rest of your skin, so they're especially vulnerable to sunburn—and prolonged redness. You should make certain to cover all exposed scars with a sunscreen with an SPF (sun protection factor) of 25 or higher whenever you head outside on a sunny day, says Stephen Kurtin, M.D., assistant professor of dermatology at Mount Sinai School of Medicine in New York City.

Sciatica

The largest nerve in your body has a very devious twist—and when you have a pain in that nerve, it can really get around.

Sciatica, pain in the sciatic nerve, can radiate from the buttocks down the back of the leg to the knee, even as far as the big toe. "People with sciatica often say their back pain is bad but their leg pain is *worse*," says Loren M. Fishman, M.D., a physiatrist and rehabilitation medicine specialist at Flushing Hospital Medical Center in New York City. Often the hip pain is far more severe on one side than the other.

When you've got pain like that, you'll need a hands-on diagnosis before anything else, Dr. Fishman says. Once the doctor has ruled out a disk problem or fracture, he may be able to find out whether tight buttocks muscles are causing your pain by compressing the sciatic nerve.

If you do have sciatica, the doctor will probably recommend a program of supervised exercises, usually with the aid of a physical therapist. Here are some of the self-care methods that could ease the pressure temporarily and bring you some pain relief.

Pick your own pocket. A bulging billfold in your hip pocket can crimp your sciatic nerve, especially if you sit on the wallet for long periods of time, says Scott Haldeman, M.D., D.C., Ph.D., associate clinical professor in the Depart-

When to See the Doctor

What *seems* like sciatic pain may be something else—hence the importance of having a proper diagnosis. You may have a herniated disk pressing against this nerve, an arthritis problem, bursitis, irritable bowel syndrome or some other back problem that requires a doctor-supervised plan of action, says Scott Haldeman, M.D., D.C., Ph.D., associate clinical professor in the Department of Neurology at the University of California, Irvine, and adjunct professor at the Los Angeles Chiropractic College.

In fact, exercises for sciatica can actually worsen a disk or arthritis problem.

Consider it an emergency if your symptoms include weakness or numbness or loss of bladder or bowel control. These problems could be related to the central nervous system and will need immediate diagnosis.

ment of Neurology at the University of California, Irvine, and adjunct professor at the Los Angeles Chiropractic College. He suggests that you put the wallet in a coat pocket or purse to make sure you don't put lopsided pressure on one buttock.

Stretch your piriformis. One of these spindle-shaped muscles lies deep inside each buttock. The piriformis is the muscle you use when you turn out your hip and raise your leg to the side—and it's often implicated in sciatic nerve pain.

To stretch the piriformis and help relieve the pain temporarily, here's what Dr. Fishman suggests.

Lie on your back on the floor and gently pull your right knee up toward your left shoulder. Grasping the instep of the right foot with your left hand, slowly draw the knee and foot across the body toward the left shoulder. Stretch for 30 seconds or more to elongate the piriformis deep in the back of the hip. Then lower your right leg, switch to the left, and repeat.

Partner up for stretches. Even better, if someone can help you with your stretches, is this routine: First lie on the floor or on a firm bed on the side that *doesn't* hurt. Lift the uppermost leg (on the side that hurts) and raise your knee to waist level as if you were taking a step. Then slowly drop the knee down toward the floor or bed. Have your partner hold this knee down with one hand while he raises the ankle of the same leg with his other hand. A cautionary note: He should raise the ankle only as far as it will go comfortably and hold for 15 to 30 seconds.

Do a butt press. You can ease sciatic pain by pressing on appropriate acupressure points, says acupressurist Michael Reed Gach, founder of the Acupressure Institute in Berkeley, California, and author of *The Bum Back Book*. First find the center of the depression at the *sides* of the buttocks. Then press both sides simultaneously and *hard*, because the acupressure points lie deep below the skin, Gach says. Keep the pressure on for a count of 15, then release.

Give your calves a seat. Assuming a position with hip joints and knees bent the best way to depress the sciatic nerve and avoid pain, says Dr. Haldeman. Here's a posture that should help: Lie on your back on the floor and place your lower legs on the seat of a chair for 10 or 15 minutes.

Seasonal Affective Disorder

'Tis the month after Christmas, the goodies long gone.
But you're still overeating—what could be wrong?
You're depressed and blue and feeling real sick
And sporting a waistline like that of St. Nick.
All winter long, the story's the same:
Too little cheer, too much mental pain.
Can't figure why you can't get it together?
A winter's surprise: It could be the weather!

Okay, so it's not the lyrics of Clement Moore, but if you identify with that . . . ahem, *poem,* you've got something in common with one in five Americans—seasonal affective disorder (SAD).

For most people, the old "winter blues" simply mean that we feel a little run-down and melancholy in the season when we *should* be jolly. But for those who experience SAD at its most extreme, the blues hit harder than a flat note on a slide trombone. "We're talking about a condition that may compromise

Lighten Up Your Mood

A surefire way to lighten up winter depression caused by seasonal affective disorder (SAD) is to undergo at-home therapy with a special lighting fixture. The most common type is known as a light box. This is a square fixture, usually a little larger than a briefcase, that stands upright on a desk or table. Other devices for treating SAD are configured as workstations, head-mounted visors or dawn simulators. Prices range from $200 to $500.

What's so special about a light box? "It's not so much that there's a magic bulb that works," explains SAD light therapy researcher George Brainard, Ph.D., associate professor of neurology and pharmacology at Jefferson Medical College of Thomas Jefferson University in Philadelphia. "What's more important is the *dosage* emitted and the fact that it's emitted at *eye level*." The dosage is about five to ten times that of normal indoor lighting, and according to Dr. Brainard, you have to *look* repeatedly at the light; just having it fall on your skin isn't enough.

"The general prescription is two hours a day at 2,500 lux—a unit of light intensity," according to Dr. Brainard. He recommends that you set the light box in a position so that you can glance for a few seconds directly into the light. Glance at the light box about once a minute over the two hours. "Alternatively, some people use a 10,000-lux box for 30 minutes a day," says Dr. Brainard.

But before you plunk down your money, one last piece of advice: "First see a qualified physician or therapist and make sure you are diagnosed with SAD," says Dr. Brainard. "These lights won't work if you're just depressed; they'll only work if you have SAD." Your health professional can also advise you about reputable mail-order companies that sell light boxes.

your life so seriously that you can't work or cope with your family, something that leaves you so lethargic that you can barely get out of bed," says George Brainard, Ph.D., associate professor of neurology and pharmacology at Jefferson Medical College of Thomas Jefferson University in Philadelphia and a researcher on the benefits of light therapy for SAD.

Research is being done on the causes of SAD, with no definite conclusions as yet, according to Norman E. Rosenthal, M.D., chief of environmental psychiatry at the National Institute of Mental Health in Bethesda, Maryland, and a pioneer in SAD research. Even though the mechanism is not known, however, most doctors are in agreement that light therapy definitely helps those who have SAD.

Symptoms of SAD may include a tendency to overeat, oversleep and even become disinterested in sex. But it doesn't have to get that far. Here's what to do to beat a major case of the blues.

Go with the glow. Although the *best* treatment for SAD is daily light therapy using a specially designed "light box," exposure to *any* type of bright light may help some people. "Flooding the room with bright, but not harsh, light actually helps some people," says Maria Simonson, Ph.D., Sc.D., professor emeritus and director of the Health, Weight and Stress Program at Johns Hopkins Medical Institutions in Baltimore. A word of caution: *Staring* into bright light emitted from lamps and overhead fixtures may harm your eyes, so don't stare at a bulb as a substitute for the light box.

Head for the Great Outdoors. The days are shorter in the winter, but you can still take advantage of what little sunlight there is. "*Any* exposure to sunlight will help," says Henry Lahmeyer, M.D., professor of psychiatry and behavioral sciences at Northwestern University Medical School and co-director of the Sleep Program at Northwestern Memorial Hospital, both in Chicago. "You should try to spend about an hour outdoors every day—even on days when it's not particularly bright and sunny."

Stroll in the dawn. "Research in Switzerland found that SAD patients who took an outdoor, 30-minute walk at sunrise showed a lot of improvement," says Dr. Brainard. "We're not sure whether it's the exercise, the sunlight or even the cold that invigorates them, but whatever it is, it seems to help."

Use your yoga. "Our research seems to indicate that some of the specific meditations in yoga may act on the pineal gland (which controls circadian and seasonal rhythms)," says Eric Leskowitz, M.D., a psychiatrist and SAD researcher at Spaulding Rehabilitation Hospital in Boston. "Yoga also provides a general energizing effect and offers great stress release. I think practicing yoga is a great way to start off the day if you have SAD."

Take milk for all its worth. A form of vitamin D called soltriol that's found in milk may help keep us in sync with the sun, according to the theory based on a study by Walter E. Stumpf, M.D., Ph.D., a researcher at the University of

North Carolina in Chapel Hill. The theory is that soltriol may trigger the release of "stimulating" hormones that keep our body clocks on track.

Keep consistent sleeping habits. "Having a regular sleep schedule and sticking to it is very helpful to all people, including those with SAD," says Alex Clerk, M.D., director of the Sleep Disorders Clinic at Stanford University in Stanford, California. "The tendency is to sleep more with winter SAD, but your body doesn't *need* more sleep. You'll be much better off keeping a consistent sleeping schedule."

Shingles

Remember your childhood case of chickenpox? You probably don't want to. The maddening itch, the red spots on your skin . . . please, never again!

People who have shingles, however, are not allowed to forget. If you have shingles (herpes zoster), it means the same virus that turned you into a giant connect-the-dots puzzle has found its way to the nervous system. In some people, that virus lies dormant in a nerve for decades, only to be reactivated when the immune system is weakened by age, disease or unmanaged stress.

With the onset of shingles, you get the itching all over again, along with severe burning pain and a blistering rash above the nerve on the affected side of your body (and sometimes on the face, back of the head or legs).

Of course, many things can cause a rash accompanied by pain and itching. So you can't be positive it's shingles unless you see the doctor and find out for sure. But if that's what you've got, here's how to zap it.

Get a helping hand from nail polish remover. For a homemade treatment that really works, crush two aspirin tablets (*not* Tylenol or another pain reliever) into a powder and mix with two tablespoons of acetone-containing nail polish remover. Stir into a solution and apply to the affected area with a clean cotton ball, advises Robert B. King, M.D., professor of neurosurgery at the State University of New York Health Science Center at Syracuse College of Medicine. To prevent possible burning, do not apply the solution to any folds in the skin where it would not have a chance to dry. Relief starts within five minutes and may last for several hours.

447

When to See the Doctor

Shingles that affect the forehead, face or anywhere near the eyes should be treated by a doctor, since there is a risk of damage to the cornea, according to Leon Robb, M.D., director of the Robb Pain Management Group in Los Angeles. Also, facial shingles may lead to temporary facial paralysis.

Since shingles is the result of a virus, doctors can usually treat it with an antiviral drug such as acyclovir (Zovirax) that slows reproduction of the virus. Steroid drugs may also be helpful, and some physicians prescribe them to prevent the pain.

You should also see your doctor if the pain is more than you can stand. Although all shingles sufferers should expect pain, superintense aching may indicate significant nerve damage.

Doctors can inject a nerve-block medication that may provide temporary relief for many people who have severe pain from shingles. And in some cases, a small implanted electrical device can help mask the pain for chronic sufferers, Dr. Robb says.

The acetone-based nail polish remover removes dead skin cells, soap residue and oil, while the aspirin desensitizes affected nerve endings. Don't use this mixture, however, if you are allergic to aspirin, as it may cause a reaction in some aspirin-sensitive people. Also, keep the mixture away from your eyes.

De-ooze with Domeboro. "When shingles blisters are oozing, the best thing to do is apply a compress of Domeboro astringent solution, an over-the-counter product that comes in tablets or powder and helps dry out the lesions," recommends David Feingold, M.D., chairman of the Department of Dermatology at Tufts University School of Medicine in Boston. Domeboro is available at any drugstore. Following the directions on the package, dissolve it in a pint of water and apply the solution to your lesions with a piece of gauze. Dr. Feingold recommends that you keep the gauze on for about 20 minutes and repeat the application several times a day.

Or calm with calamine. Another effective drying agent that stops the ooze and pain is calamine lotion. "You can apply it straight on or mix a little rubbing alcohol with it," says Bruce Thiers, M.D., associate professor of dermatology at the Medical University of South Carolina in Charleston. "But make sure it's calamine—*not* Cala*dryl,* which has antihistamines that can provoke an allergic reaction."

Revitalize your immunity with vitamins. Since a weakened immune system probably caused your shingles, you may get quicker relief if you strengthen your system with vitamins. In addition to prescribing medication, John G. McConahy, M.D., a dermatologist in New Castle, Pennsylvania, often advises his patients to rebuild the damaged structure of the nerve by taking 200 milligrams of vitamin C five times daily at the first sign of shingles. He also suggests a broad-spectrum multivitamin/mineral supplement that contains zinc, along with a B-complex vitamin supplement.

Try lysine. Some studies show that the amino acid lysine—available at most health food stores and drugstores—can help inhibit the spread of herpes zoster. Although no specific testing has been done on those with shingles, Leon Robb, M.D., director of the Robb Pain Management Group in Los Angeles, says that lysine may help and certainly won't hurt.

Protect against secondary infection. Any open sore can get infected, which would only cause more problems. If you have open sores or blisters caused by shingles, take action to prevent those secondary infections. "Probably the easiest thing to do is place an over-the-counter antibacterial ointment such as bacitracin on the lesions," says Dr. Feingold. "Hydrogen peroxide will also

Don't Be Too Hot on Hot Pepper Cream

Zostrix, an over-the-counter cream, has proven to be effective against residual pain after an attack of shingles. That's because it's made from capsaicin, a derivative of hot peppers that indirectly helps prevent "pain messages" from reaching nerve cells.

But capsaicin is the stuff that makes hot peppers hot, and the cream may also burn like the dickens. Add this extra-hot stuff to the burning pain, and it could be too much—*especially* if you have shingles blisters. Zostrix should be used to quell pain only after *all* shingles blisters have disappeared.

work fine." Don't overgoop your lesions, though, since they heal better when they're dry.

Numb the nerves. Shingles pain often continues even after blisters have healed. But you can "confuse" your own nerve endings and ease the pain by putting a plastic bag full of ice on the area that hurts. Stroke your skin vigorously with the ice bag, advises Dr. Robb.

Shin Splints

They sound like something you'd strap on your legs to keep them from going wobbly in midmarathon. But if you're a runner worth your neon green, light-as-a-feather jogging togs, you know the truth: Shin splints cause searing lower leg pain that you can definitely do without.

Of course, you don't have to have wings on your feet to suffer from shin splints. Just plain walking, especially on hills or uneven surfaces, or wearing the wrong kind of shoes can cause them. And it can happen to anyone any time he puts his underused muscles to work. The connective sheath attached to the muscles and bone of the lower leg becomes irritated, resulting in a razor-sharp pain in the lower leg along the side of the shin bone.

"The pain is your body's way of saying you've had enough," says sports injuries specialist Craig Hersh, M.D., of the Sports Medicine Center in Fort Lee, New Jersey. "If you ignore the pain and don't let up on the activity, it could result in a stress fracture. It's like bending a piece of metal back and forth over and over again—eventually it breaks."

To speed healing—or dodge shin splints entirely—work these home remedies into your workout.

Put ice on your shin. You can soothe sore shins by rubbing them for 20 minutes with ice that's been frozen in a paper cup, says Dr. Hersh. Or fill an empty bread bag with ice, wrap it in a towel, and strap the bag to the front of your shin with an elastic bandage for 20 to 30 minutes, says James M. Lynch, M.D., team physician for Pennsylvania State University in University Park. If you apply ice quickly, it reduces inflammation and eases pain, says Dr. Lynch.

Mix in massage. Although a shin massage may not produce long-term benefits, you might feel at least temporary relief, says Dr. Lynch. The best approach: gently stroking the top of the lower leg with your thumbs for 15 to 20 minutes.

Pamper with a pain reliever. Any number of over-the-counter medications such as Advil and Nuprin contain the ingredient ibuprofen, which helps take the edge off pain, says Dr. Lynch. But aspirin and acetaminophen (Tylenol) are also effective painkillers, he says. (Do not give aspirin to children because of the risk of Reye's syndrome.)

Give it a rest. But instead of sitting on the sidelines until all your symptoms have subsided, try an alternative activity, says Dr. Lynch. "I don't believe in pure rest," he says. "But if running is the offending activity, then I'd reduce that and switch to biking or swimming. Then work your way back slowly. When you're sure you're getting better, start running again."

Make a change for the familiar. What's the number one cause of shin splints among U.S. Olympic hopefuls? Change, according to Jennifer Stone, head athletic trainer at the U.S. Olympic Training Center in Colorado Springs, Colorado.

"Lower leg pain is generally caused by change, and that can be change in almost anything—your shoes, your training program, even the surface you run on," says Stone. Examine your training program—did the pain follow a change? If so, you're better switching back to the familiar routine—at least for now, she says.

See if you're a P or an S. Because the way you run has a lot to do with how your shins feel, do some simple tests to determine whether you pronate or supinate.

Overpronators roll their ankles and feet inward while they run, inequitably transferring much of the pounding into the inner portion of their lower legs, says Paul Raether, M.D., a marathoner who is a physical medicine specialist at the Kaiser Permanente Medical Center in Portland, Oregon. Supinators, however, don't turn in their ankles when they run, directing damaging stress to the outside of the legs, he says.

One way to determine your footfall tendency: Step into the tub to get your feet wet, then stand on the dry floor and look at your footprints. (To make them easier to see, step on a couple of paper towels.) If you can see your arch, you are an overpronator; if you can't, you are an underpronator (supinator), says Dr. Raether.

Then pick the proper shoes. Choose carefully. "Some shoes on the market offer more control than others," says Stone. "If you pronate, you need what's called a board-lasted shoe." To tell if a shoe is board-lasted, pull out the insole—the extra strip of material that's inside the shoe. If there's no stitching between the insole and the bottom of the shoe, it's board-lasted, just what a pronator wants. If you're a supinator, you need the other kind of shoe: Look for an insole that is stitched or stitched and glued, says Stone.

Grab some low-cost orthotics. Specially molded shoe inserts (orthotics) can often correct pronation, but they can cost a bundle. Here's an inexpensive alternative to try first: For a few dollars, get a pair of shoe inserts from the drugstore and slip them into your running shoes—they may be all you need, says Stone. If your shins are still in rough shape after using a cheap insert, see a podiatrist for the higher-priced model.

Walk before you run. It's always best to warm up the muscles of the lower legs before you go on a run, according to Stone. One way is to ride a stationary bike for ten minutes. Or take a brief walk before you break into a full-paced canter.

Pig out on hamstring stretches. Tight hamstrings—those tendons on the underside of your thighs—can literally knock you off your stride, says Stone. To keep hamstrings loose, she recommends the hurdler's stretch. After warming up, sit on the ground, extend your right leg forward, and place the bottom of your left foot on the inside of your right leg so that you're making a P with your legs. Slowly lean forward, reaching your hands to your right foot and keeping the small of your back down for a count of ten. Switch legs and repeat.

Stretch your Achilles tendons. One of the best ways to avoid shin splints is to stretch the Achilles tendon—the tendon that joins your calf muscles to your heel. Here's how: Stand about three feet away from a wall and lean against it with your hands. Start with your legs shoulder-width apart, then move your right leg forward while keeping your left leg straight. Gently lean toward the wall until you can feel the stretch on the back of your left leg and hold for ten seconds. Repeat with the other leg, says Stone.

Strengthen those shins. Shin pain is often caused by weak lower leg muscles. To build those shin muscles, Stone suggests the following routine: Sit on a table with your legs hanging over the edge. Hook one ankle through the handle of a backpack that has a book in it. Without moving your upper leg, flex your foot upward for two to three seconds. Repeat 10 to 12 times. Then switch feet and repeat. You can also strengthen your lower legs by performing basic lower leg exercises such as drawing each letter of the alphabet with the big toe of each foot in the air.

Give your calves a moving experience. Your calf muscles can use some attention, too: With your shoes off, stand erect. Slowly rise onto your toes and make like a ballerina for a count of three. Lower and repeat 12 to 15 times. If that's too easy an exercise for your calves, you can make it more challenging by performing the same exercise while standing on a step and allowing your calves to stretch over the edge of the step. Be sure to hang on to something, so you don't fall down the stairs.

Save your best stretch for last. Because research shows that your muscles are more elastic after they've been warmed up, a thorough stretch at the end of your workout will help eliminate any shin pain, says Stone. "The best time to work on flexibility problems that can cause shin splints is when you're finished exercising," she says. All exercises for hamstrings, tendons, shins and calves should be done after as well as before you begin your workout.

Shoulder Pain

Even Atlas got a break every now and then from carrying the weight of the world on his shoulders—and you can bet he didn't use his free time painting the kitchen ceiling or trying to relive his youth on a tennis court.

But you? If you're like the majority of Americans these days, you have so many responsibilities to juggle at home, at work or both that it's a wonder Ringling Brothers hasn't offered you a job. But all that stress and strain is no clowning matter: It can give you high-powered shoulder pain as a main-ring event. Along with your knees, your shoulders are the most used joints in your body—and are commonly abused and injured.

Most shoulder pain usually results from one of two causes: Muscles and tendons may be injured from prolonged overuse, as can happen when you paint or garden for too long. Or they can get pinched between bones or ligaments, a process called impingement that frequently results from activities that require power strokes or throwing, such as swimming, tennis or softball. Whatever the cause, you may get symptoms that involve a steady aching pain, with intermittent bursts of sharper pain when you're in certain positions.

Moderating or stopping the offending activity—at least for a while—is the first step on the road to recovery. But in addition, here are some other ways to ease shoulder pain and help prevent a recurrence.

Exercise *after* your workout. "Shoulder pain often results from repetitive motion—whether it's caused by your job or by playing a sport such as tennis or softball," says Robert Stephens, Ph.D., chairman of the Department of Anatomy and director of sports medicine at the University of Health Sciences–College of Osteopathic Medicine in Kansas City, Missouri. "One of the best ways to remedy this problem, and help prevent it in the future, is to perform

Try to Find the *Why*

All shoulder pain might hurt like the dickens, but not all the pain comes from the same source. To determine the probable cause of your problem, sports medicine specialist Charles Norelli, M.D., staff physiatrist at Good Shepherd Rehabilitation Hospital in Allentown, Pennsylvania, suggests you try these exercises.
- "Hold your arm out and twist your wrist as though you were emptying a soda can, then raise your arm. If this causes pain, your problem is probably tendinitis," says Dr. Norelli.
- "If the pain is in your right shoulder, grab your right elbow with your left hand and pull it across your body," advises Dr. Norelli. "If this causes pain, that might be an impingement sign—a signal that something in the bone or muscle is getting in the way." This problem may be remedied with specific range-of-motion exercises and light weight lifting.

Dr. Norelli points out that any severe shoulder pain requires professional medical attention. Heart attack pain, for example, can sometimes be transferred to the shoulder. While these quick "diagnostics" can give you a clue in many cases, if the pain is severe, be sure to see your doctor for a more thorough examination.

full range-of-motion stretching and strengthening exercises in order to compensate for these repetitive movements. For instance, if you have shoulder pain after playing tennis, perform some gentle stretching exercises such as rotating your arm inward and outward and doing slow, full arm circles (like the backstroke and crawl stroke) in both directions.

"Stretching the muscles associated with the movement that's causing you the pain may help prevent muscle imbalances and ease the tension on the joints," says Dr. Stephens.

Use heat, but don't rely on it. Applying heat to a sore shoulder will help ease your pain, but it won't cure it.

"A heating pad to shoulder pain is what a microwave oven is to a bad sandwich: The sandwich tastes better warm, but if you let it cool down again, it'll taste just as bad as it did before you warmed it," says sports medicine specialist Charles Norelli, M.D., staff physiatrist at Good Shepherd Rehabilitation Hospital in Allentown, Pennsylvania. "In other words, you'll feel better while you have heat on your shoulder, but unless you fix the problem, you'll feel just as bad once you remove the heat."

Hoist some barbells. How do you "fix" shoulder pain? Besides practicing full range-of-motion exercises, lifting weights often helps, adds Dr. Norelli. "You want to strengthen rotator cuff muscles (behind the shoulder), and lifting weights is the best way to do that," he says. "Take a two- to six-pound barbell and lift it sideways, keeping your arm straight and your thumb pointing *up*. It's important to keep your thumb pointing up, because if it points down, you could be impinging your tendon."

Wear a muffler. If you notice more shoulder pain in the winter, then Mother Nature might be more to blame than an active lifestyle.

"A lot of times, people get shoulder pain because they're breathing cold air. The pain they feel is really referred pain from the lungs taking in freezing air," says A. J. Hahn, D.C., a chiropractor in Napoleon, Ohio, who specializes in natural remedies. "The answer is to wear a muffler or scarf during the cold months."

Shyness

Maybe it's those alluring downcast eyes or that cute nervous laugh, but suitors have long considered shyness to have a certain sex appeal—at least when courting from the other side of the room.

But try to get up close and personal and what do you see? Probably nothing. The wallflower usually runs away to avoid talking to you.

Don't laugh. There's nothing funny about social anxiety—what we call shyness. It's being so worried about what you say and the impression you make that you have trouble remembering names or faces or making even simple decisions in front of other people. It's being so fearful of communication that you become a prisoner of your own insecurities.

What causes shyness? Some experts point the finger at parents who show affection only when their children "perform," rather than loving their children unconditionally. Others believe shyness is the result of traumatizing events occurring in childhood or adolescence. "There are many theories, but there is no question that a genetic factor is involved," says Warren Jones, Ph.D., a psychologist at the University of Tennessee at Knoxville and an authority on shyness. "Shyness is passed by heredity."

You can't change your genes, but even if you're somewhat predisposed to shyness, you can change some of your tactics. If you find feelings of shyness beginning to build, try these techniques.

Play Mike Wallace. "The very essence of shyness is being in a social situation and not knowing exactly what to do or say—and feeling very uncomfortable about it. But one thing a shy person can do to alleviate a lot of the negative reactions that result from this is to adopt the role of interviewer," says Dr. Jones. He gives an example of a classic situation: You're at a party where the host introduces you to a stranger and then leaves. "Confronted with this, instead of trying to wing it and worrying about 'exposing' yourself, you should take the role of *asking* the questions," suggests Dr. Jones. "Not only does that take the pressure off *you* of having to keep the conversation going, but it is also quite rewarding, since most (nonshy) people prefer to talk about themselves."

Is Your Child Destined for Shyness?

Why be shy? Good question, since nobody *wants* to be shy. Although most experts agree that genetics play a key role, early detection can help you get your children on the bold and self-confident path. Among the clues that your child is likely to suffer shyness:

- "Frantic reunions" with parents: Although every toddler objects to being left with a stranger (or anyone who isn't Mom or Dad), shy children have particularly strong reactions—especially when *reunited* with parents. "Most children will greet their parents affectionately for a short time and then get along with their business," says shyness expert Warren Jones, Ph.D., a psychologist at the University of Tennessee at Knoxville. "But children with a predisposition to shyness tend to have a frantic reunion that lasts well beyond what most parents feel is necessary."

- An obsession with the usual order of things: "Another clue is when a child shows a too-strong preference for structure and order," adds Dr. Jones. What's "too strong"? "If a routine dinner ritual like saying grace is forgotten or ignored one day, the child might object strenuously and insist on going back and doing it the way it's always done," he says.

Remember the name game. "A lot of shy people are so nervous when they're being introduced to strangers that they don't *really* listen to the person's name; they're too busy focusing on what they're going to say next," adds Dr. Jones. "A good habit to get into is to have other people repeat their names *immediately* after being introduced. (Example: 'Excuse me, you say it's Bob?') This gives you something to concentrate on instead of worrying about yourself. And more importantly, even if you missed the name completely, it's easier to admit that at the beginning of a conversation than to wait 30 minutes and have the person believe you knew his name."

Log your achievements (and they are many). "I tell people to write on one or several cards *all* the virtues they have as a person and all the achievements they've made. Then they should read that list before they give a talk, or go on a date, or do whatever activity it is that makes them feel anxious," says Christopher McCullough, Ph.D., a psychotherapist in Raleigh, North Carolina, who is the former director of the San Francisco Anxiety and Phobia Recovery Center and who specializes in the study of social anxiety. "If they have trouble making the list, then they should sit with a friend or family member who can point out all their virtues. The best way to feel comfortable and at ease is to insist on being your genuine self. And making a list of your accomplishments shows you that your genuine self isn't so bad."

Sick Building Syndrome

S ome of the most dangerous air you breathe isn't emerging from a factory smokestack or a car exhaust pipe: It's in your home. In various amounts and concentrations, you might be getting formaldehyde from plywood and other building materials, stryrene and benzene from carpets, asbestos from ceiling tiles and flooring, carbon monoxide and nitrogen dioxide from kitchen appliances and infectious bacteria and fungi from heating and cooling systems. In all, the average home has upward of 200 different air contaminants.

Talk about being homesick! Breathing these substances day after day can leave you with any of a host of ails: headache, nausea, throat or eye irritation, dizziness and fatigue as well as wheezing, sneezing, coughing and other symptoms that mimic colds, flu or hay fever. Some contaminants are even suspected of causing cancer. While it can cost thousands of dollars to "cure" a building of sick building syndrome—depending on the size of the building and severity of the problems—here are some less expensive ways to help protect yourself from ailments caused by contaminants blowing through your home.

Take a lesson from the Japanese. "Dust causes more environmental problems than any other single source, and most of the dust tracked into your home is carried in on your shoes," says Lance Wallace, Ph.D., environmental scientist at the Environmental Protection Agency Office of Research and Development in Warrenton, Virginia. "So taking off your shoes at the front door is a good way to eliminate a lot of the dust in your home that you're breathing. If you aren't going to take off your shoes at the front door, then at least use a welcome mat. In tests we conducted, we found that wiping your feet

Offices Are Even Worse

Anyone who works in an office building is likely to be exposed to indoor pollutants—and the newer the building is, the more contaminants it may have.

Buildings constructed after 1970 are particularly vulnerable, since they're most likely to be energy-efficient. Among other things, that means that you're breathing air that is largely recirculated, which *increases* your risk of developing headache, sore throat, eye irritation and other health problems associated with sick building syndrome. But here's how to protect yourself at work.

Be aware of what you wear. "The more skin you have exposed, the more likely you are to get allergies and rashes caused by indoor pollutants," says Richard Silberman, technical supervisor for Healthy Buildings International, a Fairfax, Virginia–based company that diagnoses sick buildings. "There is evidence that dust on the skin may cause some of the allergic reactions and coldlike symptoms associated with sick building syndrome. So wearing pants is better than wearing shorts or dresses, and long sleeves are better than short sleeves. Basically, the less skin you have exposed, the better off you'll be."

Don't cover air ducts. Most office buildings have centrally controlled climate control, so you can't do anything about making your office warmer or cooler. "Because of this, many people cover the air duct with tape or a piece of cardboard when they feel a draft," says Silberman. "But that should *never* be done, because that air duct is often the only source of outdoor air, and covering it prohibits fresh air from coming in."

Keep a good attitude. In studies by psychologist Alan Hedge, Ph.D., of Cornell University in Ithaca, New York, it was found that those who are most likely to suffer sick building syndrome *on* the job are literally sick *of* the job. When you're unhappy, dissatisifed or stressed out—in your job or other aspects of your life—you're a prime candidate for the physical ills caused by indoor air pollution.

Dry wet areas quickly. "If carpets get wet, be sure to clean and dry them promptly," says Silberman. "Once wet, they can have microbiotic growth that can release spores into the air. These spores can trigger sneezing, wheezing, throat and eye irritations and other problems."

on a welcome mat eliminates a lot of dust, although not nearly as much as removing your shoes."

Decorate with houseplants. Studies by Bill Wolverton, Ph.D., president and research director of Wolverton Environmental Services, a research and consulting firm in Picayune, Mississippi, show that many low-light houseplants reduce levels of benzene, formaldehyde and other contaminants, because these plants use airborne toxins as a source of food. After taking in the toxin-containing air, the plant then returns cleaner air to your home.

Generally, you need a *minimum* of one plant for every 100-square-foot (average-size) room, says Dr. Wolverton. Among the most environmentally efficient (and easiest to maintain) are bamboo, areca and other palms, peace lily, English ivy, Boston fern, corn plants, chrysanthemums and philodendron.

But make sure the plant soil is "clean." Use good-quality commercial potting soil for houseplants. "You have to make sure the soil is clean and there are no bugs or growth in it, because contaminated soil can release contaminants into the air," says Richard Silberman, technical supervisor for Healthy Buildings International, a Fairfax, Virginia–based company that diagnoses sick buildings.

Is Your Building Sick?

While all buildings have harmful contaminants, what makes some "sick"? The answer: some simple math.

"Basically, if a minimum of 15 percent of occupants in a home or an office are having the types of medical problems that seem to be linked to the building, then it's 'sick,' " says Richard Silberman, technical supervisor for Healthy Buildings International, a Fairfax, Virginia–based company that diagnoses sick buildings.

The problems include:
- Frequent headaches.
- Nausea.
- Throat or eye irritation.
- Dizziness or fatigue.
- Symptoms of colds, flu or hay fever.
- Wheezing.

Don't use air fresheners. Commercial air fresheners do nothing to freshen the air. "In fact, they're a big source of *added* indoor air pollution," according to Dr. Wallace. "Most fresheners contain chemicals that have been found to cause cancer in animals. Rather than removing odors, they just make it impossible to smell them. And it's not just aerosols that are dangerous. In tests, the solid air fresheners were found to have high concentrations of some of the nastier chemicals."

And you can't assume that air "disinfectants" are much better. "They are really nothing more than pesticides that smell good," adds Dr. Wallace. "And you certainly don't want to breathe pesticides all day."

Let your house breathe. Being energy-efficient is one thing; sealing off your house completely is another. "We've removed a lot of our homes' natural ventilation by tightening things up to save on fuel," says Thomas Godar, M.D., chief of the Pulmonary Disease Section at St. Francis Hospital and Medical Center in Hartford, Connecticut. "A tight house with a lot of insulation is like a closed box."

So open things up a little—use exhaust fans in the kitchen and bathrooms whenever possible. While storm windows and weather stripping will reduce energy costs, they can also seal off fresh air if your home is newer and built to be energy-efficient. So leave a window or two open just a crack, even in winter, if you have a newly built, completely insulated home.

Ban *all* smoke from your home. Cigarette smoke contains more than 4,000 different chemicals, including benzene, formaldehyde and carbon monoxide—possible culprits in sick building syndrome. So breathing cigarette smoke—even secondhand smoke—is bad enough. "But if you have radon or asbestos in your home—and nearly every home has radon—then you're getting even worse damage from it if there's a smoker in your house," says Dr. Wallace. "That's because radon and asbestos attach to the smoke particles you're breathing into your lungs, so you get a bigger dose than you normally would."

Leave the house after you clean it. You're probably exposed to a lot of dust—and indoor air pollution—when you're cleaning house. "That's because vacuuming picks up only maybe 15 percent of the dust," says Dr. Wallace. "Much of the dust goes right through the vacuum bag and hangs in the air for several hours." His advice: "Do your housecleaning immediately before you leave. That way, you won't be subjected to all that flying dust."

Side Stitches

What does running in the annual Hermitage, Pennsylvania, Gobble Wobble five-kilometer road race have in common with Cowboy Bob's five-second spin around the rodeo ring on the Widow Maker? Easy: In both events, the enthused contestant is in danger of contracting painful side stitches.

Pounding the pavement, riding a bucking bronco and a host of other wild and crazy antics can easily jostle your diaphragm into a sudden state of spasm.

"When you're breathing out, your diaphragm rises—and that raises tension on ligaments between the diaphragm and your other internal organs," says Owen Anderson, Ph.D., editor of *Running Research News* in Lansing, Michigan. "If your running foot hits the ground right at that moment, it creates a jolting action that temporarily upsets your diaphragm." Another theory suggests that overexertion—in a race or competition—sometimes taxes the diaphragm, sending it into spasm.

But you don't have to hang up your Keds or hobble your trusty steed to beat side stitches. Here's how to unstitch them before your competitive ambitions come unraveled.

Tone your tummy. Stronger stomach muscles help support the internal organs thought to cause side stitches. One method to get them in shape is with stomach crunches. Lie on your back with your feet on the floor and your knees raised. Fold your hands on your chest. Gently lift your torso and back off the floor about three inches and gently exhale. Then *inhale* as you slowly lower yourself back down. Repeat 20 times.

Grunt and avoid it. This technique sounds primitive, but Dr. Anderson says grunting at the first sign of a side stitch is a surefire remedy. "When your foot hits the ground and you make a forceful grunt, that helps you allow the diaphragm to be free and relaxed and release some of the tension." It's not necessary to grunt throughout the race, though—unless you want to frighten your fellow runners, says Dr. Anderson.

Go head over heels. Here's another quick fix for severe side stitches from Dr. Anderson: When you feel one coming on, stop running, lie down on your back, and pull your knees over your head. The pain should subside immediately. (If it doesn't, call a doctor, says Dr. Anderson. This kind of pain can be a signal of a heart attack.)

Start belly breathing. Rather than taking short, quick breaths, you want to breathe deeply. The best way to learn: Practice for five minutes each day. Lie down and place a book on your stomach. With every inhalation, try to raise the book before expanding your chest, says Dr. Anderson. That action of your diaphragm automatically creates deep breathing.

Don't eat and run. If you're prone to getting side stitches, avoid eating or drinking for a couple of hours before you go on a run or a bumpy ride. A full stomach pulls on the diaphragm more forcefully, creating greater tension and, as a result, side stitches. "Lots of extra fluids are needed during the longer races such as marathons, but you should be able to get by without them in ten-kilometer races and shorter competitions," says Dr. Anderson. By experimenting with amounts, however, you may find that you're able to tolerate some fluids. The only caution: If you're going to run in the heat for an hour or more, you need to drink about 1¾ cups of water (14 ounces) before starting. After that, drink 3 to 4 ounces every ten minutes, if possible, whether you're prone to side stitches or not, he says.

Stay away from carbonated beverages. Some experts believe that one reason side stitches occur is because gas is trapped from bubbly drinks, says Susan Perry, a physical therapist specializing in sports medicine at the Fort Lauderdale Sports Medicine Clinic in Fort Lauderdale, Florida. As a result, it's best to avoid any carbonated drinks within a few hours of participating in the activity, she says.

Moderate your pace. Slowing down may keep your stitches from knocking you out of the race, says Dr. Anderson. "A lot of times, a runner who feels a stitch coming on can simply slow down a bit, try to relax and change breathing patterns. In five minutes, he won't even know he had that initial stitch."

Switch your specialty. If you've tried *everything* and painful side stitches continue when you run, you might consider riding a bike or walking to get your exercise. "There's much less jolting with biking and walking," explains Dr. Anderson.

Sleep Apnea

When it comes to comedy, whether it's Dagwood Bumstead's sofa antics or the Three Stooges and their sleeping sound effects, snoring has always given us a good laugh—and the louder the snarfing, gurgling and harrumphing, the louder our yuks.

But shake-the-walls snoring could be a sign of a potentially life-threatening condition called sleep apnea, in which the throat relaxes and closes during sleep. Sleep apnea affects nearly one of every ten Americans—primarily middle-aged to older men who are usually overweight.

"The difference between regular snoring and sleep apnea is that with sleep apnea, you actually *stop* breathing, anywhere from ten seconds up to three minutes," says Peter Hauri, Ph.D., co-director of the Mayo Clinic Sleep Disorders Center in Rochester, Minnesota. "And these stoppages are frequent—a minimum of at least 15 per hour. Usually the person stops breathing for 30 or 40 seconds and then gasps for air (making the snoring sound) and resumes breathing. For your bed partner, it can be most terrifying." And it could be dangerous as well—since people with sleep apnea have a much higher risk of heart attack.

If your doctor has diagnosed you with sleep apnea—and that can happen only after a thorough examination of your sleeping habits—you probably have been made aware of the risks. But here are some remedies you should also note.

Solve it with spray. One way to cut your congestion is with an over-the-counter saline spray that will moisten mucous membranes and help make breathing easier. You can mix your own saline nasal spray by dissolving no more than ½ teaspoon of salt (⅓ teaspoon if you're hypertensive) in eight ounces of warm water. Collecting the solution in a nosedropper, tilt your head back and sniff the spray into each nostril. Spit out the water and blow your nose. *Note:* Don't overdo the salt—too much can burn your nostrils.

Lighten your load. It's no wonder that nearly *all* those with sleep apnea are overweight. "Often, losing weight *alone* is enough to solve the problem," says Dr. Hauri. That's because fat deposits in the obese—particularly men—are at the base of the tongue. The extra fatty tissue blocks an already clogged air passage, making nighttime breathing more difficult.

Say no to nightcaps. Drinking in the evening is never a good idea for snorers, but it's particularly dangerous for those with sleep apnea. Research by Merrill Mitler, Ph.D., director of research for the Division of Chest, Critical Care and Sleep Medicine at the Scripps Clinic Sleep Disorders Center in San Diego, found that drinking can *double* your episodes of sleep apnea compared with going to bed sober.

"You should limit alcohol for at least six hours before going to sleep," says Bernard DeBerry, M.D., a Laguna Hills, California, surgeon who specializes in procedures related to snoring and sleep apnea and who is clinical associate professor of surgery in the Head and Neck Division at the University of California, Irvine, College of Medicine. "Alcohol is a central nervous system depressant, and as such, it decreases control of muscles in your upper airway." The more "relaxed" those muscles are, the more snoring—and the greater chance that the person with sleep apnea will stop breathing.

Avoid allergenic foods. "People with food allergies should avoid the foods that cause a reaction, because those foods can add to their congestion," according to Dr. DeBerry. "The more congested you are, the more clogged your airway, and the greater the risk of sleep apnea. So if you know that eating a certain food will cause your nose to block up, by all means, don't eat that food—especially in the hours before bedtime."

Ban the butts. "Smoking irritates the upper respiratory tract and makes sleep apnea worse," says Thomas Roth, Ph.D., director of the Henry Ford Hospital Sleep Disorders and Research Center in Detroit and president of the National Sleep Foundation. Besides, smoking also contributes to congestion.

Don't nosh at night. A midnight snack may help cure insomnia, but it can spell disaster for those with sleep apnea. "Eating just before sleep can add to congestion," says Dr. DeBerry.

Sleepwalking

If wakewalkers are people who wander around lethargically during the day with a glazed look in their eyes, what do you call people who do it at night? While they're *asleep?*

Of course, the term *wakewalking* hasn't been widely accepted yet. But *sleepwalking* has, perhaps because as much as 15 percent of the population—as many as 30 million Americans—are sleepwalkers. This most-joked-about medical condition is most prevalent between ages 6 and 12 and usually ends by age 14. (If sleepwalking continues beyond age 18, doctors advise seeking counseling at a sleep disorders center.)

So what if you wake up one night to find a member of your household sleepwalking around? Here are some doctor-recommended tips on how to deal with sleepwalkers.

Don't wake them suddenly. There's no truth to the rumor that waking up a sleepwalker is dangerous to the walker. But if you do, stand clear. "If you wake a sleepwalker abruptly, you can startle him and may wind up with a black eye,"

When to See the Doctor

In adults, sleepwalking is associated with excessive stress, so dealing with the stress in your life is a good way to control or eliminate sleepwalking," says Peter Hauri, Ph.D., co-director of the Mayo Clinic Sleep Disorders Center in Rochester, Minnesota. (And don't use alcohol and other sedatives as stress relievers, because they interfere with sleep quality.) Dr. Hauri and other doctors recommend treatment at a sleep disorders center if you are over the age of 18 and have a problem with sleepwalking.

says Gary Zammit, Ph.D., director of the Sleep Disorders Institute at St. Luke's–Roosevelt Hospital Center in New York City. "The best thing to do with a sleepwalker in your house is to *gently* guide him back to bed and encourage him to lie on his back. You can talk to him, but it should be in a soothing and gentle manner."

Protect them. "While you shouldn't intervene with a sleepwalker, you should take measures to protect him from injury," adds Marc Weissbluth, M.D., director of the Children's Memorial Hospital Sleep Disorders Center in Chicago and author of *Healthy Sleep Habits, Happy Child.* "That means locks on doors, gates on stairs, bolting down windows and removing sharp-edged toys. As long as they're protected from injury, they'll be fine. Either they will go back to bed by themselves or they'll sleep somewhere else."

Make sure they get enough sleep. Being overtired or not getting enough sleep—the culprit behind sleep terrors and bed-wetting—can also cause sleepwalking in some children, says Dr. Weissbluth. "Often the answer is simply to make sure the children get more sleep."

Snakebites

Ever since that unfortunate episode in the Garden of Eden, snakes haven't exactly been characterized as the Albert Schweitzers of the animal kingdom. Aside from their snake-in-the-grass reputation, the infamy of their poisonous bites has grown far and wide—even to places where there are *no* poisonous snakes.

True, there are some 45,000 snakebites every year in the United States, but fewer than one-sixth of them involve poisonous snakes. "And a significant number of bites from poisonous snakes are dry bites," says wilderness medicine specialist Kenneth W. Kizer, M.D., M.P.H., professor of emergency medicine at the University of California, Davis. If you have a dry bite, Dr. Kizer explains, it means the snake doesn't deposit any venom into the bite wound or deposits such a small amount that you probably won't become seriously ill from it.

While the average person has about as much chance of dying from a snakebite as of getting struck by lightning, you should never take snakebites lightly—so see your doctor immediately. If possible, try to get a good look at the snake—and be able to describe it—so your doctor has a better idea if it's poisonous. (Do whatever you can to identify the snake without endangering yourself or others.) If the snake was not poisonous, the doctor probably will just clean the wound and apply a topical antibiotic ointment to prevent infection. You will need to keep an eye on the wound for the next few days: The doctor will advise you about watching for signs of infection.

In the meantime, here are some emergency treatment tips that will tide you over until you get to a hospital or doctor's office.

Don't play TV medic. Forget that old advice about marking Xs on the bite with a razor blade and trying to suck out the venom. "Most people do more damage to themselves than they do good when they try to 'cut and suck,'" says Dr. Kizer. "You can really hurt yourself if you don't know what you're doing. At best, you'll extract only about 5 percent of the venom anyway." And that wouldn't save anyone except a very small child.

Keep the wound away from ice. Soaking a bitten hand or foot in a bucket of ice water usually does more harm than good. It is likely to cause frostbite. Since pit-viper venom makes tissues very temperature-sensitive, icing can lead

---

Is It Poisonous or Not?

Even if you don't have a merit badge in snake identification, it helps to be able to recognize the most common poisonous snakes.

Pit vipers—rattlesnakes, copperheads and cottonmouths—are responsible for the majority of venomous snakebites in North America. These snakes have triangular heads. There are distinctive "pits" between the nostrils and eyes on *both* sides of the head. The eyes have elliptical pupils. And they also have (need we mention?) two fangs.

The coral snake, another poisonous one, has no facial pits, but it's easily recognized. It is ringed with white or yellow bands touching red and black rings. Coral snakes are generally found in the southern United States. Not *all* varieties are poisonous, but you'd need that merit badge to tell the difference. So err on the side of caution.

to serious damage—even loss of an otherwise salvageable limb, says Earl Schwartz, M.D., chairman of the Department of Emergency Medicine at Bowman Gray School of Medicine of Wake Forest University in Winston-Salem, North Carolina.

Stay calm and stay put. "Fear is the biggest thing to worry about with snake-bite," says Dr. Kizer. "The best advice I can give is to remain calm." After all, if you've been bitten by a North American snake—even a poisonous one—the risk of death is very low. He recommends that you send someone for help, then "sit down somewhere." The area of the bite should be below heart level when you're seated. If you do move, go slowly. If you're alone when you get bitten, walk, *don't* run, when you go for help. "The more quickly you move, the harder your muscles work," says Dr. Kizer. As a result, the venom will get into your circulation more rapidly if you start running.

Splint the bitten area. Putting a splint on the snakebitten area helps prevent muscle contractions from spreading the poison any faster. "Fashion a splint out of anything that's stiff and straight—branches work very well," notes Dr. Kizer. Wrap a towel, T-shirt or pair of socks around the splint to hold it on—but tie it loosely. You don't want to cut off blood supply to the bitten area.

Forget about tourniquets. In the old days, some first-aiders believed you should tighten a cloth around the arm or leg, making a tourniquet that cuts off the blood supply. Don't try it, warns Dr. Kizer. Tourniquets can cause serious injury and should not be used.

Sneezing

Don't feel dopey and try not to be grumpy if you achoo on cue. You're just sneezy, so there's nothing to be bashful about. Without dwarfing the size of the problem, you should be happy to know that within limits, you can be your own doc in stopping those noisy nose fits.

"A sneeze is usually a response to an allergic nasal irritant," says Howard J. Silk, M.D., a physician at the Atlanta Allergy Clinic and assistant professor of pediatrics at the Medical College of Georgia in Augusta. "And you must always guard against common household allergens such as dust, mold, mildew, pets and dust mites."

But don't hold your breath—literally or figuratively. After taking all cleaning and allergic precautions, "don't expect miracles right away," Dr. Silk says. "It could take six months to significantly reduce all the allergic materials in your house." Start with patience, and add the following actions.

Muffle your mattress. Beds often harbor mites that feed on dead skin cells, Dr. Silk says. Sheathe mattresses and box springs in an airtight, noncotton cover, then wash the sheets regularly in water at least 130°F. That temperature is hot enough to kill the microscopic monsters that cause so many sneezes.

Down with down. Though comfortable and natural, down pillows have a big minus: They hold dust and mites, Dr. Silk says. Instead, choose a washable,

---

Sneeze . . . And Blow

Although some people try to stifle their sneezes, the best response is to go with the blow, according to Gailen D. Marshall, Jr., M.D., Ph.D., assistant professor and director of the Allergy and Clinical Immunology Division at the University of Texas Medical School at Houston. "It may be socially acceptable to stifle a sneeze, but it's potentially extraordinarily dangerous," he says.

The peril is in the eustachian tubes, which connect nasal passages to the middle ear, regulating air pressure on both sides of your eardrums. If you suppress a sneeze, mucus from your throat and nose could be thrust into the middle ear or sinuses.

Since the mucus is nonsterile, Dr. Marshall says, "it's very possible to create a sinus infection from sneezing improperly. You can potentially precipitate a middle ear infection as well." At the very worst, if the snuffed-out sneeze is forceful enough, the backed-up pressure may rupture an eardrum.

As for the best way to blow your nose: Close one nostril and blow gently through the other into a tissue, Dr. Marshall says. Force out air and mucus in several puffs, not one all-or-nothing blow. Alternate nostrils until your nose, at least for the time being, is clear.

hypoallergenic polyester pillow. Wash it every few weeks, again in water hot enough to kill any mites that might pervade the polyester.

Stuff the stuffed animals. They're cute and cuddly, but stuffed animals and dolls collect dust and dust mites. To safeguard your sneezing snout, Dr. Silk says, you may have to give your teddy bear to the family archivist. It doesn't belong in your room anymore.

Don't get your pet's dander up. People who have allergic reactions to dogs or cats are usually reacting to dander, the small flakes and scales of the animal's skin, according to Dr. Silk. Cat saliva and urine can also be allergens. "If you're allergic to pets, don't keep them," says Dr. Silk. "If you have them and don't want to get rid of them, keep them outside or at least out of the bedroom."

Always wash your hands immediately after petting any cat or dog, he recommends, and bathe your pet once a week.

Be pro-antihistamine. "If the sneezing spell is short and seasonal, people can try an over-the-counter antihistamine to see if it provides some relief," says Horst R. Konrad, M.D., chairman of the Division of Otolaryngology/Head and Neck Surgery at Southern Illinois University School of Medicine in Springfield. Topical nasal sprays containing cortisone are the most effective medicine for reining in sneezing fits and allergies, according to Dr. Konrad. But these are available only by prescription.

Let the grass grow. If plants send your sneeze control haywire, limit your time outside. "Don't mow the lawn," Dr. Konrad says. "Talk someone else into doing it." And keep the windows closed when the grass flies.

Don't make a move. You may think relocation is the answer to your allergies, but there are always going to be allergens, no matter where you move. "Obviously, it's hard to avoid spring," says Mark Loury, M.D., assistant professor in the Department of Otolaryngology/Head and Neck Surgery at Johns Hopkins University Hospital in Baltimore. "In the spring, it's tree pollen. In summer and early autumn, sagebrush and tumbleweed pollinate throughout the western United States. In the fall, regardless of location, ragweed and molds are just about everywhere." Dust, of course, is unavoidable year-round, no matter where you live.

Snoring

The purpose is to *sleep* like a log, not sound as though you're *sawing* one. Yet soon after they hit the sheets, nearly half of all folks play nocturnal lumberjack at least occasionally.

But the reason for all that nighttime noise has more to do with Sir Isaac Newton than Paul Bunyan—especially if you, like most problem snorers, sleep on your back. Snoring is often caused by gravity acting on loose tissue in the upper airway, says Peter Hauri, Ph.D., co-director of the Mayo Clinic Sleep Disorders Center in Rochester, Minnesota. When you're lying on your back, either the tissue or your tongue "falls" into your throat and obstructs your airway.

Excess weight and nighttime drinking are commonly associated with snoring. "The best advice I can give to anyone who snores is lose weight. And don't drink—since alcohol plays a role in snoring most of the time," says Thomas Roth, Ph.D., president of the National Sleep Foundation and director of the Henry Ford Hospital Sleep Disorders and Research Center in Detroit. In addition, consider these methods of reducing the rasp of sawing wood to the whispered hiss of sound sleep.

Beware the drowsiness drugs. Booze isn't the only sedative that turns up the snoring volume. "Any sleeping pills and tranquilizers should be avoided—and that includes allergy medicine with antihistamine," according to Bernard DeBerry, M.D., a Laguna Hills, California, surgeon who specializes in procedures related to snoring and sleep apnea and who is clinical associate professor of surgery in the Head and Neck Division at the University of California, Irvine, College of Medicine. "If you must take allergy medication, talk to your doctor about one that produces less sedating side effects, such as terfenadine (Seldane) for hay fever. In general, if your medicine makes you feel sleepy during the day, then you shouldn't be taking it, especially if you have problems with snoring."

Snooze on your side or stomach. It's no coincidence that most problem snorers sleep on their backs. "Basically, when you're on your back, your tongue falls back like a wet rag into your throat," says Dr. DeBerry. "That's not exactly helpful in maintaining a clear airway." That's why *all* experts say sleeping in another position—preferably on your stomach—usually helps decrease both the volume and incidence of snoring.

Stop nighttime racket with tennis balls. To *keep* you off your back, try this old favorite remedy. "Get an old T-shirt or pair of pajamas and sew a long pocket in the back. Then place several tennis balls in that pocket and wear it to bed," says Rosalind Cartwright, Ph.D., director of the Sleep Disorder Service and Research Center at Rush–St. Luke's–Presbyterian Medical Center in Chicago. "If you roll on your back, the tennis balls will be so uncomfortable that you'll move to another position."

Get more sleep. "It's not a well-known fact, but sleep loss causes snoring," says Dr. Roth. "If you're snoring and not sleeping enough, you may be able to fix the problem by going to bed an hour or so earlier or sleeping later."

Sleep on a firm mattress. If your mattress is soft or saggy, get a new firm one. A flat, firm mattress helps keep your neck straight and reduces obstructions in your airway, according to Portland, Oregon, otolaryngologist Derek S. Lipman, M.D., author of *Stop Your Husband from Snoring*.

Elevate your bed. "Body position plays an important role in snoring. If you can avoid lying flat, you're much better off, because the tissue won't vibrate so

When to See the Doctor

Heavy-duty snoring is sometimes associated with sleep apnea—which means that a person literally stops breathing for a period of time. This condition is particularly prevalent among overweight, middle-aged men, and it can be life-threatening. So see your doctor if snoring is persistent or if somebody has observed that you frequently stop breathing during sleep.

Also, frequent snoring can lead to other serious medical problems such as high blood pressure or irregular heartbeat as well as headaches, excessive fatigue and personality changes—all good reasons to see the doctor if snoring persists.

much," says Dr. Roth. Some experts recommend getting an adjustable bed that raises your torso, but an easier method is to place some bricks or blocks of wood under your headboard to raise the front of the bed.

Add some pillows. "Placing additional pillows under your head to prop yourself up will also help by changing your sleeping angle," adds Dr. Roth. "Two pillows are better than one pillow, and three pillows are better than two."

Or *remove* all pillows. Pillows can be more of a hindrance than a help, however, if they only kink your neck, says researcher Earl V. Dunn, M.D., of the University of Toronto's Sunnybrook Health Science Centre. The pillows should adjust your entire torso angle to bring you higher. If they elevate only your neck, you're better off without them.

Stop the smoke, stop the snore. Doctors agree: If you smoke and snore, the smoking has to stop. Smoking causes changes in the tissue of your respiratory system that can contribute to snoring, says Dr. Lipman. Specifically, the demon weed increases congestion in your nose and throat and causes swelling of the mucous membranes of the throat and upper air passages. And it reduces oxygen uptake by the lungs.

Exercise regularly. "People who exercise regularly are much less likely to form congestion in the upper respiratory tract," says Dr. DeBerry. Besides, regular aerobic exercise improves cardiovascular health and strengthens overall breathing and lung capacity, which may offset problems that lead to snoring. But exercise should be avoided just before bedtime, since it can "leave your body too charged up to sleep," he adds.

Sore Throat

It feels as though someone's holding a lit match at the back of your throat. That raw, burning sensation seems to radiate to your whole head. And you know what that means: at least a few more days of discomfort, as your sore throat takes it course.

A sore throat is often the earliest symptom of a cold or the flu. But you can also get a sore throat for a lot of other reasons—from viral or bacterial infections, dry air, smoking, exposure to irritants or too much cheering at a hockey game.

A persistent, recurrent or severe sore throat, or one accompanied by fever, needs medical treatment. But many sore throats can be soothed by the simple remedies given here and should disappear within a week.

Suck on soothing lozenges. "I simply suggest sugar-free vitamin C such as N'Ice," says Michael Benninger, M.D., chairman of the Department of Otolaryngology at Henry Ford Hospital in Detroit and chairman of the committee on Speech, Voice and Swallowing Disorders of the American Academy of Otolaryngology. If you want a lozenge with actual pain-numbing power, look for one that contains benzocaine, such as Cēpacol or Chloraseptic, adds Arthur Jacknowitz, Pharm.D., professor and chairman of clinical pharmacy at the West Virginia University School of Pharmacy in Morgantown. But don't rely on these lozenges for more than two or three days, Dr. Benninger warns. "While they relieve pain, they don't do anything to address the real cause of your pain, whether it be an infection or the abuse of your vocal cords."

Or try zinc gluconate tablets. Some people swear by these, and in one study at the Clayton Foundation Biochemical Institute at the University of Texas at Austin, they did prove to be effective relievers of sore throat and some other cold symptoms.

"The trick is to let the dissolved zinc bathe your throat for a while," says Donald Davis, Ph.D., the study's main researcher. "Don't just swallow the tablet." The lozenges should be used for no more than seven days, he adds, because large amounts of zinc can interfere with your body's ability to absorb other minerals.

Sip something hot. Try decaffeinated tea or herbal tea with honey, suggests Dr. Benninger. "A number of the performing artists I see use that, and it appears to work for them. I don't know why, but it is very soothing."

Tip your head back and roar. While gargling won't kill off the germs causing your sore throat, it will moisturize and temporarily soothe your upper throat, Dr. Benninger says. And while there are many possible gargles on the market, such as Listerine, salt water is as good as any, and it's cheap, he adds.

Mix one teaspoon of salt (no more or you'll dry out your throat!) in a pint of warm (never hot) water. To gargle, start by taking in a deep breath. Pour a small

When to See the Doctor

At the first sign of *sore* throat, most doctors suspect *strep* throat, a very painful form of sore throat caused by the streptococcus bacteria. It's a serious concern, since strep throat, if left untreated, can lead to problems such as rheumatic fever and rheumatic heart disease.

"With strep throat, the pain is really bad, and it hurts to swallow," says Michael Benninger, M.D., chairman of the Department of Otolaryngology at Henry Ford Hospital in Detroit and chairman of the committee on Speech, Voice and Swallowing Disorders of the American Academy of Otolaryngology. If small children are in this kind of pain, you can usually tell: "They scrunch their faces when they swallow, they cry, and they drool," says Dr. Benninger. And children with strep throat usually run a fever as well.

So if you suspect that you or your child *does* have strep throat, be sure to see a doctor as soon as possible. There are prescription antibiotics that can usually cure the condition quickly.

Also have your sore throat checked by a doctor if it's accompanied by any of the following.
- Trouble breathing, swallowing or opening your mouth
- Joint pains
- Earache
- Rash
- Fever above 101°F
- Blood in the phlegm or saliva
- A persistent lump in the throat
- Hoarseness that lasts more than two weeks

amount of salt water into your mouth and tilt your head back. Let air bubble out slowly to create the garling effect. If it's noisy, it's right. Gargle as often as you like.

Indulge in garlic. "When a sore throat is caused by a virus infection, as opposed to bacteria, eating garlic can bring quicker relief," suggests Yu-Yan Yeh, Ph.D., associate professor of nutrition at Pennsylvania State University in University Park and a researcher on the healing properties of garlic. "Garlic has been shown to have antiviral and antifungal activities."

Try an eye-opening cocktail of tomato or mixed vegetable juice, two garlic cloves and a dash of Worcestershire sauce. Run it through a blender and drink. Or simply add garlic to your favorite dishes. "It doesn't matter whether it's fresh or powdered garlic," Dr. Yeh says.

Avoid tobacco smoke. "To avoid a sore throat in the future, don't smoke and don't expose yourself or your children to sidestream smoke," says Dr. Benninger. Smokers are much more likely than nonsmokers to have chronic throat irritation. And their children have more throat infections than the children of nonsmokers.

Keep indoor air cool and moist. During the cold winter months, the extreme dryness of heated indoor air may cause a recurring mild sore throat, especially in the morning and especially if a stuffed-up nose is making you breathe through your mouth, Dr. Benninger says. "A humidifier on your furnace is okay as long as it's working well, but most people don't keep the house humid enough. Indoor air should be at 35 to 40 percent relative humidity. If you can't achieve that with your furnace humidifier, keep a humidifier in your bedroom, and close the bedroom door at night."

Keeping the temperature of your house on the cool side—65° to 68°F—will reduce your need to add moisture and will also help keep inflammation down.

Trade in your toothbrush. "Lingering sore throats may be traceable to bacteria on a toothbrush," says Richard T. Glass, D.D.S., Ph.D., chairman of the Department of Oral Pathology at the Colleges of Dentistry and Medicine at the University of Oklahoma in Oklahoma City.

If you're having chronic problems, he suggests you trade in your toothbrush for a new model every two weeks. "It's also a good idea to throw your toothbrush away at the beginning of an illness, when you first start feeling better two or three days later and then when you feel completely well."

Splinters

Getting a splinter can be a real thorn in your side. And unfortunately, trying to *remove* it can often be just as troublesome. All that digging around with a needle can smart like the dickens and make mincemeat of even the toughest hide. And besides causing pain, that tiny splinter of wood (or sliver of glass or metal) can also cause infection if it's not removed cleanly and carefully.

Here's what the pros recommend for painless splinter removal, to keep that itsy-bitsy invader from causing mightier problems.

Let warm water do the work. Before you go probing for that splinter with a needle, give the affected area a good soak. "Often a 10- to 15-minute soak in warm water will cause the wood to swell, which causes the splinter to pop out on its own," says Marian H. Putnam, M.D., a pediatrician in Boston and clinical instructor of pediatrics at Boston University School of Medicine.

Ice away the pain. If a warm soak doesn't do the trick, try putting an ice cube on the splinter. "Many people claim that it numbs the area, so it doesn't

When to See the Doctor

Although most splinters can be treated at home, there are times when a doctor's expertise is needed.

"If the splinter is deeply embedded or occurs in a sensitive area such as the face or underneath a nail, I think it's best handled by a doctor," says Kathy Lillis, M.D., a pediatric emergency medicine physician at Children's Hospital of Buffalo in Buffalo, New York. "Or if a child has a splinter and is extremely terrified, it's probably better to have a doctor remove it, even if it's a small splinter." The pediatrician may be able to give a local anesthetic before removing the splinter, she points out.

hurt as much when they try to remove the splinter," says Kathy Lillis, M.D., a pediatric emergency medicine physician at Children's Hospital of Buffalo in Buffalo, New York.

Get the right tweezers. If you must remove the splinter the old-fashioned way—by digging it out with a pair of tweezers—make sure you have the right tools for the job, says Dr. Lillis. "You should have tweezers with ridged edges, which are available at most drugstores. And you can grip more easily if they have flat ends, as opposed to curved ones."

Cleanse those tweezers. Always wash tweezers in isopropyl rubbing alcohol before you use them, doctors say. You should then apply a liberal dose of hydrogen peroxide to the splinter itself. "The peroxide helps clean the wound to prevent any infection, and it can wash away any flecks of debris, so you'll have a cleaner removal," says Dr. Putnam. After removing the splinter, wash the area with hydrogen peroxide, then with a liquid hand soap.

Give yourself a facial. If you have a few cactus plants on your windowsill, you've probably gotten a spine in your skin more than once. A mask of gel should help get it out. "Just spread the gel over the area. When it dries, you can peel it off like a sheet—and the cactus spine usually comes right out," according to Dr. Putnam. In some cases, several applications of gel may be needed. A really stubborn spine may require tweezers to remove. While the mask technique works well for cactus needles, she adds that it may not remove other splinters as easily. (Glue, incidentally, is not a recommended method of removing cactus spines or splinters, according to Dr. Putnam.)

Sprains

Step off the curb the wrong way, or lose your balance in stiletto heels, and *ooof!* . . . you sprain your ankle. Hold your hand out to catch yourself from a fall and *yowww!* . . . sprained wrist.

Sprains occur because of excessive stretching or tearing of a ligament, which is one of those tough bands of elastic-like tissue attached to a joint.

Treat Strains with Heat, Not Cold

There's a difference between *sprains* and *strains*. Sprains affect ligaments (or joints). Strains occur when a *muscle* is stretched or partially torn. If you have a strain, you can tell, because it won't get swollen or black and blue like a sprain. And the treatment is different. You'll heal faster from a strain if the area around the injured muscle is heated slightly, says John Rabkin, M.D., assistant professor of surgery at the Oregon Health Sciences University in Portland.

Heat works better for strains because it increases blood flow and the influx of oxygen to muscles, which speeds production of collagen, a crucial step in the healing process. Just put a hot water bottle or heating pad on the affected area for 15 to 30 minutes four to six times a day. But don't rub on Ben-Gay or another ointment before applying heat; the skin can absorb so much of the cream that it can cause deep blistering.

You'll feel pain for sure, but there's usually another sign as well: The area may be swollen and black and blue. If you suffer a sprain, all that pain and swelling are sure to send you to a doctor, who may prescribe a compression air cast. But most sprains are minor, and with proper R and R, you'll fully recover in a few weeks. To help yourself along, try these measures.

Eat pineapple. "You can speed recovery and get rid of any bruising from a sprain by eating a lot of pineapple—especially right after your injury," says Steven Subotnick, D.P.M., a sports podiatrist in Hayward, California, and author of *Sports and Exercise Injuries*. "That's because pineapple has bromelain, an enzyme that helps heal bruises and speed healing." (The only drawback is that bromelain can cause dermatitis in some people, so take the pineapple off your diet if your skin begins to feel itchy.)

Use ice and elevate. Most experts recommend *immediate* icing for sprains, followed by elevating the sprained joint above heart level. The cold deadens the pain and decreases blood flow, which lessens swelling. Keep the ice on for 15 to 20 minutes, then take it off for an equal amount of time, four or five times daily for at least two days. Be careful not to place an ice pack *directly* on your skin. Instead, wrap it in a towel. By elevating the joint, you also help keep blood flowing *away* from that area, which reduces pain and swelling.

Wrap it. "Wrapping the sprained area in an elastic bandage helps keep the joint in position and prevents further injury," adds Dr. Subotnick. "Wrap it so that it's snug, but not so tight that you're cutting off circulation."

Get the right shoes. If you repeatedly sprain your ankles, here's a way to avoid it in the future: Wear the shoes specifically designed for your activity. They provide the support, traction and cushioning needed, which can greatly reduce your risk of reinjury. Generally speaking, high-top sneakers are best if you're prone to ankle injuries.

Or get new shoes. If you're a runner, you should replace running shoes every 500 to 750 miles, suggests Joseph Ellis, D.P.M., a sports podiatrist and consultant for the University of California, San Diego. Running shoes take a beating, and after a while, they don't protect your feet as well. Beyond the 500-mile mark, "shoes have lost much of their ability to absorb shock, increasing risk of injury," says Dr. Ellis. (Other doctors suggest replacing running shoes as often as every 300 miles.)

Stiff Neck

Maybe it's just to remind us that our lives are full of stress. Or it could be a punishment for sleeping with the windows open on a cool autumn night. Or because we didn't fix the shocks on the car, now we have to pay the price in aches and pains.

Sometimes the proverbial pain in the neck does have a physical basis. Stress—physical or otherwise—tenses the muscles in your neck, and you wake up one morning with a neck that sends complaint messages flashing through your nervous system.

A stiff neck is a common, usually harmless, problem that lasts just a few painful days. Whether you already have a stiff neck or you've had it before and want to avoid an encore, try these helpful hints.

Roll a towel into a collar. "Take a dry towel, roll it up, fasten it with a safety pin in the front or back, and use it as a soft collar to support your head," says

When to See the Doctor

If neck pain gets worse or doesn't improve within 24 hours and is associated with headache, drowsiness, confusion or fever, people really need to be seen by a physician," says Christa Farnon, M.D., associate director of Occupational Medical Services for SmithKline Beecham, a pharmaceuticals company in King of Prussia, Pennsylvania. "Sometimes a stiff neck is a sign of meningitis, a very serious illness that is treated with high dosages of antibiotics.

"Also, if the pain radiates into an arm and the arm becomes numb and increasingly dysfunctional, a stiff neck could be an indication of a slipped disk," Dr. Farnon adds.

Christa Farnon, M.D., associate director of Occupational Medical Services for SmithKline Beecham, a pharmaceuticals company in King of Prussia, Pennsylvania. "This supports your head in place and limits the movements that you make with your neck." If you would prefer a ready-made collar, check with a medical supply store; ask for a soft cervical collar.

Dunk a terry towel. Dr. Farnon recommends a moist, hot compress, using a towel. "Dunk the towel into hot water, wring it out, and apply it to the back of your neck," she says. "It's better than dry heat." If a moist compress is impractical, a hot water bottle or heating pad works almost as well. Place the bottle or pad on your neck for 30 minutes three or four times each day.

Shower away pain. "A hot shower will also help relieve the tension in your neck muscles," says Ron Plamondon, D.C., director of member services for the American Chiropractic Association in Arlington, Virginia. The hot shower gently massages your neck muscles while providing deep heat.

Try a pain reliever. Reach for the aspirin: Two pills every four hours will reduce the swelling and pain of a stiff neck. If aspirin doesn't agree with your stomach, try another pain reliever recommended by your doctor. Also remember not to give aspirin to children because of the risk of Reye's syndrome.

Sleep on your back. To avoid morning neckaches, try to fall asleep on your back, with a pillow under the curvature of your spine, suggests Joseph J.

Building a Better Neck

Strength and flexibility training isn't only for your arms. Even your neck can benefit from these exercises to prevent and treat neck pain, if you remember two simple rules: Never exercise if the pain is intense, and never allow someone else to twist your neck for you.

Go isotonic. Isotonic exercise strengthens your muscles and prevents injury. Take your right hand and hold it against your right temple, then press your head against the palm of your hand, tightening the neck muscle. Hold for five seconds, relax, and repeat. You can move your hand to the left, front and back of your head, putting pressure on different sides to strengthen the neck muscles all around.

Increase flexibility. Let your head hang forward so that the weight of your head draws your neck into a curve, suggests Bill Connington, board chairman and president of the American Center for the Alexander Technique in New York City. This position will gently stretch the muscles in the back of your neck. When you are finished, imagine that you are building the neck up again, vertebra by vertebra, until your head is balanced on top of your spine. Next, watch yourself in a mirror as you let your head tilt toward one shoulder. Bring your head straight, then let your head tilt toward the other shoulder. Don't force it; allow the weight of your head to do the work.

Try out your range of motion. Allow your neck to relax so that your head is poised on top of your spine. Move your head slowly from side to side as if you're saying no. Keeping your neck relaxed, nod your head up and down as if you're saying yes. If you find that there are places where it is harder to move your head, keep breathing evenly and remind yourself to relax the neck.

Practice releasing and relaxing. Lying on the ground with your knees bent, your feet flat and a paperback book underneath your head for support, try this relaxation technique: Imagine your muscles releasing and your head unlocking from your spine. Ask the muscles at the base of your skull to soften. Let your back spread out against the floor, and feel your breathing deepen. A few minutes each day will ease chronic neck pain.

Biundo, Jr., M.D., professor of medicine and chief of physical medicine and rehabilitation at Louisiana State University Medical Center in New Orleans.

Avoid the draft. Older people are especially prone to stiff necks caused by open car or bedroom windows, says Dr. Farnon. Do not sleep in a draft, and when driving, keep the window closed on your side.

Fix your car's shocks. The condition of your car may be playing a role in your stiff neck. Good shock absorbers will make both your car and your body run more smoothly, says Susan Zahalsky, M.D., former director of medical services at the Comprehensive Spine Center at Midway Hospital Center in Los Angeles.

Walk around. Is your workplace giving you a pain in the neck? If your muscles are "locked" in the same position, you'll begin to ache. "If you're doing desk work every day, get up every 20 minutes or so and walk around to keep your muscles alive," says Deborah Caplan, a physical therapist and founding member of the American Center for the Alexander Technique in New York City. She suggests stretching exercises: Make large circles with your arms to extend your muscles, and look around the room—up, down and to the side—to get the kinks out of your neck.

Look forward to your work. Computers and reading materials should be placed directly in front of you, at eye level. For computer users, Dr. Zahalsky suggests purchasing an Easy Reader, but any book stand will do and can be bought at an art supply store. If you are in a jam, a pillow placed under your book may also work.

Keep your phone off your shoulder. The telephone is often the greatest pain in the neck for workers. If you spend time on the phone, Caplan recommends getting a headset that will hold it in place.

Stomachache

You've long since graduated from using stomachache as an excuse to get out of having to go to school. But you're probably still learning a thing or two about how to avoid this brand of midsection misery—such as bypassing the blue plate special during your next visit to the local diner.

Actually, food is only one cause of stomachache. "In fact, you're probably more likely to get a stomachache when your stomach is empty, as the result of stomach acid," says Michael Oppenheim, M.D., a Los Angeles family practitioner and author of *The Complete Book of Better Digestion*. He points to stomach acid as one cause. "Anxiety is also another common cause, especially among children," he adds.

For the stomachache, doctors say it's okay to simply gut it out. But there are some things you can do to stop your bellyaching a bit quicker.

Take an antacid. "If the pain occurs when your stomach is empty, food can't be the cause," says Dr. Oppenheim. "Most likely, it's stomach acid—so taking an antacid is the answer."

When to See the Doctor

Most stomachaches are minor and don't require a doctor's assistance," says William B. Ruderman, M.D., chairman of the Department of Gastroenterology at the Cleveland Clinic–Florida in Fort Lauderdale. "But if pain becomes intolerable or there's vomiting, fever, excessive nausea or abdominal cramping in an otherwise healthy person, you probably should notify your doctor." This could indicate food poisoning or a more severe abdominal condition such as appendicitis or stomach ulcers.

If stomachache lasts longer than 24 hours, call your doctor for advice, adds Dr. Ruderman. Prolonged pain could be a sign of something more serious.

Almost any antacid can help neutralize stomach acid, but it can also have other effects on digestion, depending on the kind you choose. "The basic thing to look for in an antacid is the amount of calcium or magnesium it contains," says William B. Ruderman, M.D., chairman of the Department of Gastroenterology at the Cleveland Clinic–Florida in Fort Lauderdale. "If you tend to have trouble with constipation, then pick a brand that lists magnesium first on the label. If you're more prone to diarrhea, pick a brand listing calcium first."

Have a snack. A light snack can also absorb stomach acid if your stomachache isn't the result of overeating.

"A bland diet with soft foods is best—things such as bananas or crackers," says Dr. Ruderman. "Apple juice is an excellent choice. But stay away from overly sweet juices such as strawberry or raspberry as well as acidic beverages such as orange juice." He points out that the acidic drinks can actually *aggravate* stomach acid.

Drink to burp. If that stomachache is the result of overeating, then a good burp is usually the quickest way to get relief. Adults may turn toward a product like Alka-Seltzer, but children usually prefer a better-tasting remedy.

"My approach to treating mild stomachache is the same as what my mother did—with flat ginger ale or cola," says Perri Elizabeth Klass, M.D., a pediatrician in Boston and author of *Baby Doctor.* "The carbonation in the soda helps stir things up, so you burp and feel better. And I believe that if soda is a little flat, it has a slightly medicinal taste, which probably helps on a psychological level."

What Causes Stomach Gurgling?

A rumbly stomach may get your attention, but should it demand your concern? "You can't do much about stomach gurgling—and there's no need to," says William B. Ruderman, M.D., chairman of the Department of Gastroenterology at the Cleveland Clinic–Florida in Fort Lauderdale.

"To understand this condition—called borborygmus—think of your stomach as a giant mixmaster. When you eat, your stomach grinds up and mixes the food you've eaten to help digestion. The gurgling you hear is the noise created as the intestines squeeze this solution through."

Hey, relax. Mom was only half right when she suggested a nice hot cup of tea. "Tea, particularly peppermint tea, can calm down your stomach, but it should be warm—not hot," says Dr. Ruderman. "You're also better off with lukewarm beverages. Something too hot or too cold can induce a spastic response in your stomach, which increases pressure and pain."

Feast on fiber. Studies show that the incidence of stomachache was halved among a group of children who ate high-fiber cookies at the first sign of stomachache. "Popcorn is also an effective source of fiber," says William Feldman, M.D., head of the Division of General Pediatrics at the Hospital for Sick Children in Toronto. "Eating prunes, and fruits in general, can help a lot," adds Dr. Klass.

Stomach Cramps

Most of us have had a muscle cramp somewhere in our body at one time or another. A calf muscle may tighten up into a hard knot, a hand may "freeze." Even your little toe can cramp up if you stretch your foot the wrong way.

The point is, muscle cramps can happen anywhere you have muscles, and that includes your stomach, where a cramp may be mistaken for a "generic" bellyache, indigestion, upset stomach or side stitch.

Muscle cramps can occur when a muscle isn't getting enough oxygen-carrying blood to meet its needs. Your stomach can become the fall guy for cramping when stress, overindulgence or heavy exercise after a big meal sets the stage. Your first line of defense? Stomach-soothing over-the-counter drugs. Your best long-term strategy? Avoid tummy-knotting situations. Here's what you need to know.

Try a smooth coating. Several over-the-counter drugs are designed specifically to relieve the stomach pain that's caused by overindulgence, says Thomas Gossel, Ph.D., R.Ph., professor of pharmacology and toxicology and associate dean at Ohio Northern University College of Pharmacy in Ada.

"For first-line treatment, I'd recommend Pepto-Bismol, a liquid coating that relieves many minor stomach upsets," Dr. Gossel says. Antacids and sodium

When to See the Doctor

Pain that seems to be in your stomach can be caused by countless things, including some that don't have anything to do with your digestive tract, says John C. Johnson, M.D., director of Emergency Medical Services at Porter Memorial Hospital in Valparaiso, Indiana, and past president of the American College of Emergency Physicians.

If your "stomach cramp" persists for more than 30 minutes, or if it seems to be increasing in intensity, see a doctor. You may have an obstruction, a twist in your intestines or inflammation.

Heart attacks are often mistaken, early on, for attacks of indigestion. That mistake can be fatal. If your pain includes a feeling of pressure, nausea or vomiting, sweating, chest pain or trouble breathing, don't wait to see if it goes away. Get to an emergency room fast!

bicarbonate (Alka-Seltzer) may also help some people, he adds, especially if the cramping is compounded by heartburn.

Forgo feeding frenzies. Eat slowly, chew your food well, and don't guzzle down drinks. Does that sound like your mother talking? Well, she has a chorus of agreement: It's what stomach experts recommend, too. Food that's chewed well first, and mixed with saliva, is easier to digest, according to John C. Johnson, M.D., director of Emergency Medical Services at Porter Memorial Hospital in Valparaiso, Indiana, and a past president of the American College of Emergency Physicians.

Need help slowing your chomper speed? Try changing your eating environment. Instead of eating over the kitchen sink, set a place at the table. Add soft music and candlelight and you can't help but slow down.

Graze, don't gorge. Stomachs are very sensitive to overstuffing. "A distended stomach can cause sharp pain and can be very uncomfortable for some people," says Dr. Johnson. If you're one whose stomach cramps up when you just dig right in, try eating smaller, more frequent meals.

Hold off on eating if you're upset. Anxiety and eating don't mix. "When you're tense, the blood supply to your digestive system is reduced, making it hard to digest food," says Steven Fahrion, Ph.D., a clinical psychologist and director of the Center for Applied Psychophysiology at the Menninger Clinic in Topeka, Kansas. While there are many ways to relax, one of the fastest and easiest is with deep, slow, deliberate breathing, Dr. Fahrion says. As you exhale, imagine tension leaving your body.

Stick with noncaffeinated drinks. Coffee and colas make a tense stomach only worse, Dr. Johnson says. Try water, fruit juices or a tummy-taming herbal tea.

Go easy on cold fluids. Leave chugalugging for the fraternity boys. Too much of your favorite icy cold beverage, downed too fast, can send your stomach into temporary but painful spasms.

Fill up on fiber. In one study of bellyache-prone kids, two high-fiber cookies a day (providing ten grams of fiber daily) cut episodes of stomach pain in half.

"Fiber helps food move through the digestive system more quickly and so may reduce stomach and intestinal cramping," says William Feldman, M.D., head of the Division of General Pediatrics at the Hospital for Sick Children in Toronto.

Give your guts a time-out. Allow a half-hour or more for big meals to move through your stomach before you engage in heavy-duty activities, recommends Dr. Johnson.

"Exercise diverts blood from your digestive system to your arms and legs, increasing your chances for stomach and intestinal cramps," he explains.

Then speed things up with a little walk. If you're feeling full after a sumptuous repast, try "walking it off" before you resort to antacids. Light exercise, especially walking, helps speed the movement of digested food through your bowels. "This may reduce stomach cramps by allowing the stomach to empty faster," Dr. Johnson says.

Stress

I f you've been sick lately, suspect stress. Some doctors say that as many as *nine of ten* visits to the doctor may be related to stress. That includes everything from allergies and asthma to herpes and heart disease.

Now if that little bit of news isn't stressing enough, there are also those angst-inducing traffic jams and long lines, jerky bosses and inept workers, too much to do and too little time to do it. And let's not forget unemployment, pollution, crime and your home's lousy plumbing.

If all these small annoyances and big frustrations push your stress button, it's worth doing something about, because uncontrolled stress can lead to burnout—that dragged-out, done-in feeling that you just can't move ahead or get anything done. Although "job burnout" is the common phrase, when stress goes wild, your health and home life as well as your work are affected.

How can you reduce stress and avoid burnout? You've probably heard all about the stress-busting effects of (now take a deep breath) relaxation therapy, massage, biofeedback, positive imaging, prayer, support groups, yoga and regular exercise—and still your collar feels hotter than Texas asphalt in August.

But instead of staying burned up and burned out, why not try some of the tactics experts recommend for staying cool?

"Audit" your stress. To control stress, you have to first determine what *is* the stress in your life, says Paul J. Rosch, M.D., clinical professor of medicine and psychiatry at New York Medical College in Valhalla and president of the American Institute of Stress in Yonkers. "To do that, sit down and list *all* the things in your life you find especially stressful. Then separate them into two categories: things you can do something about, and those you cannot control and must learn to accept." This process will enable you to allocate your time where it'll do the most good—and to stop worrying about things you can't do anything about.

Look for the silver lining. "The key to controlling stress is to monitor and challenge your negative thinking," says psychologist Richard Blue, Ph.D., a stress management specialist with the Behavioral Institute of Atlanta. "When you look for the positive side of what's causing you stress—and usually you *can* find some positive things about it—you'll see that it's probably not as stressful as you're making it out to be."

To train yourself to think more positively, begin each sentence with "at least" whenever you're stressed out, advises Dr. Blue. *Examples:* If you work for a jerky boss, remind yourself "At least I have a job." When you're stressed out because of a leaky kitchen faucet, tell yourself "At least I own a house."

Reevaluate your role in life. "In most cases, stress burnout (whether triggered by job, home life or whatever) is the result of a mismatch between your personality or goals and the realities of a situation," says Dr. Rosch. That means asking yourself some hard questions and giving yourself honest answers—about your work ethic, talents and true desires. "Find the right match between your job and your personality and the odds are you'll never suffer job burnout," says Dr. Rosch.

Bust a Gut to Bust Stress

It seems laughter *is* the best medicine, at least when it comes to beating stress. That's because laughter—like exercise—makes the body produce endorphins, the body's natural physical *and* emotional painkillers.

Endorphins produce a feeling of well-being that makes you more resistant to stress. There are other physical benefits as well, many to the cardiac and circulatory systems—where stress does its most harm.

To add more yuks when you feel yucky, you need to make a serious effort to find humor on a regular basis, suggests Steve Allen, Jr., M.D., clinical assistant professor of family medicine at the State University of New York Health Science Center at Syracuse College of Medicine and son of comedian Steve Allen. Dr. Allen, who specializes in laughter therapy, suggests you go so far as to imagine how your "snags" might be handled by the producers of a TV sitcom.

Example: "Here I am, stuck in traffic for the rest of my life. Guess my kids will grow up, get married, have kids and grandkids, forget me and get stuck in the same traffic jam a few miles back before I get out of this gridlock."

Rate your responses. "Most of our stress is the result of 'catastrophizing,'" says Allen Elkin, Ph.D., a practicing psychologist and program director at the Stress Management and Counseling Center in New York City. One way to stop catastrophizing is to rate the importance of your stressor on a simple 1 to 10 scale. If you miss the subway, you may give yourself a 4; if you lose your wallet, an 8. Then think of some *real* stressors—a heart attack, losing a job, a death in the family—and go back and *re*rate the missed subway and lost wallet. "Over time, you'll recognize when you're catastrophizing situations and get some more balance," says Dr. Elkin.

Take a Zen-second relaxation break. "One thing that's very effective at helping with stress is a method I call rapid relaxation, which takes about 10 or 20 seconds," says Dr. Elkin. "You take a deep breath, deeper than normal, and hold it in until you notice a little discomfort. At the same time, squeeze your thumb and first finger together (as if you were making the okay sign) for six or seven seconds. Then exhale slowly through your mouth, release the pressure in your fingers, and allow all your tension to drain out. Repeat these deep breaths three times to extend the relaxation. With each breath, allow your shoulders to droop, your jaw to drop and your body to relax. I recommend doing this several times throughout the day, particularly when you begin to feel stress building."

Soak yourself. A warm—*not* hot—bath helps reduce stress by increasing peripheral circulation and relaxing muscles, which causes a calming effect. Soak for no more than 15 minutes in water 100° to 102°F. This is an effective time and temperature for stress relief.

Hit the sheets. When sex is good, it's very good for easing stress. Orgasm is a great relaxer, and even nonorgasmic sex helps calm you, according to Joshua Golden, M.D., director of the Human Sexuality Program at the University of California, Los Angeles. Sex also helps emotionally to establish or reaffirm meaningful bonds and to build self-esteem.

Get a pet. Research by Alan Beck, Sc.D., professor of ecology at Purdue University School of Veterinary Medicine in West Lafayette, Indiana, and author of *Between Pets and People,* shows that when people pet an animal, their blood pressure, heart rate and *stress* drop almost immediately. "I think one reason is because touching an animal is one of the few socially acceptable opportunities for many people to show outward affection—and people *do* have a need for touch.

"Even looking at fish in an aquarium has similar effects. The eyebrows become less furrowed, there's a more relaxed smile and sometimes even a slight drooping of the eyes—all facial expressions that indicate being at ease and less stressed," he says.

Stretch your body. "Stretching can help you feel more peaceful and relaxed," says Dean Ornish, M.D., director of the Preventive Medicine Research Institute in Sausalito, California, and author of *Dr. Dean Ornish's Program for Reversing Heart Disease.* Whenever you get a break during the day, do some easy stretches. "Just as your mind affects your body, your body can affect your mind," says Dr. Ornish. He suggests that you practice your stretches with slow, fluid movements. (And wear loose, comfortable clothing that *allows* you to stretch easily.)

Press your head. Applying light pressure on your temples with a circular motion helps massage nerves, which in turn relaxes muscles throughout your body, says Emmett Miller, M.D., medical director of the Cancer Support and Education Center in Menlo Park, California.

Have a good cry. It's one of the oldest and most effective responses to stress—and it still works as well now as when Adam and Eve shed a tear over the stress of buying a new home. Not only crying but yelling and other emotional outbursts may help release pent-up frustration and stress, suggests Dr. Miller. But choose wisely where to yell—in an auto works well.

Stretch Marks

Since life is a series of trade-offs, it stands to reason that with every joyous event comes some downside: Experience the miracle of childbirth and you're bound to pay for it in some way—other than Junior's college tuition.

Stretch marks are as much a part of motherhood as Hallmark greeting cards, but even so, you don't necessarily have to carry them for the rest of your life. These cosmetic curses (particularly annoying come bikini season) are just

When Retin-A Works, When It Doesn't

Retin-A, which is available only with a doctor's prescription, has been getting a lot of attention for downplaying those nasty stretch marks. But there's a catch.

"The best time to use it is when the stretch marks are new—when they are pink and a little painful," says Melvin L. Elson, M.D., medical director of The Dermatology Center in Nashville, Tennessee, and the researcher who made the Retin-A/stretch mark connection. "If you wait until the marks become white, the success rate plummets from 80 percent to around 10 percent."

That means the prescription drug *must* be used within 6 to 12 weeks *after* getting the stretch marks—no later than three months after having a baby or losing a lot of weight. And Retin-A *cannot* be used during pregnancy or while you're breastfeeding.

As it does when used for wrinkles, the drug produces some initial skin irritation, peeling and redness at the application site. It works because it causes the "generation" of collagen, that all-important protein substance in the skin, Retin-A essentially performs a repair job, but you need to wait until the peeling and redness go away before you'll see its benefits. If a doctor does prescribe Retin-A, be sure to follow instructions carefully.

harmless reminders that the human body isn't made of Play-Doh. And while pregnancy takes most of the blame for stretch marks, anyone can get them. Puberty, obesity and even weight loss are all common causes. Any time the body goes through drastic-enough physical changes, a skin protein substance called collagen can pull apart from the skin's elastic fibers, and that's when the telltale marks appear.

"They're basically nothing more than scars," says Stephen M. Purcell, D.O., chairman of the Department of Dermatology at Philadelphia College of Osteopathic Medicine and an assistant clinical professor at Hahnemann University School of Medicine in Philadelphia. So—what can you do about them?

If you go the doctor's prescription route, there's tretinoin, a topical derivative of vitamin A marketed as Retin-A and best known for its effectiveness at erasing wrinkles. But for some people, home remedies *without* prescription might also get results.

Butter them up. "Although there's no scientific proof backing it up, some of my patients claim that rubbing on cocoa butter helps reduce or eliminate stretch marks—particularly in dark-skinned people," says Dr. Purcell.

Try hands-on healing. "We do know that massaging scars after surgery is beneficial, since it stimulates blood flow and distributes collagen more evenly—resulting in a less noticeable scar. So maybe that could work for stretch marks as well," says Dr. Purcell. "That could be the explanation behind cocoa butter." In other words, maybe it's the *massaging* action, rather than the cocoa butter, that gets rid of stretch marks.

Stuffy Nose

It doesn't take much to get a stuffy nose. With every breath you take, you subject your nasal membranes to everyday irritants such as pollen, dust, cat dander and particles of air pollution—all of which can clog things up faster than rush-hour traffic. In fact, just about *any* substance in the air can stuff a sensitive nose. And of course you already know what a cold can do to block up your nasal passages. Did you know that you come face-to-face with more than 100 different cold germs daily?

Well, breathe easy—or at least easier. Because there are plenty of ways to unblock that stuffiness. Here are some of the most effective.

Sniff an onion. "Basically, the only thing you get from rubbing on menthol or other decongestants is some irritation that stimulates the nose to run and unblock the stuffiness," says Venice, Florida, otolaryngologist Hueston C. King, M.D., visiting professor at the University of Texas Southwestern Medical Center at Dallas. "You can get the same effect from smelling an onion."

Go heavy on the spice. The cure for a stuffy nose is to make it runny, and few things make it run faster than spicy meals. "Hot and spicy foods trigger a reflex response to make your nose runny," says Gordon Raphael, M.D., an allergist and a former researcher at the National Institute of Allergy and Infectious Diseases in Bethesda, Maryland. "Eat some hot chili peppers and your nose will immediately start running." This running helps break up congestion and remove irritants that may be causing the stuffiness, adds Dr. King.

Try Mom's chicken soup. Or any other hot liquid taken from a cup. When you drink anything hot, the steam of the liquid helps unclog nasal passages, and the fluid itself helps dilute mucus in the nose and makes breathing easier, says Varro E. Tyler, Ph.D., professor of pharmacognosy at Purdue University in West Lafayette, Indiana, and author of *The Honest Herbal*. Besides soup, hot tea with lemon and even hot water are excellent decongestants.

Hit the showers. Breathing the steam from a hot shower is probably the easiest way to cut mucus and keep it from getting thick—a common cause of stuffiness, says Douglas Holsclaw, M.D., professor of pediatrics and director of the Pediatric Pulmonary and Cystic Fibrosis Center at Hahnemann University Hospital in Philadelphia.

Run a humidifier. A humidifier certainly helps put moisture in the air, but it can be counterproductive if it also spreads water impurities, spores and germs. "Use distilled water to fill the humidifiers and you won't have impurities," advises Alvin Katz, M.D., an otolaryngologist and surgeon director at Manhattan Eye, Ear, Nose and Throat Hospital in New York City. And clean the unit

When to See the Doctor

Stopped-up nasal passages can harbor sinus infections. "The question is not *if* a blocked sinus will get infected but *when*," says Gailen D. Marshall, Jr., M.D., Ph.D., assistant professor and director of the Allergy and Clinical Immunology Division at the University of Texas Medical School at Houston. Once infection does occur, he points out, you'll have to make a trip to the doctor.

What are the warning signs of sinus infection? Before the infection hits, you'll feel pain radiating from your nose to the blocked sinuses, either under the eyes or beneath the forehead. You may even think it's a headache. If the sinuses remain clogged, you may develop a fever, a nasty taste in your mouth or bad breath.

"Any of those three symptoms may lead to the conclusion that you have a full-blown sinus infection," Dr. Marshall says.

weekly by circulating a solution of half water, half white kitchen vinegar. The solution should be run through the unit for 10 to 15 minutes near an open window to avoid the persistence of a vinegar odor. Then discard the vinegar solution and fill the unit with fresh distilled water. The unit can run for up to a week without cleaning again. Keeping open pans of water near the stove and radiators can also help humidify, but the water needs to be changed frequently.

If you use a decongestant spray, use it sparingly. You should use a decongestant spray no more than twice a day for a maximum of three or four days in a row, according to Gailen D. Marshall, Jr., M.D., Ph.D., assistant professor and director of the Allergy and Clinical Immunology Division at the University of Texas Medical School at Houston. Then take an equal amount of time *off* the medication. When the relief it provides begins to wane, or when you notice that its effectiveness lasts for a shorter time, "there's a good chance you're becoming dependent, and it's time to stop," says Dr. Marshall.

Over-the-counter nasal spray decongestants are among the most potentially addictive of all drugs, Dr. Marshall says. "Person after person innocently gets hooked on them."

Among other effects, the sprays can also damage the cells lining the nose, says Stephen Goldberger, M.D., an otolaryngologist at the Grand Forks Clinic in Grand Forks, North Dakota. "The sprays can cause these cells to lose their microscopic hairs, or cilia, which are crucial for keeping the normal mucous coating in the nose moving," he says.

"It's difficult to wean yourself from nasal sprays, because the resulting congestion is so bad," Dr. Marshall says.

Spritz with saline. Unlike decongestant spray, nasal saline spray may be used indefinitely, according to Dr. Marshall. With saline versions, you just moisten the membranes in your nose, which helps you breathe easier. And you don't need to buy the spray at a pharmacy: You can mix a batch of home brew by dissolving ¼ teaspoon of table salt and ¼ teaspoon of baking soda in about eight ounces of water. With a small atomizer or nosedropper, spritz one or two droppers of the solution up your nostrils as often as necessary.

Although saline soothes, it doesn't provide extended relief. "It'll moisten and clean out things that are aggravating the congestion," Dr. Marshall says. But the saline itself doesn't clear up congestion.

Swallow some relief. Any of the over-the-counter oral decongestants usually are fine to take for a stuffy nose. But they should be used with caution by people with heart problems, high blood pressure or urinary tract problems,

A Stuffy Nose Makes For a Stressed Baby (and Parent)

When a newborn gets a stuffy nose, it can be particularly irritating—for both parent and child. "Babies under three months are what we call obligatory nose breathers, which simply means they won't breathe through their mouths. So when a baby gets a stuffy nose, it's inordinately stressful," says Douglas Holsclaw, M.D., professor of pediatrics and director of the Pediatric Pulmonary and Cystic Fibrosis Center at Hahnemann University Hospital in Philadelphia.

"Many parents come rushing into the emergency room or their pediatrician's office because their baby won't eat or sleep and is cranky all the time. It's because the baby's nose is stuffed. A baby cannot suck on a bottle or feed if he can't breathe through his nose."

To relieve an infant's stuffy nose, first use a bulb syringe or nasal aspirator to clear the nose of as much mucus as you can. Then fill a medicine dropper with saline solution. Holding the baby in your arms, positioned so that his head is slightly below the rest of his body, drop the saline into each nostril. You're doing it right if the saline hits the top of the baby's mouth, says Dr. Holsclaw. Immediately after spraying, hold the baby upright. Be sure to give one *quick* squirt in each nostril—so you don't "flood" the baby's nose with the saline.

Dr. Marshall warns. Oral decongestants may aggravate an irregular heartbeat and can counteract medications to reduce high blood pressure, he says. And people with urinary tract problems may find themselves having difficulty urinating if they take an oral decongestant.

Keep booze in the bottle. Substances in fermented alcoholic beverages can clog your nose as easily as they cloud your mind. "Almost anyone who gets recurrent colds or sinus problems has congestion problems when he drinks wine, beer and cordials," according to Alexander C. Chester, M.D., clinical professor of medicine at Georgetown University Medical Center in Washington, D.C. But they may be able to tolerate scotch, gin or distilled spirits, he notes.

Watch out for milk . . . and wheat. A number of people have an allergy to milk that is different from lactose intolerance: It congests the ducts in the nose.

If that's causing your discomforts, you can see a fairly dramatic response to the elimination of milk products, Dr. Chester says. "Probably about 10 percent of the people can feel enormously better." A sensitivity to wheat may also cause congestion.

Treat it with zinc. "Zinc seems to have a specific effect on the nose," says Dr. Chester. Zinc supplements have been used to treat people whose sense of smell has diminished, and zinc may improve congested sinuses as well. Take a 50-milligram supplement daily, Dr. Chester suggests. Continue to take the supplement if you notice an improvement.

Get relief with vitamin C. Vitamin C has been advocated for the common cold, but it could spell relief for people with stuffed-up noses in general, whether or not they have colds. "Vitamin C in varying doses may bring relief to a congested nose," Dr. Chester says. But you shouldn't take more than 500 milligrams daily without a doctor's consent.

Raise the head of your bed. Lying on your back tends to build up the pressure of nasal fluid, according to Dr. Chester. Try raising your head by placing a few books under the bedposts or sleeping on more than one pillow. "Both help the nose to drain," he says. And don't lounge around in bed when you're congested. That gives mucus more of a chance to pool in your head rather than drain, according to Dr. Chester.

Work out to work it out. "Exercise is a natural decongestant for common nasal stuffiness," Dr. Chester says. Walking helps: When you walk, you stimulate better breathing and better blood circulation. Walking also helps shrink nasal membranes, and besides, you get a good breath of fresh air.

Stuttering

We all get a kick out of watching Porky Pig's animated arsenal of sputters, misfires and f-f-f-false starts. But if you, your spouse or your child is among the millions of Americans whose speech is laden with hesitations, prolongations, repetitions and blockages, then you know firsthand that stuttering is *not* as amusing as a Looney Tunes cartoon.

About 4 percent of all children between the ages of two and seven will develop a stutter—but there will be far more boys than girls. Although most of the children who stutter will outgrow the problem by puberty, a small percentage (less than 1 percent) carry it into adulthood.

As yet, no one knows what causes stuttering, and there is no cure. "Our best guess is that it is due to a combination of psychological, neurological and genetic factors," says Barry Guitar, Ph.D., professor of communication science and disorders at the University of Vermont in Burlington. But they do know that it is habit forming and is usually related to stress, according to Martin F. Schwartz, Ph.D., executive director of the National Center for Stuttering in New York City.

When a child is learning to speak, or when an adult has to speak in stressful situations (before a large audience, for instance), that stress focuses tension on the vocal cords, closing and locking them. The person struggles to speak but can't do so easily: The struggle becomes a stutter. "If the vocal cords can be kept open and relaxed, however, the stuttering can be stopped immediately," says Dr. Schwartz.

If you or your child does stutter, try these techniques.

Pause a second. If you're stuttering, maybe it's because you're trying to speak as fast as or faster than others—and you just don't need to. "Slow down to a normal rate and set your own relaxed pace," says Edward G. Conture, Ph.D., chairman of the Program of Communication Sciences and Disorders at Syracuse University in Syracuse, New York. "When someone asks you a question, pause one to two seconds before responding, then answer at a rate that is comfortable for you."

Nip stutter starters in the bud. The moment before a stutter begins, you may grimace, twist your face or purse your lips without being conscious of these movements. R. Gregory Nunn, Ph.D., a clinical psychologist and president of R. G. Nunn and Associates, a private clinic in San Diego, suggests using *competing behaviors* when you feel these stuttering precursors come on.

When muscles tense up, for instance, let your arms, shoulders, chest and stomach slump and relax. If your lips are pursed, open them slightly. Or loosen your tight throat by letting out a little air through your mouth before saying just one word per breath, gradually increasing the number until you feel comfortable.

Record your stuttering. Keep a personal log of all your stuttering episodes, noting what takes place prior to and during the stutter, says Dr. Nunn. "When you become aware of situations and behaviors that contribute to your stuttering, you can catch them in advance and prevent stuttering before it starts." If you always stutter on the phone, for instance, be prepared to use some competing behavior techniques even before you dial.

Practice natural breathing. "A stutterer tries to superimpose speech over short, rapid, uneven breaths or speak while holding his breath," explains Dr. Nunn. "We want him to get used to natural speech breathing." Take a relaxed breath through the mouth, filling your lungs with a comfortable amount of air, and let it out slowly and easily, producing a deep, hollow sound. Practice this breathing pattern daily. Then try to maintain the deep breathing while you speak, letting the words come out easily as the smooth, even breath is being exhaled.

Synchronize your airflow. Dr. Schwartz recommends the following method to take tension off the vocal cords. First relax. Take a short, easy breath through your mouth. Just before speaking, let the air flow passively through your mouth, opening up the locked cords. Slow the first word a bit, easing into the first syllable, gliding to the next. Then proceed at a comfortable pace. Do this with each sentence, stopping and starting at natural pause points. Stuttering should stop right away. Practice this technique for 15 minutes three times a day, and try to integrate it into all your conversation. Four months of daily practice should make this behavior a habit.

Nix cola and coffee. Caffeine, sugar and other stimulants encourage muscle and vocal tension, says Dr. Schwartz. They should be eliminated or greatly reduced.

When to See the Doctor

How do you know whether to help a stuttering child at home or to see a speech specialist? Martin F. Schwartz, Ph.D., executive director of the National Center for Stuttering in New York City, provides these guidelines.

If you are the parent of a child who stutters and someone in the immediate family also stutters, there's a chance your child's habit may continue into adulthood. Note whether there's a lot of struggling with words or at midsentence and also whether the stutter occurs every day and the child reacts by acting unhappy or refusing to speak. When stuttering is this persistent, you should definitely go to a speech specialist.

By adulthood, the habit is ingrained, and a good bit of one-on-one counseling may be needed to overcome it. The help of a licensed speech therapist may be necessary before you can change the habit.

Also, if stuttering should develop *for the first time* in adulthood or very suddenly in an older, normally fluent child, it may be the result of a neurological condition, a head injury or an event that has been very upsetting. See a doctor immediately.

Skip the sweets. Sugar reduction alone has completely eliminated stuttering in some children, says Dr. Schwartz. You may observe rapid improvement in your child's speech simply by decreasing his consumption of cakes, cookies, candy and soda.

Set the pace. "When kids try to speak as fast as or faster than adults, they often stutter," says Dr. Conture. "If you speak slowly and evenly to your child, he'll soon get the picture and slow down naturally." Other pacemaking tips from Dr. Conture: Pause one to two seconds before responding to your child's questions. Try not to finish the child's sentences, talk over him or interrupt. And don't tell him to speak slowly while *you* proceed rapidly.

Take a listening break. A fast-paced, hectic environment where it is difficult to speak and be heard may increase stuttering in children, says Dr. Conture. When talking with a child who stutters, turn off the TV and radio as often as possible, or keep the volume low, so the child doesn't have to verbally compete with background talking. It's ideal if you can set aside time for family discussions and then give everyone a chance to speak in turn without undue interruption. And if your child talks to you while you are doing things that require your concentration, take a time-out. "Assure him you are listening and then *do* listen," says Dr. Conture.

Sunburn

E ven before there was a hole in the ozone layer, going to the seashore could leave you sea-sore. But now, with more harmful ultraviolet rays peeking through, limiting your sun exposure is essential, particularly between the sizzling summer hours of 10:00 A.M. and 3:00 P.M. The best prevention is also a wise precaution: Wear sunscreen with an SPF (sun protection factor) of 15 *all* the time.

Okay, but maybe you forgot. And now you're in pain. Well, you can try those old standbys aloe and over-the-counter hydrocortisone cream. Even an extra moisturizer can help a lot. But when you have too much fun in the sun, here are some *other* ways to take the fire out of sunburn pain.

Just add milk. "Dip some gauze into milk and apply it to your sunburned skin," says dermatologist John F. Romano, M.D., clinical assistant professor of medicine at The New York Hospital–Cornell Medical Center in New York City. The milk should be about room temperature or slightly cooler but not refrigerator-cold. "Milk is an excellent remedy for any kind of burn," notes Dr. Romano.

Keep this milk compress on the burn for 20 minutes or so, and repeat every two to four hours. Since milk can leave skin smelling "sour," be sure to rinse yourself off with cool water afterward.

Be soothed by vegetables. Boil some lettuce in water, then strain it and let the liquid cool for a few hours in the refrigerator before applying it to your skin with cotton balls, recommends Lia Schorr, a New York City skin care specialist and author of *Lia Schorr's Seasonal Skin Care*. Other vegetables that produce results? Thinly sliced pieces of raw cucumber, potato or apple can be placed on sunburned areas such as the forearm. The coolness from the vegetables is soothing and might help reduce inflammation.

503

Get Jolly Green skin care. Wrapping a bag of frozen corn or peas in a towel and applying it to the burned area also helps cool the pain, says dermatologist Frederic Haberman, M.D., a clinical instructor of medicine at Albert Einstein College of Medicine of Yeshiva University in New York City. But be sure to wrap it first, so you don't place the icy package directly on your skin.

Double your dosage of pain reliever. "Probably the best thing you can do is to take *two times* the recommended amount of ibuprofen (Advil) or another pain reliever for the first two doses and then go to the recommended dose," advises Dr. Romano. Doubling the usual dosage of ibuprofen or aspirin helps block a chemical in your body that causes pain. But check with your doctor, since some people have a reaction to aspirin. And remember not to give aspirin to children because of the risk of Reye's syndrome.

Eat for vitamin E. A regular dose of vitamin E is thought to do a host of good, providing protection from a variety of things from heart attack in men to fibroid tumors in women. "It also decreases the inflammation you can get from sunburn," says Karen E. Burke, M.D., Ph.D., a dermatologist and derma-tologic surgeon in New York City who has studied the effects of vitamin E. Good food sources of vitamin E include whole grains such as wheat germ, vegetable oils—especially sunflower and soybean oil—and nuts.

If you choose to purchase vitamin E supplements, be sure to read the small print: You should get only the natural form. But check with your doctor before taking vitamin E or other vitamin supplements.

What about rubbing vitamin E on your skin? Although you can also treat sunburn with a direct application of vitamin E by opening a vitamin E acetate

When to See the Doctor

An everyday case of sunburn may hurt like the dickens, but it usually doesn't require medical help. However, get yourself to a doctor if you experience chills, nausea, fever, faintness or fatigue, warns dermatologist Rodney Basler, M.D., assistant professor of internal medicine at the University of Nebraska Medical Center in Omaha. And be sure to get help immediately if your burn is accompanied by purple blotches or discoloration, excessive blistering or intense itching. These symptoms may indicate internal complications.

To Make Matters Worse . . .

Some diuretics, antibiotics, tranquilizers, birth control pills and diabetes medications can add more salt to your sunburn wounds. They can make you sun-sensitive. So can some medicated soaps, perfumes and Retin-A, the wrinkle "remover." So if you use any of these medications or products, doctors advise you to take extra precautions when exposing your skin to the sun.

capsule and rubbing the liquid directly on your skin, it's more effective to take it internally to decrease sunburn pain, suggests Dr. Burke.

Soak yourself in diluted vinegar. "Pour one cup of white cider kitchen vinegar into a tub of tepid water and soak yourself in it," recommends Harry Roth, M.D., clinical professor of dermatology at the University of California, San Francisco. "It's very soothing to your skin and helps relieve the pain of sunburn."

Or try baking soda and cornstarch. Another recipe for relief, also from the kitchen cabinet: Mix ¼ cup of baking soda and ¼ cup of cornstarch into a tub of tepid water and soak yourself, adds Dr. Roth.

Heal with oatmeal. If you find the smell of vinegar or milk too intense, you can wrap dry oatmeal in some gauze or cheesecloth and run cool water through it, suggests Dr. Haberman. Wring out the excess water and apply the cloth for 20 minutes every two to four hours.

Don't be *too* clean. While you have sunburn, stay away from highly fragrant bubble baths, soaps, colognes and perfumes, according to Thomas Gossel, Ph.D., R.Ph., professor of pharmacology and toxicology at Ohio Northern University College of Pharmacy in Ada. They may be too drying and irritating to your already parched skin. Stick with mild soaps and don't scrub too hard when you wash.

Sweaty Palms

I f your palms sweat more than a stool pigeon under police interrogation, you have a condition that doctors know as hyperhidrosis—excess sweating of your palms. In nonmedical language, you might call it just plain embarrassing. But here's how to get quick, hands-on relief.

"Shock" yourself dry. "The best treatment out there is a low-level electrical current called iontophoresis," according to Norman Levine, M.D., chief of dermatology at the University of Arizona College of Medicine Health Sciences Center in Tucson. Dr. Levine recommends a device called the Drionic that administers the low-level current.

How it works: The Drionic uses a 9-volt battery—not enough to harm you but enough to plug up overactive sweat ducts and keep them plugged for about six weeks. To remedy a sweaty palm condition, simply place your palm on top of the device for a few minutes. Further information about the Drionic is available from General Medical Company, 1935 Armacost Avenue, Los Angeles, CA 90025.

The "Obvious" Solution Is Not the Best

W hy not dry those clammy hands with baby powder? After all, it seems like the cheapest dry-all solution.

"Baby powder might be the first thing people turn to. But rubbing powder on your palms is one of the worst things you can do, unless you have a very mild case," says Stephen M. Purcell, D.O., chairman of the Department of Dermatology at Philadelphia College of Osteopathic Medicine and an assistant clinical professor at Hahnemann University School of Medicine in Philadelphia. "As the powder absorbs the perspiration, it will cake up, leaving you with sweaty, caked-up hands instead of just sweaty hands."

Treat your palms as underarms. For a mild case of hyperhidrosis, the solution may already be in your medicine chest. "Some people find relief by rubbing underarm antiperspirant on their palms," says Stephen M. Purcell, D.O., chairman of the Department of Dermatology at Philadelphia College of Osteopathic Medicine and an assistant clinical professor at Hahnemann University School of Medicine in Philadelphia. But check the label: The kind of antiperspirant that works on clammy hands should contain aluminum chlorohydrate, the active drying ingredient.

Manage your stress. "One effective way of remedying hyperhidrosis is through stress management," says Dr. Levine. "Learn biofeedback or practice some other stress control treatment, since this condition is at least partially brought on by stress or nervousness."

Swelling

E yes, nose, thumbs, toes—just about any body part can swell up. It happens for lots of different reasons, and the sensations that go along with swelling can be painful, itchy or annoying. And while there are many general remedies for swelling, some body parts require their own special treatments.

Swelling often accompanies injury, for instance, as fluid normally flowing through blood vessels seeps out into the surrounding tissue. That may happen when blood vessels are injured by a bump, by a muscle or ligament tear or by a fracture.

Swelling can also happen slowly, without an injury, as the result of pooled blood in an arm or leg. Through a process called effusion, fluid seeps from the blood vessels into tissue. It's this kind of swelling that occurs when you notice your hands puffing up while you walk or if your feet get a shoe size bigger when you've been standing around for a long time. (Because varicose veins impede the return of blood to the heart via the veins, they can cause this kind of swelling.)

Hives, welts and the itchy bumps caused by mosquitoes and other blood-sucking parasites are other examples of swelling. So are the stuffy, runny nose and scratchy, puffy eyes that accompany hay fever.

When to See the Doctor

Many injuries that cause swelling deserve a doctor's prompt attention. That's because ligament or muscle tears, fractures or cartilage damage may be hiding under all that puffiness.

If you think you might have an ankle, foot or leg fracture, don't try to remove your shoe. Let the doctor do that. First-aid treatment is different for each kind of fracture, but generally you want to keep the limb from moving around until the doctor can treat it.

Also, if swelling is the result of an insect bite or sting and is accompanied by severe reactions such as chest tightness, dizziness or fainting, seek medical help at once. These are signs of potentially deadly anaphylactic shock.

"The more a body part swells, the more blood circulation is slowed. And poor blood circulation slows healing," says Clayton Holmes, an athletic trainer and assistant professor of physical therapy at the University of Texas Health Science Center at San Antonio. For serious injuries, you'll want to see the doctor and follow his recommendations. But here are some all-purpose ways to keep swelling down.

Try an over-the-counter antihistamine. These drugs help counteract the swelling caused by insect stings and many kinds of allergic reactions, says Thomas Platts-Mills, M.D., Ph.D., head of the Division of Allergy and Clinical Immunology at the University of Virginia Health Sciences Center in Charlottesville. Antihistamines are contained in some liquid medications, but Dr. Platts-Mills recommends the faster-acting chewable tablet. "Take the dosage suggested on the box as soon as you are stung," he says. (That way, the drug gets into your system quickly.) Take the antihistamine at recommended intervals as long as the swelling continues. *Note:* Antihistamines are useless for injury-related swelling.

Remember RICE. Not the long-grain variety but a proven first-aid method for injured ankles, knees and elbows: rest, ice, compression and elevation. "The sooner you do all four, the better," says Holmes.

If you want to reduce swelling in a leg, for instance, do RICE in this order. Wet a four- to six-inch-wide elastic bandage in ice water. Firmly wrap it a few times around the injured ankle or knee, providing compression, then apply two quart-size plastic bags of crushed ice, so they completely surround the joint. Continue wrapping, using the bandage to hold the ice in place. Leave the ice on for no longer than 20 minutes. Take off the ice and rewrap the injury. Wait an hour before you ice again.

While you're icing, elevate the injured part above the level of your heart.

Rest the injured part by immobilizing it. If it's an ankle or knee that's hurt, don't try to hobble around. Get some assistance when you walk, or else use crutches.

Step in place. Standing motionless for long periods of time may cause swelling. That's because up to a quart of blood pools in your legs and feet, and fluid may seep out of blood vessels into tissue. That not only makes your legs feel like lead, it makes your feet a size bigger. So walk in place, lifting your knees and pointing your toes downward. That helps your muscles pump blood upward. If you must stand still, keep your knees slightly flexed. Don't lock them, experts say.

Stay active after exercise. If you stop suddenly after hard exercise, blood can pool in your legs, resulting in swelling and sometimes low blood pressure as well. Instead of stopping abruptly after a run or swim, cool down with lighter activity for ten minutes or so. That keeps your circulation going but at a less intense pace, suggests John Duncan, Ph.D., associate director of the Exercise Physiology Department at the Cooper Institute for Aerobics Research in Dallas. This gradual slowdown is especially important for people taking heart medications such as beta blockers.

Bend and pump. Swinging your arms while you walk is a good way to loosen up, but the centrifugal force it creates can make blood pool in your hands, causing swelling. "Try bending your arms 90 degrees at the elbows, and use them as pistons," suggests Dr. Duncan. "Raise them up higher than you normally would and swing with the cadence of your walking gait." While you're doing that, keep your hands loosely open. Although you can occasionally clench your hands to squeeze out fluid, continual clenching interferes with the flow of fluid through the arm and will make your lower arm swell.

Keep a loose grip on your bike. Do your lower arms swell when you're bicycling? Unless you're barreling down some potholed road, you shouldn't have to grip the handlebars of your bike so tightly that you cut off circulation in your arms. But that's exactly what some people do, even while they're riding

Stuck Ring? Dental Floss to the Rescue!

A ring may be a symbol of wedded bliss, but it can pose real danger when it's stuck on a swelling finger. Because it can cut off blood circulation just as surely as a tourniquet, that band of gold has got to come off—the sooner, the better.

If your knuckle has swollen and is already too big to slip the ring over, try this trick using dental floss. (Better yet, use waxed dental tape.) Used by emergency medical technicians, the technique is recommended by John C. Johnson, M.D., past president of the American College of Emergency Physicans and director of Emergency Medical Services at Porter Memorial Hospital in Valparaiso, Indiana.

Take a long piece of floss (two to three feet is not too long). Starting at the tip of the finger, closely wrap the floss around the finger, spiraling down toward the ring. Keep the encirclements ⅛ inch apart or less. When you get to the ring, slip the end of the floss under the ring and pull it toward your palm. Lift that end of the floss over the top of the ring and pull up toward the tip of your finger. As the floss unwinds, it will ease the ring up and off the finger.

To make this even easier, grease the floss-wrapped finger with petroleum jelly before you remove the ring.

stationary bicycles indoors, Dr. Duncan says. "A healthy person might not notice it, but someone who already has circulation problems will see his lower arms swelling," he says. So keep a loose grip, he suggests, and shift from the upper to lower bars occasionally. Or simply move your hands. Padded gloves can help, too.

Swimmer's Ear

Call it swimmer's ear, jungle ear, ear fungus or otis externa—it's all the same thing: an infection that flourishes in warm, moist ear canals (the outermost tubes of the ears where sounds go in).

Everyone has bacteria in his ear canals, and most of the time these bacteria present no problem. But when the ear canal gets waterlogged and irritated, these bacteria start to multiply, and the result is a stuffed-up, itchy ear that feels swollen and tender.

Swimmer's ear isn't reserved *just* for swimmers. Anything that traps moisture in the ear canal can trigger this condition. Bacteria can get a foothold behind earplugs, hearing aids or abundant earwax. Dust and dry skin can aggravate swimmer's ear, and it's likely to be worse if you have narrow ear canals. If swimmer's ear is a recurrent problem for you, here's how to stop bacteria from launching an attack.

Get the drop on bacteria and fungi. Get an eyedropper-style bottle from the pharmacy and fill it with a mixture of half white kitchen vinegar and half rubbing alcohol. After swimming or showering, tilt your head and put in enough drops to fill the ear canal. Then tilt your head the other way to let the solution pour out. Growth of fungi is inhibited in this acidic environment, says Stephen P. Cass, M.D., assistant professor of otolaryngology at the Eye and Ear Institute of Pittsburgh.

If the skin of the ear canal is irritated, use half vinegar and half *water* (instead of alcohol) to reduce the sting, says Nancy Sculerati, M.D., assistant professor of otolaryngology and director of pediatric otolaryngology at New York University Medical Center in New York City.

Take your ears to the drugstore. Over-the-counter antiseptic ear drops—such as Auro-Dri and Swim Ear—also make life hard for bacteria and fungi. For treatment, follow directions on the package and bottle.

Stop the pain. "If swelling makes your ear hurt, take aspirin or acetaminophen (Tylenol)," says Dr. Sculerati. But don't give aspirin to children, because it increases the risk of Reye's syndrome, a life-threatening neurological condition.

Bathtub Advice: Keep Your Head above Water

People who never even twiddle their toes in a puddle can get swimmer's ear. The biggest culprit may be bathtubs, suggests Robert A. Dobie, M.D., chairman of the Department of Otolaryngology at the University of Texas Health Science Center at San Antonio.

"Bathtub water is loaded with all the germs from your body in a very small amount of water," he says. A dunk that puts your ears underwater could create a soggy situation and lead to infection. So even if you've put your body in the tub for a good long soak, keep your ears high and dry.

Dry up. You can dry up the bacteria's soggy homestead by draining and drying your ears after swimming. First lean over sideways and pull on your ear to straighten the canal and let water drain out, says Jerome C. Goldstein, M.D., executive vice president of the American Academy of Otolaryngology/Head and Neck Surgery in Alexandria, Virginia.

For an additional drying out, use rubbing alcohol. "Put a few drops in the ear canal and let it run all the way in," says Anthony J. Yonkers, M.D., chairman of the Department of Otolaryngology/Head and Neck Surgery at the University of Nebraska Medical Center in Omaha. "Then turn your head over and let it run out. The alcohol mixes with water and carries it out."

Blow-dry your ears. "If you use a hair dryer to dry the ears, you'll avoid stagnant water in the ear canal," says Robert A. Dobie, M.D., chairman of the Department of Otolaryngology at the University of Texas Health Science Center at San Antonio. Set the dryer on warm or cool, and hold it about 18 inches away from your ear for a minute or so.

Turn to oil. Repeated soaking and drying removes protective oil from the ear's tissue-thin skin, which can lead to other problems. To avoid that, "put two or three drops of baby oil in your ears *before* you go in the water," says Dr. Goldstein. And if dry skin is very severe, a few drops of baby oil or vegetable oil applied with a dropper at bedtime will restore missing oil, says Dr. Dobie.

Try a hydrocortisone cure. "If the ear canal starts to dry out and itch, people may start to scratch and pick at it," says Dr. Dobie. To eliminate the itch, he suggests using an over-the-counter 1 percent hydrocortisone cream. Apply it with your fingers at the recommended dose for about two weeks. If the irritation remains or worsens in that time, check with a doctor about more potent treatments.

Create a moisture seal. Silicone putty earplugs can help protect infection-prone ears, says Dr. Sculerati. "Make a ball of silicone bigger than the entrance to the ear canal and mush it so that it covers the opening but does not go deep inside," Dr. Sculerati says. Don't use hard plugs on tender ears, because they can abrade the skin and *cause* infection, she warns.

Teething

After your baby reaches the age of six months, you may notice the precocious tyke trying to whittle the crib with his mouth. This is the age when he begins to gnaw on just about *anything* within gumming distance. It's not only a tender age—it's an age when *gums* are tender and teeth are pushing through, and all this eager-beaver gum work is an aggressive way to help teeth break through the gums.

"Teething is really more fretful than painful," says Lewis Leavitt, M.D., professor of pediatrics at the University of Wisconsin Medical School in Madison. "The baby may be very fretful, but usually he's consolable."

Tell that to Junior! As those new choppers are pushing through, your child may fuss and cry for hours on end. Parents can't do much to change the scenario, but they can do a thing or two about those overworked gums. Here's how.

Become a crooner. "Probably the best thing a parent can do is to soothe his child," suggests Dr. Leavitt. "A good place to start is by singing or humming to the baby while holding him." Rocking in a rocking chair at the same time can also help soothe and distract your teething child.

Cool those gums. Chewing rings and teething toys do help a child who is teething, but they seem to be even more effective when they've been refrigerated.

"Anything that's cold and hard to bite will help," says Becky Luttkus, head instructor of the National Academy of Nannies in Denver. "A wet washcloth placed in the refrigerator—*not* the freezer—is an excellent choice. The best choice is a white rather than a color-dyed washcloth—that way, baby won't get any dyes into his system."

Try a rubdown. Simply massaging the baby's gums with your finger is easy and often helpful. And if you place a small gauze pad on your finger, you can kill two birds with one stone—you'll relieve teething pain and help clean the baby's mouth, says John A. Bogert, D.D.S., executive director of the American Academy of Pediatric Dentistry in Chicago.

Temporomandibular Joint Disorder

*T*emporomandibular joint disorder is quite a mouthful—hence, doctors and patients alike refer to it as TMD. But if you've got it, *pronouncing* TMD is about the easiest thing your jaws can manage.

TMD (formerly known as TMJ) is best known for its intense and debilitating pain in the temporomandibular, or jaw, joint, located in front of your ears (where sideburns are). But other ailments fall under the rubric as well: "TMD is actually a broad description for a lot of different problems in the entire facial area," says Wilmington, Delaware, dentist Barry Kayne, D.D.S., clinical assistant professor at the University of Pennsylvania School of Dental Medicine and Temple University School of Dentistry, both in Philadelphia, and a TMD specialist. "More frequent symptoms include pain in the temple, in the cheeks, behind the eyes, in the back teeth or in the throat. There may also be a popping or clicking of the jaws, neck stiffness, stuffiness in the nasal passages, ringing in the ears and migrainelike headaches . . . really bad pain throughout the entire face."

Whether brought on by growth problems, arthritis or trauma (whiplash, a sock in the jaw or other types of stretching and pummeling), TMD is common: As many as one in three people have it in some form. Sometimes TMD causes occasional jaw pain. For other people, it may be the root cause of earaches or unexplained headaches. Many people with full-fledged TMD suffer from headache—the kind of headache that creates a terrible pain in the sideburn area. If you suspect that you have TMD, here's how you may ease your discomfort.

Give your jaw R and R. "The best home remedy for TMD is to manage your jaw as you would manage a bad knee that's been injured: Provide as much rest for the area as possible, and avoid aggravating the area," says Dr. Kayne. That means you should avoid *all* unnecessary jaw movements when you're talking or eating. And you should avoid the extensive jaw movements that go along with singing or even yawning.

Stop that yawn. If you feel a yawn coming, restrict it by placing your fist under your chin, advises Andrew S. Kaplan, D.M.D., director of the TMJ/Facial Pain Clinic at Mount Sinai Hospital and associate clinical professor of dentistry at Mount Sinai School of Medicine, both in New York City.

Protect yourself from Old Man Winter. "You should always wear a scarf and hat during cold weather," says Dr. Kayne. "You want to keep your head and neck as warm as possible in order to maintain good blood flow." With good blood flow, he points out, there's less inflammation and less muscle pain.

Unclench your teeth. If you clench your teeth, as do many people who have TMD, practice this tactic: Place your tongue behind your top front teeth so that it rests against the roof of your mouth, suggests Owen J. Rogal, D.D.S., director of the Pain Center, a multidisciplinary medical center in Philadelphia, and past executive director of the American Academy of Head, Facial and Neck Pain. This position helps separate your top and bottom teeth and relaxes your jaw.

Here's why it helps: Many people react to stressful situations by clenching their teeth, according to Dr. Kayne. "Although stress doesn't cause TMD, it certainly aggravates it," he says. "Making a conscious effort to keep your lips together and your teeth apart in stressful situations certainly helps if you have TMD." (For more tips on how to stop clenching or grinding your teeth, see page 534.)

Position a pillow . . . so you sleep on your back. Sleeping on your side or stomach puts pressure on one side of your jaw—and that causes TMD pain, says Dr. Kayne. He recommends a special cervical pillow that will help keep

TMD No-No's

The things that most of us do unconsciously with our jaw can spell disaster to someone with temporomandibular joint disorder (TMD). Among some well-practiced habits that need to be broken, here are things to avoid.

Don't:

- Cradle a phone between your neck and shoulder.
- Hang heavy bags or pocketbooks on your shoulder when you walk.
- Carry children or heavy objects.
- Prop your head or chin on your hand for long periods, à la Rodin's *Thinker.*
- Lie on your stomach with your head tilted to one side.
- Lie on your back with your head propped forward to read or watch TV.
- Grit your teeth or clench when lifting weights or other heavy objects (if you must lift weights, be aware of this!).

you on your back. "A doctor or physical therapist can tell you the best thickness for you; for most people, it's medium," says Dr. Kayne.

Try the rolled towel insurance. Here's another way to make sure you sleep on your back: "Take a bath towel, fold it up several times, and put it behind the bend of your knees," suggests Dr. Kayne. That way, your knees are bent. "It's a good way to help ensure you're sleeping on your back," says Dr. Kayne.

Straighten your posture. Desk jockeys are particularly vulnerable to TMD neck pain, because they often sit at their desks with their chins jutting forward, Dr. Rogal observes. He advises that if you have a desk job or do a lot of sitting, you should stand up every hour of so and straighten your posture.

Take a pain reliever. Aspirin is a "marvelous" drug for any muscle or joint problem—including TMD, says Harold T. Perry, D.D.S., Ph.D., past president of the American Academy of Craniomandibular Disorders and professor of orthodontics at Northwestern University Dental School in Chicago. Ibuprofen products such as Advil are also recommended. "If you go that route, take aspirin or ibuprofen three or four times a day for 10 to 20 days," says Dr. Kayne.

"But be consistent. Once you start, don't interrupt taking the pain reliever unless you notice stomach irritation. And also take a pain reliever *after* a meal." (And remember not to give aspirin to children because of the risk of Reye's syndrome.)

Eat soft. Whenever TMD acts up, your diet should calm down. "Don't eat anything chewy, crunchy or hard for 6 to 12 weeks," says Dr. Kayne. "That means *everything* you eat should be cooked or baked. Eat only *very* ripe fruits and vegetables. No gum, nuts, pizza, bagels, rolls, steaks—nothing that works your jaw." After ten days on a soft diet, you should notice some relief. However, Dr. Kayne advises continuing for a full 12 weeks. "If your condition doesn't improve substantially after that, see your doctor," he says.

Get heated up. When your jaw, head or neck feels achy, apply a heating pad to ease pain. The heat increases blood flow and helps break up muscle pain, according to Dr. Kayne.

Or cool down. When the pain comes along in hard spasms, icing the area is the prescribed therapy, says Dr. Kayne. "Put an ice bag on for ten minutes, then remove it for ten minutes—and continue this process for an hour," he says. Make sure that the ice bag is wrappd in a towel. *Note:* A bag of frozen vegetables works just as well.

Tendinitis

Your brother says that it's a pulled muscle, your spouse claims that you have tendinitis, and your neighbor is sure that you have bursitis. But all you know is one thing: You've played a little too much basketball, and now your knee feels as though it will never move again.

How do you know that your soreness is actually tendinitis, and what can you do to ease the pain? Tendinitis is an inflammation of the tendon—the cord that attaches the muscle to the bone. "So that's where you would feel the pain," says Robert E. Leach, M.D., professor and chairman of the Department of Orthopedic Surgery at Boston University Medical Center and chairman of the U.S. Olympic Committee on Sports Medicine and Sports Science. A pulled muscle, on the other hand, occurs in the "belly" of the muscle, which hurts only when you stretch it.

If you find yourself with tendinitis, take a break and try these tactics to make it feel better.

Put on an ice pack. "Ice decreases inflammation by decreasing blood flow to the injured area," says Steven F. Habusta, D.O., of Parkwood Orthopedics in Toledo. "There is no such thing as too much ice."

You can buy an ice pack made of gel, or you can make a pack by putting ice in a sealable plastic bag. Another alternative: Use a bag of frozen vegetables. Dr. Habusta suggests, however, placing a terry cloth towel between your skin and the ice pack to prevent burns or blisters.

Stretch it. "Careful stretching of the affected muscle and tendon so that it doesn't get too tight is important in both the treatment and prevention of tendinitis," says Dr. Leach. "But don't stretch so much that you cause pain. Pain usually means that you are tearing tissue." Stretch your sore muscle every day, using smooth and slow motions.

Down an anti-inflammatory. "Aspirin and ibuprofen (Advil) are immediately available to most people," says Dr. Leach, "and they're both anti-inflammatory. Take either of them (but not both) a couple of times a day." But pay attention to the amount that you take each day. "If you notice that you are not getting better

When to See the Doctor

Does the pain get worse every time you hit a tennis ball? Is it getting more difficult to open that jar of mayonnaise?

If the pain is getting worse or lasting a long time, you should see a doctor, according to James A. Nicholas, M.D., director of the Department of Orthopedics at Lenox Hill Hospital in New York City. He recommends seeing the doctor if the pain interferes with your ability to do whatever it is that you want to do (and that could be something as simple as climbing the stairs).

Dr. Nicholas notes that tendinitis can have many origins, some more serious than others: "It could be caused by injury, by gout, by rheumatoid arthritis or by certain metabolic disorders."

or that you've been increasing the amount, it's obvious that you should be doing something else," says Dr. Leach. Also, do not give aspirin to children because of the risk of Reye's syndrome.

Smooth on some heat. "Sometimes we use liniments over the area, such as Ben-Gay," says James A. Nicholas, M.D., director of the Department of Orthopedics at Lenox Hill Hospital in New York City. When a liniment is rubbed lightly on the skin over the sore tendon, it may ease your pain. Don't use more than the label recommends, though: In excess, these products can burn your skin. *Note:* Don't use a heating pad with liniments, as this may result in a very painful burn.

Try warm compresses. "When we treat chronic injuries in athletes, we use wet heat," says Dr. Nicholas. To produce an application of wet heat, dampen a towel, completely cover one side with a double layer of plastic or cellophane, and place a heating pad on top of the plastic. The damp towel side should be held against the skin for an hour and a half each day. Dr. Nicholas says this procedure is a convenient way to provide continuous wet heat. "Make sure that the heat is not so high that you burn yourself," he warns.

Elevate it. If you can rest the painful limb or joint above heart level, you'll ease the swelling that often accompanies tendinitis. If you have tendinitis in your leg, for instance, rest with your leg raised on top of a pile of pillows.

Sling it. For tendinitis in your shoulder, you can place the arm on the affected side in a cloth sling as you would a broken arm. The idea is to keep the arm immobile, so the shoulder doesn't move around.

Pamper yourself with a massage. Not only is massage very soothing, it also helps by relaxing the muscle and tendon, so they can be stretched very easily, says Dr. Leach. Although a massage is no cure, it will help you feel more comfortable while the inflamed tendon is healing.

Talk to your shoe salesperson. Certain shoes can help prevent the tendinitis that occurs in the Achilles tendon, just above your heel. Carol Frey, M.D., chief of the Foot and Ankle Service and associate clinical professor of orthopedic surgery at the University of Southern California School of Medicine in Los Angeles, says your best bet is to ask a salesperson for a shoe with a small heel wedge and a molded Achilles pad. If you explain that you have tendinitis, the salesperson should be able to direct you to an appropriate pair of shoes.

Listen to your body. Tendinitis plagues even the most well trained athletes, but you can prevent it somewhat if you avoid overexercising and overtraining. "The basic problem is overuse of the muscle/tendon unit," says Dr. Leach. He points out that this can happen even when people train and stretch properly but get a little overenthusiastic about exercising. It seems the body has a point when it says "Wait! That's too much!" According to Dr. Leach, the best precaution is to give your body a rest.

Build your muscles. "After your tendinitis heals, you'll want to strengthen the muscle area," says Dr. Leach. "It gets weaker, and when it's weaker, it's more likely to have trouble again." Strong muscles can also help *prevent* tendinitis. Dr. Leach recommends regular lifting exercises with weights (or even phone books) to help prevent tendinitis.

Make stretching a daily routine. Having adequate stretching ability and elasticity will help you prevent tendinitis, says Dr. Nicholas. Slowly stretch your muscles in the morning and before exercising. Not only will you feel better, you will protect your tendons from injury. But be sure to stretch nearby muscles as well as those that are afflicted. If you have Achilles tendinitis, for example, you should stretch the thigh muscle as well as the calf muscle. And if you have tendinitis in the elbow (tennis elbow), you need to stretch shoulder muscles as well as biceps and triceps.

Tennis Elbow

Whether your racket is tennis, toting a briefcase or tiddlywinks, *any* strain of the forearm tendons can make your elbow feel like you've just been beaten by Boris Becker in straight sets.

But why be aced by an easily treated ailment when the right racquet, exercises and therapy can have you swatting up a storm before you can say game, set or match? Before you say goodbye to all games involving the elbow, take some hints from the masters of arms.

Let your elbow rest. If swelling and soreness have already set in, your elbow needs at least three weeks' rest from playing tennis, says Susan Perry, a physical therapist specializing in sports medicine at the Fort Lauderdale Sports Medicine Clinic in Fort Lauderdale, Florida. And while you're resting it, take some other measures to relieve the pain.

Put a cap on it. Made from a derivative of hot peppers (capsaicin) and commonly used for shingles, Zostrix is extremely effective at zapping elbow pain, says Craig Hersh, M.D., a sports injuries specialist at the Sports Medicine Center in Fort Lee, New Jersey. This topical over-the-counter ointment, available at most drugstores, works as a temporary anesthetic when rubbed on the sore area, he says. "It doesn't work on inflammation—it works at the nerve level, blocking the transmission of pain."

Cool down that elbow. You can soothe that sore elbow by rubbing it with a paper cup filled with ice (fill the cup with water and freeze it) or a resealable plastic bag filled with ice cubes and wrapped in a towel. "Just don't leave the ice on any longer than 10 to 20 minutes," says Perry. Apply the ice no more than four times a day, with at least an hour between icings, she suggests.

Give peas a chance. A bag of frozen peas (or other small vegetables) also works well as a reusable elbow ice pack, says Perry.

Do You Have Briefcase Elbow?

Here's a hot new excuse for *not* taking out the trash: "Honey, it gave me tennis elbow." Actually, you may be right. If you repeatedly carry a heavy garbage bag one-handed, holding it far in front of you, a case of tennis elbow could be trashing your ability to do this home chore.

Okay, but what about *briefcase* elbow?

Possible, says Susan Perry, a physical therapist specializing in sports medicine at the Fort Lauderdale Sports Medicine Clinic in Fort Lauderdale, Florida.

"A lot of business professionals get tennis elbow because they're lifting their briefcases with their arms extended—and that pulls the forearm tendon," says Perry. If you often tote a bulging briefcase, she suggests holding the case close to your side when you lift it from floor to desk: A similar technique works with the garbage bag, too.

Prepare by stretching. Before playing a tennis rematch with your club's top seed, consider using proper forearm stretching and strengthening techniques. Here's what Perry suggests: Extend your right arm in front of you until your elbow is straight. With palm down, slowly bend your wrist until your fingers are pointing toward the ground. Using your left hand, gently press the top of your right hand until you feel a tension stretch on the top of your forearm. Without any movement, hold for 15 seconds. Repeat with the other arm.

Now extend your right arm in front of you with the palm up. Using your left hand, gently press as if you wanted to push your right wrist down. But don't move the arm: Hold for 15 seconds, keeping up the pressure. Repeat with the opposite wrist. This exercise stretches the bottom of your forearm, says Perry.

After stretching, try strengthening. After you've stretched your forearms, help strengthen them with these exercises: Place your forearm on a desk with the wrist over the edge, palm up. Grip the handle of a hammer in your extended hand. (You can also use a two-pound can of vegetables or soup.) Slowly curl your hand up, then down, flexing the wrist, repeating 20 times. Change hands and repeat.

Get stronger still with swivels. Swiveling your arm while holding a heavy object is another way to build strength. Holding a hammer in your right hand, sit up straight, with your right elbow against your side. Lift your forearm until it's parallel with the floor. Now, still holding the hammer, twist your wrist 20 times, as if you were turning a doorknob. Repeat with the other hand.

Check your swing. "If you play tennis and have tennis elbow, you probably have a poor backhand technique," says Perry. Instead of leading with your elbow on your backhand, Perry says you should get your racquet in front when you hit a backhand shot. "If you can't find the problem yourself, take a tennis lesson from a professional and have him check out your swing," Perry adds.

Change your frame. Using a metal racquet? If you've got tennis elbow, you're better off switching to a different kind, says Allan Levy, M.D., director of the Department of Sports Medicine at Pascack Valley Hospital in Westwood, New Jersey, and team physician for the New York Giants professional football team and the New Jersey Nets professional basketball team. While metal frames transmit the shock of ball contact to your poor, beleaguered elbow, other kinds better absorb the blow, he says. "Wooden racquets are better than metal, but you just can't buy them anymore."

Next best? "A composition racquet or one made with graphite will certainly help, as long as it's not too large or strung too tightly," says Dr. Levy. Also, be on the lookout for new experimental ceramic racquets, which are supposed to eliminate tennis elbow. But if you're unwilling to part with your metal racquet, slightly loosening the strings should help, says Dr. Levy.

Thinning Hair

Father Time gets most of the blame for thinning hair. The average person loses about 100 strands per day (while the average hair grows only ½ inch per month). So the more days you live, the more hairs you lose.

But heredity is also a factor. In some families, there's a pattern of male baldness. (To a lesser degree, women in the same family can also have thinning hair.)

While you can't stop time or heredity, you can do something about the way your hair appears, even if it's thinning. Here's how.

Alter your hair hue. "Coloring your hair makes it look thicker, because as part of the coloring process, you actually 'rough up' the hair," says John Corbett, Ph.D., vice president of technology for Clairol, based in Stamford, Connecticut. He explains that it's easier to retain the appearance of fullness "because hairs don't slide over one another and lie flat against one another."

If you have extremely thin hair, go for a lighter color. "Dark colors show more of a contrast between hair and your scalp, whereas lighter colors—particularly shades of blond—hide the scalp more easily," says Dr. Corbett.

Go for the curly look. Getting a permanent wave also makes hair appear thicker, because the surface is altered (as it is in coloring) and because the "wave" in the perm makes hair appear fuller.

Blow it dry. "Using a blow dryer can make hair look two to three times thicker than styling it with water or styling oils—and it *doesn't* harm the scalp, as some people believe," says Douglas D. Altchek, M.D., assistant clinical professor of dermatology at Mount Sinai School of Medicine in New York City. "When you blow-dry your hair, you plump it up, so it looks higher." Like hair coloring, blow-drying also roughs up hair shafts, so they appear thicker and fuller.

But hold the dryer more than three inches away from your hair, so you don't cause excessive dryness to your tresses. It's also a good idea to use conditioner after your shampoo when you regularly blow-dry your hair.

Wash it daily with protein shampoo. When hair is oily, it gets stringy looking. "Washing hair every day gets the oils out of it. Daily shampooing also gives hair more body, so it looks thicker right off the bat," says Harry Roth, M.D., clinical professor of dermatology at the University of California, San Francisco. "When you wash your hair with shampoo containing hydrolyzed animal proteins—also called thickeners—it actually gives hair *more diameter*."

Adds Dr. Altchek: "These hydrolyzed animal proteins coat hair so that each hair shaft is two to three times as full as it usually is. They also make hair more fluffy, which makes it appear fuller."

Use a "kitchen" conditioner. One of the best conditioners for those with thin hair is white vinegar—that's right, the same kind you use in cooking. Mix one tablespoon of white kitchen vinegar in a pint of water and massage it into your hair after shampooing, says Dr. Roth. "It changes the chemical balance of your hair to be slightly more acidic; for some reason, that makes hair appear thicker and gives it more shine. The vinegar *doesn't* leave an odor in your hair," he adds. (But of course, be sure to rinse it out before you step from the shower.)

Be an egghead. Another kitchen item that can contribute to thicker hair is the lowly egg. Simply crack an egg over your hair before shampooing, and toss away the shell. "Massage it in for five minutes and then rinse it out," adds Dr. Roth. Since egg is basically animal protein (albeit *non*hydrolyzed), it has the same effect as the specially formulated shampoos.

Go light on commercial brand conditioners. Commercial conditioners do a good job of making hair look fuller, as long as you don't overuse them. "Most people use way too much conditioner, which makes hair limp and more likely to nap together—and that makes it look even *thinner*," says Dr. Altchek. Don't use more than a teaspoonful each time you wash—that's just a dab in the palm of your hand. "Anything more is wasted and can actually make your hair look worse," according to Dr. Altchek.

Manage with mousse. A daily application of styling mousse is another way to make hair look fuller. "Since mousses have resins, they coat the hair and add diameter to it," says Dr. Corbett. Mousse lifts the hair off the scalp, which also adds to the appearance of fullness.

Thumb-Sucking

N early half of all children suck their thumbs sometime between birth and adolescence. And nearly *all* parents worry about it—maybe a bit too much. Granted, if Junior fails his driving test because his thumb is in his mouth instead of on the steering wheel, you might want to spend money on professional help instead of driver's ed. But if he's still in preschool, thumb-sucking comes with the territory.

"If your child is under five, there's no reason to knock yourself out with worry," says Stephen J. Moss, D.D.S., professor and chairman of the Pediatric Dentistry Department at New York University College of Dentistry in New York City. "Most thumb-sucking occurs between birth and age three, and it does *nothing* to harm the teeth. It's not until a child is six or seven and getting his permanent teeth that it can cause damage that might later lead to braces. And the type of damage done by thumb-sucking is the easiest and least expensive to fix."

Still, thumb-sucking is one of those transitional things. And if it's high time to speed along that transition, here's how to go about it.

Make Junior conscious of the habit. "A habit is a series of unconscious movements that are repeated, so in order to stop the habit of thumb-sucking, you have to bring it to a conscious level," says Dr. Moss. "The way I recommend is just to remind the child, in as neutral a way as possible, that he is sucking his thumb. Say 'Oh, I see you're sucking your thumb' or 'Did you know you were sucking your thumb?' *Don't* say 'Don't suck your thumb' or he'll feel bad about it. The purpose is to make the child conscious of this unconscious act, not to make him feel guilty."

Chart the progress. Some pediatric dentists recommend that parents keep a calendar to chart the progress of quitting the habit. The calendar should be placed in a conspicuous place. Place a sticker or gold star on the calendar

Should You Worry?

What's the best advice for parents of preschoolers who suck their thumbs?

"Close your eyes," says Mitchell C. Sollod, M.D., a pediatrician in San Francisco. "Eventually they will stop, and worrying about it isn't going to make them stop any sooner. Most parents can drive themselves crazy over thumb-sucking, when the truth is, it's harmless. It doesn't mean there's anything psychologically wrong with your child or that he's not maturing the right way. It just happens to be one of those things that brings a lot of pleasure."

You should talk to your child about quitting if he is still sucking his thumb at age six or seven or when he has begun to get his permanent teeth. "By that age, however, most kids know it's time to stop," says Stephen J. Moss, D.D.S., professor and chairman of the Pediatric Dentistry Department at New York University College of Dentistry in New York City.

each night a child goes without sucking his thumb. (Nothing is done when the child does suck his thumb.) This method is recommended by pediatric dentist Monica Cipes, M.D., an assistant professor at the University of Connecticut School of Dental Medicine in Hartford who has studied the effectiveness of using such calendars.

Plan a reward. If you're keeping a calendar of nights without thumb-sucking, let the child know how well he's doing. "We usually suggest parents give the child a reward if he goes five nights without sucking his thumb," says Dr. Moss. "With this method, many children will stop sucking their thumbs within two weeks."

Cover their hands. "All the tricks used to stop thumb-sucking—covering their thumbs with socks, nail polish, bandages or rubber bands—*will* work, but only *after* the child is made conscious of thumb-sucking," adds Dr. Moss. "Don't even try these methods until you've made the child conscious of the habit through frequent 'reminders.'"

smother it w/ vasaline

Tick Bites

Ticks are a lot like unwanted dinner guests: They're no bother until they start feeding at *your* expense. Fido may be living a dog's life because of these little buggers, but it's not until they burrow their tiny heads into *your* skin and slurp up *your* blood that you get...well, really ticked off.

There are two types of ticks to watch out for, with a sizable difference between them. The common dog tick is an eight-legged creature with a round abdomen about the size of a pinhead. It's easy to find—and brush off—before it burrows its head into your skin for a meal. The deer tick, on the other hand, is harder to spot, because it's smaller. You'll have to look closely to find these tiny round critters crawling around your legs or clothing.

Actually, most tick bites go unnoticed or cause just a little scratching. But occasionally, these tiny terrors can cause big-time trouble: Depending on what, if any, bacteria and viruses they may be harboring, ticks can spread

When to See the Doctor

If you find a tick walking on your body, it hasn't bitten you yet and can safely be removed. But if the tick is attached and you remove it, keep alert for signs of redness around that area. A bull's-eye rash can appear even *one month* after the encounter. It will have a clear center and red circles of inflammation as much as 15 inches in diameter. (A rash may also develop away from the site of the bite.)

Another warning: flulike symptoms that include headache, fever, swollen glands, stiff neck and general fatigue. These symptoms suggest Lyme disease, which must be treated with doctor-prescribed antibiotics.

Avoid Ticks with an Ounce of Prevention

If you're spending any time outdoors from spring to fall, especially in wooded or high-grass areas—even grassy dunes—take the following precautions to avoid getting nicked by a tick.

- To determine if you're in tick country, tie a piece of white flannel to a string and drag it through the grass or underbrush. Examine it frequently. If ticks are present, they will cling to the cloth.
- Whenever you're in a wooded area, leave as little skin exposed as possible. That means wearing long sleeves, long pants and high socks (with pant legs tucked in). Disrobe outdoors whenever possible and *immediately* wash clothing after your hike.

Rocky Mountain spotted fever, Colorado tick fever, tularemia (also known as deer fly fever), Lyme disease and other ailments ranging from undesirable to downright dangerous. So the first thing you want to do is get that tick off.

Be tick-alert. Check your clothes, skin and hair after you've been strolling through long grass or walking in the woods. If a tick is removed before it "digs in," there's no chance you'll get sick.

Ease it out. If you do find a visitor with its head dug into your skin, here's how to coax it off: Using a pair of tweezers, grab the tick as close to your skin as possible and pull it straight out, without jiggling or twisting. *Don't* use your fingers, since bacteria from the tick can penetrate right through the skin of your fingers.

Some advice about tweezing: "Don't pull too fast," cautions Herbert Luscombe, M.D., professor emeritus of dermatology at Jefferson Medical College of Thomas Jefferson University and senior attending dermatologist at Thomas Jefferson University Hospital, both in Philadelphia. "And if you're not having success, you might try applying a little heat to the tick's back. Blow out a match and carefully touch the tick with the tip, taking care not to burn your skin. The heat may encourage it to let go."

Clean up. Once you've removed the tick, wash the bite area thoroughly with soap and water, says Claude Frazier, M.D., an allergist in Asheville, North Carolina. Then apply iodine or another antiseptic to guard against infection.

Stop 'em before they start. Ticks aren't insects (they're acarids), but some over-the-counter insect repellents will also repel ticks. If you really want to spoil a tick's appetite, spray your clothes with any repellent containing DEET (diethyltoluamide)—especially before you go walking in the woods. Keep this stuff away from your eyes, however, as it can sting fiercely. And DEET-containing repellents should be used sparingly on exposed skin, especially on children.

Tinnitus

For most people, the rhythmic sound of ocean waves caressing the shore is as soothing as a mother's lullaby. But if that splish-splash-hiss-crash is *inside* your ears, it's a different story. Tinnitus, or "ringing in the ears," is the name of *that* lullaby. And it's anything but soothing!

Tinnitus is not a disease, and it doesn't cause hearing disorders. It's any kind of swishing, hissing, whirring, ringing, whistling, buzzing or chirping that goes on *inside* your head.

The causes? Tinnitus can be a sign of hearing loss, or it can result from head injuries, ear infections or diseases that range from the common cold to diabetes. People who work with noisy equipment, such as power tools, can also get it. Or tinnitus may be initiated by a single loud noise, such as a gunshot or an explosion.

Sometimes tinnitus is only temporary. If you have a ringing in your ears for only a few days (perhaps after listening to loud music), take it as a warning sign. Tone down your listening habits or tinnitus may become permanent.

Even when tinnitus moves in to stay, there are still things you can do about it. The first move is a medical checkup. After that, here are some ways to make it easier to live with.

Tone down sound around you. "*Never* expose your ears to loud sounds, because they simply make tinnitus worse," says Jack Vernon, Ph.D., professor of otolaryngology at Oregon Health Sciences University and director of the Oregon Hearing Research Center, both in Portland. "If you have to raise your voice to be heard, then the sound around you is too loud. That includes vacuum cleaners, dishwashers, lawn mowers and so forth."

So wear earplugs whenever noise abounds. Pharmacies carry foam, rubber and moldable wax plugs as well as headphones you wear like earmuffs.

Try a little night static. Some people don't notice their tinnitus in the daytime, but as soon as the lights go out, they're up to their inner ears in bells and buzzers. "For those folks, I recommend detuning an FM radio to static *between* stations," says Dr. Vernon. If you keep the radio near the bed, just loud enough to be audible, the static near your head will mask the sounds *in* your head and let you fall asleep. Other sounds that might be the key to dreamland: a fan running all night or a bit of soft music.

Play that shower! In the "mask that sound" department: "Some people can't hear their tinnitus when they take showers," says Dr. Vernon. Of course, you can't stay in the shower all day, but you *can* carry shower sounds around with you. Dr. Vernon suggests making a long-playing tape of a running shower. When the tinnitus gets bad, listen to the tape through headphones, he recommends. (The idea is to find a band of tones that includes your tinnitus tone but is more acceptable to listen to.)

Breathe deeply to dismiss distress. "Reducing stress often reduces tinnitus," says Robert E. Brummett, Ph.D., a pharmacologist at the Oregon Hearing Research Center. Deep, slow breathing is one safe way to ease tension any time you feel it creeping up on you, according to Dr. Vernon. But he cautions that this may not be enough. See a counselor if you're having difficulty dealing with stress in your life and your tinnitus is becoming worse because of it.

Skip the smokes and drinks. "Restrict the nicotine, alcohol, tonic water and caffeine you consume," Dr. Brummett suggests. If you find that it helps to cut out one or all of these, consider a permanent vacation from the noise provoker.

Don't take aspirin. People with tinnitus who take aspirin daily (for arthritis, for example) should try a different anti-inflammatory drug if possible, suggests Dr. Brummett. Aspirin can cause or worsen tinnitus. Some of the other anti-inflammatory drugs can also cause or worsen tinnitus, but not in everyone. By working with your doctor, you can try some of the alternative drugs until you find one that you can tolerate.

Give yourself a dose of distraction. "Getting distracted from tinnitus surely will help," says Dr. Vernon. "Focus on some outside things: Help other people.

Join some volunteer groups. Don't retire!" he suggests. "People with tinnitus need to enrich rather than restrict their lives."

Toothache

On the Registry of Pain, toothache is right up there with listening to a 5,000 kazoo concert or clobbering your thumb with a hammer. It's the kind of pain that makes you want to yowl.

Most toothaches are due to bacteria and decay that have penetrated the tissue at the tooth's center, according to Kenneth H. Burrell, D.D.S., director of the American Dental Association's Council on Dental Therapeutics in Chicago. The subsequent inflammation causes pressure, which causes pain. These bacteria can also create localized areas of infection, called abscesses, at the root tip. Both situations can produce a deep, sharp throbbing sensation and extreme sensitivity. (If it's just a sharp "burst" of pain that quickly vanishes, you probably have sensitive teeth rather than a toothache.) In addition, gum disease, failed restorative work, tooth fractures—even sinus infections and heart ailments—can produce intermittent bursts or a constant stabbing pain that'll drive you up the wall.

This long day's journey into excruciation can easily be avoided by practicing a daily routine of brushing and flossing and seeing your dentist twice a year. But that probably doesn't mean too much if your molar is already beating like a bass drum. When the pain is on the march, you'll soon be marching to the dentist. But in the meantime, here are a few things you can do to grin and bear it.

Rinse with warm salt water. Hot or cold water will only aggravate an already sensitive tooth, but swishing some warm salt water will relieve a lot of the pain, says William P. Maher, D.D.S., assistant professor of endodontics at the University of Detroit Mercy School of Dentistry.

Just mix two to three teaspoons of salt in a glass of water. The salt draws out some of the fluids causing the swelling and have a general soothing effect. The saltwater rinse also cleans the areas around the infected tooth. Even unsalted lukewarm water (about body temperature) can flush out an irritating piece of rotting food and provide some relief.

When to See the Doctor

Make an appointment with your dentist as soon as you feel a toothache—and *keep* that appointment, no matter what.

"If you have a toothache and the pain goes away, you should not assume you are cured," says William P. Maher, D.D.S., assistant professor of endodontics at the University of Detroit Mercy School of Dentistry. Have your teeth checked by a dentist. "The condition could actually worsen with no outward symptoms at all."

The problem is that the pulp can go dead even while the bacteria are still very active. The bacteria may be working under the crown, but after the pain dissipates, "you wouldn't even know it, because your early warning system has been removed," says Dr. Maher. But unless you have the underlying problem taken care of, you may risk losing the tooth.

Take an analgesic. "Anything you would take for a headache you can take for a toothache," says Dr. Burrell. That old standby, aspirin, works wonders to tame toothache pain and inflammation. If you have adverse reactions to aspirin, try ibuprofen (Advil or Nuprin). Ibuprofen has even more anti-inflammatory power, and it's gentler to the stomach than aspirin.

If you do use aspirin, never put it directly on a tooth or gum, warns Dr. Burrell. It will only produce a painful acid burn. Also, don't give aspirin to children because of the risk of Reye's syndrome.

Find relief in the freezer. "Ice will shut down some of the superficial nerves," says Thomas Lundeen, D.M.D., co-director of the Clinical Pain Program at the University of North Carolina in Chapel Hill. It is particularly helpful with bruises or other traumatic injuries to the tooth or mouth, since ice can greatly reduce swelling. But don't apply ice directly to a tooth: Use an ice pack wrapped in a towel outside the mouth.

Try some oil of cloves. Eugenol (oil of cloves) is available over the counter and provides exceptional temporary relief, especially for toothaches that are temperature-sensitive. Such pain is usually due to problems of the pulp, the tooth center, says Martin Trope, D.M.D., chairman of the Department of Endodontology at Temple University School of Dentistry in Philadelphia. Most drugstores sell eugenol toothache kits. You can even mix liquid eugenol with zinc oxide to create your own temporary fillings for painful cavities. A few drops on the tooth surface or in a cavity or crack should do the job until you can get to the dentist.

Numb it with benzocaine. "Benzocaine is a local, over-the-counter anesthetic that works well if there is a large cavity or damage to the tooth surface," says Dr. Maher. "It numbs things. The closer you can get it to the pulp, the better it works."

Several easy-to-apply, brand-name oral gels and ointments contain this numbing agent. Dab the gel on the entire tooth surface and surrounding gum with your finger or a cotton swab. If you have a visible cavity, try to get the gel inside the cavity area.

Don't get all heated up. Keep heat away from your teeth, warns Dr. Trope. In fact, avoid both temperature extremes. Very cold or hot drinks may increase the pain when they hit your nerve endings. Extremely salty or sugary foods and drinks can have the same effect, he adds.

Use some more ice on your hand. Here's a neat trick developed by pain researcher Ronald Melzack, Ph.D., of McGill University in Montreal, Quebec. Rub a piece of ice on the V-shaped area between your thumb and forefinger for five to seven minutes, until that area goes numb. This treatment significantly eases tooth pain by sending impulses along the same pathways that toothache pain travels. The impulses close the gate on incoming pain messages—in effect, shutting off the ache.

You may want to exercise . . . or not. "Most people with a throbbing toothache just want to sit still—and that is probably best," says Dr. Lundeen. "On the other hand, physical activity, especially of the aerobic type, may produce enough endorphins (the body's natural pain relievers) that the pain will be greatly reduced." If you can, try a brisk walk or jog. But don't force yourself to keep going if the pain gets worse.

Breathe deeply—and listen up. "Soothing music and deep breathing bring about a relaxed state, which can help alleviate some toothache pain," says Dr. Lundeen. Researchers at the University of Washington in Seattle have discovered that slow rhythmic music effectively reduces your awareness of much acute pain, including dental pain, by distracting your attention and generating pleasant moods and images. So sit back, turn on the stereo, and let the dulcet tones of your favorite crooner chase away your toothache blues.

Put out that cigarette. "Tobacco is associated with a great number of dental and oral problems and can really irritate sensitive gums," says Dr. Lundeen. "Snuff and chewing tobacco are especially damaging." Tobacco stimulates adrenaline, which sensitizes us to pain. And the nicotine in tobacco blocks endorphins.

Tooth Grinding

When your life's a grind all day, your teeth are bound to grind all night. Pent-up stress is the usual cause of tooth grinding—also known as bruxism—a common and potentially ruinous process of nighttime gnashing or daytime jaw clenching.

Whether it's a daytime habit or a nighttime problem, you may be unaware of what you're doing to those pearly whites until they literally "grind down" in size. Besides affecting looks, untreated bruxism makes it harder for you to eat, since all that grinding erodes tooth enamel to the point where teeth become more sensitive to hot and cold foods and drinks. Often bruxism causes severe headaches and facial and jaw pain—especially when chewing and just after waking up.

If these symptoms have a familiar bite, here are some remedies to chew on to stop your gritting.

Handle the stress in your life. You're more prone to bruxism if you let stress get to you before you get to it—one reason why hard-driving, stressaholic, Type A personalities are particularly susceptible to tooth grinding, says Neil Gottehrer, D.D.S., director of the Craniofacial Pain Center in Abington, Pennsylvania. "Many sublimate frustration or aggression into jaw clenching or tooth grinding."

His advice: Squeeze a tennis ball when you feel stressed, or practice a *regular* stress reduction technique such as meditation, listening to music or another pastime that helps you unwind and release stress before it takes up permanent residence in your gut.

Change your sleeping position. If you sleep on your side or stomach, you're more likely to have bruxism, *even* if you control the stress in your life, says Tom Colquitt, D.D.S., a dentist and bruxism researcher in Shreveport, Louisiana.

How to Stop Tooth Grinding in Children

Children feel pressure, too, and half-pints often take the full brunt of stress right in the jawbone. That's one reason why nighttime bruxism is *more* common in kids than adults.

Failing to nip childhood tooth grinding can do devastating damage to primary teeth and take an irreversible toll on a youngster's permanent choppers. So if your child has a nighttime tooth-grinding habit, here are some ways to help nip it in the bud, from bruxism researchers Alexander K. C. Leung, M.D., and W. Lane M. Robson, M.D., both of the University of Calgary and Alberta Children's Hospital in Calgary.

- Make bedtime enjoyable and relaxed by reading to and talking with children. This gives them an opportunity to review some of their fears and angers of the day.
- Give your kids ample opportunity and space to play throughout the day. With preschoolers especially, it's important to have toys and games suited to their stage of development. With older children, encourage them to pursue activities like organized sports that release pent-up energy.
- Be patient, sympathetic and understanding about the troubles they're having—whether it's potty training or schoolwork. Threats and punishment only raise the stress level and are likely to make bruxism worse.

But even with these precautions, you should definitely take your child to a dentist or pediatric dentist if the child has significant bruxism, according to Dr. Leung and Dr. Robson. They point out that most pediatricians look for cavities and missing teeth, but only dentists regularly check for signs of bruxism. And it takes a dentist to prescribe a special dental appliance that prevents teeth from being worn down.

You can take some pressure off your teeth and reduce tooth grinding if you just change your nighttime position. Sleep on your back, advises Dr. Colquitt.

Or get a contoured pillow. If you *must* sleep in the fetal position, place a contoured foam pillow under your face, adds Dr. Colquitt. Then place another ordinary pillow between your arms, as if you were hugging it. When you sleep in this position, the contoured pillow reduces strain on your neck and jaw, and the other pillow helps prevent you from rolling over onto your face. You can purchase a contoured foam pillow, which ranges in price from about $35 to $50, at most surgical supply houses.

Munch on crunchy food before bedtime. Eating raw apples, cauliflower, carrots or celery helps tire out jaw muscles, so they'll be too tuckered to gnash at night, says Harold T. Perry, D.D.S., Ph.D., a past president of the American Academy of Craniomandibular Disorders and a professor of orthodontics at Northwestern University Dental School in Chicago.

Just say no to nightcaps. If you are looking for an excuse to "numb" your jaws, look somewhere *besides* your liquor cabinet. "Studies have shown that alcohol actually makes you clench *more*," says Jeffrey P. Okeson, D.M.D., director of the Orofacial Pain Center at the University of Kentucky College of Dentistry in Lexington. "My guess is that alcohol disrupts the sleep cycle and influences increased muscle activity in your jaw." If aching jaws are troubling you, Dr. Okeson recommends two ibuprofen (Advil) tablets.

Try the 60-minute solution. A regular workout for at least 20 minutes three times weekly helps relieve pent-up stress *and* releases endorphins, the body's natural painkilling substances. "Participating in some sort of physical activity each day is a healthy way to release stress and may be helpful in solving your nighttime tooth-grinding problem," says Dr. Okeson.

Guard your gnashers. Many dentists prescribe specially made acrylic mouthguards to prevent or minimize nighttime tooth grinding. As an alternative, you might have success with the kind of mouthguard that's available at a sporting goods store, according to Sheldon Gross, D.D.S., a past president of the American Academy of Craniomandibular Disorders and a lecturer at Tufts University in Medford, Massachusetts, and at the University of Medicine and Dentistry of New Jersey/New Jersey Medical School in Newark. Look for a sports mouthguard that can be "custom-fitted" by placing the mouthpiece in hot water and biting down. "Try it—and if it works, fine. If it doesn't, check with your dentist for a prescription," suggests Dr. Gross.

Practice proper jaw posture. "There are only three times when your lower teeth should be touching your upper teeth—when you chew, swallow and speak," says Dr. Okeson. "At all other times, your teeth should *not* be touching." To make sure your jaws are in their proper position, sit up straight and blow a little air through slightly parted lips. In this position your teeth are slightly separated—just where you want them. "With practice, your jaw will assume the correct posture automatically," says Dr. Okeson.

Heat up your jaws. Applying wet heat to the sides of your face helps relax clenching jaw muscles, says bruxism specialist Kenneth R. Goljan, D.D.S., of Tulsa, Oklahoma. Soak a washcloth in very hot water, wring it out, and place the cloth on your jaws as often as possible—especially right before bedtime.

Tooth Sensitivity

You take a swig of cold water. Or perhaps you eat something sweet. Or you're just brushing your teeth. Suddenly you are zapped with a burst of pain like a discharge from a car battery. It really hurts! But unlike a toothache, it's gone as quickly as it came.

Although it may feel like Dr. Frankenstein just gave your mouth a jolt, the real story is not quite so horrifying. You're suffering from a condition called hypersensitivity. It's not a toothache but a painful response to an outside stimulus. While extremely discomforting, it's easily treatable and usually not serious.

"Tooth sensitivity results from the exposure of dentin—the layer just below the surface of the teeth—and roots," says Thomas Lundeen, D.M.D., co-director of the Clinical Pain Program at the University of North Carolina in Chapel Hill. "It's usually caused by a receded gum, worn enamel, small cracks in the teeth or overzealous brushing. When these things occur, they can expose microscopic tubules, little holes leading from the dentin directly to the sensitive pulp tissue at the tooth's center."

At first there may be no pain—until these tiny tubules come in contact with air, cold, heat, sugar or another physical stimulus. These stimuli transmit signals directly to the pulp, and *zap!* Get ready for a shock wave of pulp pain you wouldn't believe! But unlike the constant pounding of a toothache, this sensation vanishes as soon as the stimulus is removed. And also unlike a toothache, the pulp of a sensitive tooth is usually not infected or inflamed.

When to See the Doctor

If tooth sensitivity persists for longer than a month despite your attempts to remedy the situation, or if it is really interfering with your daily activities, see your dentist, says William P. Maher, D.D.S., assistant professor of endodontics at the University of Detroit Mercy School of Dentistry.

You may actually have a cavity or bad filling, but only your dentist can make that decision. If it is, in fact, a case of severe hypersensitivity, the dentist can nix it with fillings, crowns, fluoride treatment, bonding agents or, in a few cases, root canal surgery.

"Hypersensitivity feels a lot worse than it really is," says William P. Maher, D.D.S., assistant professor of endodontics at the University of Detroit Mercy School of Dentistry. "Most tooth sensitivity will go away in time. The teeth are very sensitive at first, but after a month or so, the pulp will react by laying down some hard tissue from inside the tooth, like a wall, to protect itself."

If the sensitivity persists, see a dentist. In the meantime, these simple tips can keep your tender teeth in check.

Use a toothpaste designed for sensitive teeth. "Keeping the tooth clean and plaque-free with a fluoride toothpaste will stimulate the tooth to fill in the tubules," says Dr. Lundeen. "Try to avoid toothpastes with whiteners—they're harsher and more abrasive. Your best bet is a desensitizing toothpaste such as Sensodyne or Denquel, which contain ingredients that help block up the tubules."

Brush up and down. Bad brushing not only can cause hypersensitivity, it can undo all nature's repair work. Instead, brush with a gentle up-and-down motion. Be extra careful near the gum line—that's where most sensitivity occurs.

Switch to a soft-bristle brush. "Stiff, hard brushes can scrape and strip away enamel and cause gums to recede, especially for someone using excessive pressure when he brushes," says Kenneth H. Burrell, D.D.S., director of the American Dental Association's Council on Dental Therapeutics in Chicago. "Softer bristles are less likely to irritate sensitive teeth and will not expose underlying tubules."

Avoid extremes of hot and cold. "Naturally, if you have a sensitive tooth, you guard it from any stimulus," says Dr. Maher. "Serve hot or cold foods at temperatures close to room temperature, and try to avoid biting into foods of different temperature extremes at the same sitting." (Breathing through your mouth in very cold weather can also give your sensitive teeth a chilly shock.)

Oil up with eugenol. "A few drops of an over-the-counter preparation containing eugenol provide exceptional relief for all pulp-related pain," says Martin Trope, D.M.D., chairman of the Department of Endodontololgy at the Temple University School of Dentistry in Philadelphia.

Skip the salt water. "A saltwater rinse is fine for a regular toothache, but in the case of hypersensitivity, it will just cause a movement of the fluids within the tubules, which will stimulate more pain," says Dr. Trope.

Don't eat acidic foods—or sweets. Lemons, tomatoes and other foods with high acid content can eat away at your tooth enamel and hinder your tooth's natural healing process, warns Dr. Lundeen. And for some people, eating sweets causes a flare-up of pain, according to Dr. Maher—so just avoid them.

Tooth Stains

About the only thing that shines on game shows more than those fabulous showcase prizes are the smiles of the hosts. But while Wink and Chip and Skip and the rest of the hosts have a staff of makeup artists to make sure their smiles are whiter than the Arctic landscape, the rest of us regular folks have only ourselves to keep our teeth stain-free.

And sometimes, that can be harder than Double Jeopardy. Some stains can be handled only by a professional—specifically those caused by the use of certain antibiotics, a high fever or quirks in metabolism. But if you just have day-to-day problems with stained-looking teeth, there are everyday things you can do to improve them.

"Stained teeth are caused by a lot of the things we like: coffee, tea, colas, smoking, even the foods we eat. The obvious suggestion is to give up those things, but that's easier said than done for most people," explains Barry Dale, D.M.D., an Englewood, New Jersey, cosmetic dentist and assistant clinical professor at Mount Sinai Medical Center in New York City. "Even things we *don't* do can lead to staining. Teeth get more yellow as part of the natural aging process."

But some of the staining can be avoided or removed if you follow this advice.

Make water your chaser. Since coffee, tea and cola—some of our most consumed beverages—cause most of the staining in our diets, caffeine consumers can offset some of the discoloration by swishing water *after* each cup or glass. "Ideally, you can prevent many stains from forming by brushing after each meal or snack," says David S. Halpern, D.M.D., a dentist in Columbia, Maryland, and a spokesdentist for the Academy of General Dentistry. "But since most people don't do that, I advise my patients to take a cup of water and swish it around after they drink coffee or another staining beverage. Besides diminishing the initial film stain of coffee, it also helps keep their breath relatively fresh."

"Bleaching" Kits Clean Wallets More Than Teeth

Thinking about using one of those tooth polishes advertised on TV that promise you a mouthful of pearly whites? If you go ahead and spend your money for those products, you're being shucked like an oyster.

"Some are so abrasive that while they may initially appear to whiten your teeth, they can make them even darker, because they strip away the enamel—leaving the darker dentin exposed," says Barry Dale, D.M.D., an Englewood, New Jersey, cosmetic dentist and assistant clinical professor at Mount Sinai Medical Center in New York City. "What happens is that you turn your slightly yellowed teeth a darker color."

And dark teeth are only the beginning of your problems if you use these polishing gels, pastes and other "bleaching" kits. New evidence suggests that they can be harmful to your health. "Some studies suggest they may potentiate other cancer-causing agents," says Dr. Dale. "That means if you smoke, for instance, using bleaching kits may enhance the risk of mouth cancer."

Eat a lot of crunchy foods. "Consuming apples, celery and other crunchy foods that rub against the teeth helps dislodge debris that can cause staining," adds Dr. Halpern. "I notice there is more of a staining problem in patients who eat a lot of sticky foods."

Keep peroxide for cleaning wounds, not teeth. True, dentists use a peroxide solution to bleach stained teeth. But that doesn't mean you can do it yourself with store-bought varieties. "What we use is a special 35 percent peroxide solution that's very strong," says Dr. Dale. "There's no evidence that rinsing with the 2 percent peroxide you buy at the drugstore will help keep teeth white."

Don't brush too hard. Logic might suggest that the harder you brush, the cleaner you'll get your teeth. But reality says otherwise. "Brushing too vigorously can actually strip some of the enamel off teeth, exposing the darker inner layer called the dentin," says Dr. Dale. *His advice:* Brush your teeth firmly but not vigorously—and use only soft-bristle brushes, not those with medium or hard bristles. "If you can't remove the stain with regular brushing and toothpaste, then you won't remove it by brushing harder."

Triglyceride Control

Think of triglycerides as too much of a good thing. Along with cholesterol, triglycerides are the major source of fat circulating in the blood. And just as cholesterol is needed to protect nerves and build strong cells and hormones, triglycerides are necessary for producing your body's energy. But that doesn't mean they're always beneficial.

On the contrary, when triglycerides get too high, you increase your risk of heart disease, because there's too much fat in your blood. High triglycerides also have a bad rep because they have been associated with lower levels of high-density lipoprotein (HDL), the "good" cholesterol.

If you're wondering whether your triglyceride level is too high, your doctor can tell you. In general, you need to get the level down if your triglycerides are over 500 milligrams per deciliter (mg/dl). But any level between 250 and

500 mg/dl is considered borderline, and most doctors think it's best to keep levels below 150. Here's how.

Gobble up garlic. Studies show that eating as little as one clove a day can lower triglyceride production. And the more you eat, the better the effect. "Studies on lab animals show that a diet made of 2 percent garlic—the equivalent of three to five cloves per day for the average American—can reduce triglycerides 25 to 30 percent," says Yu-Yan Yeh, Ph.D., associate professor of nutrition at Pennsylvania State University in University Park and a researcher on the healing properties of garlic. "What garlic does is lower production of triglycerides as well as reduce their release from the liver into the blood." (It can also reduce cholesterol as much as 15 percent, he notes.)

Fresh or powdered? It doesn't even matter. *Any* garlic is good garlic.

Feed on fish. Besides garlic, a diet rich in certain fish has been shown to lower triglyceride levels in some people. "We did a fish oil study and found that even people with low or below-normal trigylcerides saw a reduction after eating a lot of fish oil, which is rich in omega-3 fatty acids," says Beverly Clevidence, Ph.D., research nutritionist at the U.S. Department of Agriculture Human Nutrition Research Center's Lipid Lab in Beltsville, Maryland. For best results, however, you need to consume about 15 grams of fish oil a day—the amount in eight ounces of salmon, mackerel or herring, the best sources of omega-3's.

Don't light up. Although often overlooked, smoking is one of the biggest contributors to excessive blood fats. It does damage indirectly by reducing HDL cholesterol, which helps take triglycerides from the blood back into the liver for excretion. "With fewer HDLs, there are more of the undesirable blood fats, including higher levels of triglycerides," says Dr. Clevidence.

Go easy on alcohol. Even in small amounts, booze has a damaging effect. "That's because the liver often converts alcohol into blood fats," explains Dr. Clevidence. "Something like one in three people who have high triglycerides can lower them by staying away from alcohol."

Make your carbs complex. There's no question that simple carbohydrates such as candy, sugars and other sweets boost triglycerides. Besides, they provide "empty" calories that are high in fat but low in nutrition. For effective dieting and triglyceride control, Dr. Clevidence suggests replacing fat with complex carbohydrates: "You get a lot of vitamins and nutrients for the calories." That means eating a lot of grains and pasta dishes as well as plenty of fresh fruits and vegetables.

Lose weight—even if you don't need to. Although it's well established that overweight people are usually at greatest risk of high triglycerides, "some normal-weight people can lower their triglycerides by losing weight—even if it's just a few pounds," says Dr. Clevidence. "We're not exactly sure why it occurs, but for some people, it does."

If you're overweight, dieting is probably the *best* way to reduce triglycerides. Along with a regular exercise program—one hour of exercise at least three times a week—it's best to limit total dietary fat intake to about 20 percent of total daily calories. But even if fat intake is around 30 percent, you'll probably see some benefits, says Robert DiBianco, M.D., associate clinical professor of medicine at Georgetown University in Washington, D.C., and director of the Cardiac Risk Factor Reduction Program and cardiology research at Washington Adventist Hospital in Takoma Park, Maryland.

TV Addiction

I t's been called everything from the plug-in drug to the electronic baby-sitter, and with good reason. Studies show that people watch amazing amounts of television; in fact, children often spend more time in front of the set than in school. So what can you do if you fear that the tube is invading your life?

"One of the major predictors of how much television people watch is how much time they spend at home," says Aletha Huston, Ph.D., professor of human development at the University of Kansas in Lawrence. Obviously, taming television addiction is easier if you get out of the house and find other hobbies, sports and entertainment. But, especially if you have young children, this can be difficult. So try these tips to unglue your family members from their seats in front of the screen.

Plan ahead. Make use of a weekly TV schedule. Look through it and decide which shows you truly want to watch, suggests Robert A. Mendelson, M.D., a pediatrician in Portland, Oregon, and immediate past chairman of the Committee on Communications of the American Academy of Pediatrics. To reach agreement on a schedule, Dr. Mendelson recommends holding a family meeting each Sunday. Each person can choose one to two hours per day of programming for the family to watch. Write the showtimes on a calendar and make a policy of "No channel flipping!" At other times the TV is dark.

Set weekly limits. "If you are going to set viewing limits, consider doing it by the week," says Washington, D.C., psychologist Diana Zuckerman, Ph.D., a former member of the American Psychological Association's Task Force on Television and Society. Think about how many hours per week family members are now watching, and slowly reduce the number of hours until you reach a "target" allowance.

See shows together. Our experts agree that watching television with your children is a good idea. "If a parent is there to interpret what the child is viewing, everything can be a learning experience," explains Dr. Mendelson. Gather around the set, ask questions, and encourage responses to what is being shown.

How Much Do You Really Watch?

How do you determine if the amount of television you are watching is too much?

One way, of course, is to compare yourself with others. On average, adults watch three to four hours of television per day, and adolescents watch a little less. But you may not realize how much you are actually watching until you keep track for a week.

"Once you keep a diary of the amount of television that you watch, you may find that you are actually within the norm," explains Aletha Huston, Ph.D., professor of human development at the University of Kansas in Lawrence. "Most people watch more than they think they do."

Though three to four hours each day may be average, our sources agree that this is generally too much. "If you find yourself regretting that you've watched so much television—and wishing that you'd done something else—it's a sign that you're not using your time very well," says Dr. Huston.

Give your kids dinner chores. Instead of enlisting the television as babysitter while you prepare dinner, assign the kids to help. "Even the littlest child can put napkins on the table. The more they can help, the more autonomy they feel, and the more they feel like a part of the family," says Lottie M. Mendelson, a pediatric nurse practitioner in Portland, Oregon, and an expert on children and television.

Shut the fridge. If the television is on, keep the refrigerator door closed. "There's no question about the correlation between television watching and obesity," says Dr. Mendelson. "It is not that obese children watch TV but that children who watch a lot of TV become obese."

This is also true of adults. When you always combine watching and eating, "it sets up a system where when you eat, you think about watching television, and when you watch TV, you think about eating," says Dr. Zuckerman. "In the end, you eat too much, and you watch too much TV."

Let them pay to watch. One way to delay children's TV watching is to insist that they get their homework done first. But kids can also "pay" for their viewing time by reading, doing chores around the house or playing with a younger sibling, Dr. Zuckerman says.

Type A Personality

You know the Type A person all too well. He's the guy in line behind you at the supermarket who fumes as you fumble through your pockets looking for the exact change. She's the woman who rages when you arrive five minutes late for an appointment. He's the fellow who glares at you if you beat him playing golf.

By now you've probably figured out the *A* in Type A stands for anger. But there are other Type A traits that many researchers believe increase your risk of suffering a heart attack, including hostility, competitiveness and impatience.

"Trivial things—like waiting a few extra moments for an elevator—that don't bother a calm Type B get some Type A's very angry," explains Meyer Friedman, M.D., a cardiologist who is director of the Meyer Friedman Institute in San Francisco and author of *Treating Type A Behavior and Your Heart.*

If your Type A outbursts are getting you frazzled and ruining your health, here are some ways to keep your feelings under control and soften your image as a raging bull.

Be a good actor. Ask yourself what personality traits you'd like to shed in the next year. "If you want to be less hostile, then just for a day pretend that you are a person who isn't hostile," Dr. Friedman says. "Do the things that the person you want to be a year from now would do. Then keep doing them day after day. By the end of the year, you may find you're no longer pretending."

Create a thinking spot. "Find a place where you can think out loud," says Joanne Babich, Ph.D, a psychologist in Phoenix. "By talking out loud to yourself, you learn to take a second look at your reactions to situations, and it will teach you a lot about what you're really feeling."

Jot down your feelings. Keeping a record of times and situations in which you typically get angry helps you realize how frequently in a day you blow your stack. It also helps you sort out the real cause of that anger, which often is something you have no control over.

"The elevator may be slow, so you get angry because you think that a person on a floor above you is deliberately holding it up. But in reality, you can't possibly know that. If you write down that feeling, it may help you talk yourself out of your anger," says Redford Williams, M.D., professor of psychiatry and director of the Behavioral Medicine Research Center at Duke University Medical Center in Durham, North Carolina, and author of *The Trusting Heart: Great News about Type A Behavior.*

Don't take the bait. Imagine that you're a fish that swims downstream each day, says Lynda Powell, Ph.D., an epidemiologist at the Yale University School of Medicine in New Haven, Connecticut. "When you wake in the morning, there is clear water ahead of you, but as you start swimming downstream, all of a sudden, a hook drops," she says. The "hook," she points out, could be any annoying event—like getting in your car in the morning and discovering it's on empty because your teenage son was driving around the night before. That's a hook—and you can make a conscious decision whether you're going to bite it or just swim by it.

"Life is a series of hooks—unexpected minor things—that you can choose to tangle with or pass by," says Dr. Powell. You can expect that these unforeseen but irritating events will occur every day. Type A people really can choose to shrug off those irritants.

Hostility and Your Heart

Sure, many classic Type A's are time-pressured, hard-driven workaholics who juggle six projects at once. But when it comes to heart disease, not all Type A's are created equal.

"There are some very specfic characteristics of some Type A's that seem to be associated more strongly with heart disease," explains Pierre Dion, Ph.D., a clinical psychologist in Ottawa, Ontario. "The time-urgent, hostile person who bangs on the steering wheel and swears when the car in front of him slows down is more at risk for heart disease than other Type A's who aren't as hostile."

Hostility and fast talking that interrupts other people are two Type A behaviors that were linked to high blood pressure—yet another risk factor for heart disease—in a study of 218 men and women at the Toronto Hospital.

For all "hostile" Type A's, regular exercise can be a bridge to better health. "Many studies have shown that aerobic activity such as bicycling, running, fast walking and swimming is protective against heart disease," Dr. Dion says.

Pick the longest lines. It may seem odd, but one good way to cure a short-fuse temper is to stand in the longest lines at grocery stores, post offices and banks. "It teaches you patience and that the world won't come to an end if it takes a few minutes longer than you expected," Dr. Babich says. "It may even give you a chance to strike up a conversation with someone."

Check your image. Look at your facial expressions in a mirror several times a day. Do you look cheerful, or are you scowling? "Looking at yourself in a mirror gives you an idea what kind of image your face is projecting to the world," Dr. Powell says. "So if you're scowling, practice smiling. That will give you a chance to sense what a smile really feels like, and you'll also see how much better an image you project by doing it."

Keep your cool. It's true that counting to ten or deep breathing can do wonders to reduce anger. "I'm treating an executive who loses his temper quickly. So whenever he feels himself getting angry, he has learned to take several deep breaths," Dr. Babich says. "After each breath, he says to himself

'I'm feeling a little more calm than I did a moment ago.' Then he is able to face the situation with a new perspective."

Practice saying "I'm wrong." "Type A people have difficulty apologizing, because it would mean that they would have to admit they are wrong," according to Dr. Babich. "Some mental health professionals require that Type A's apologize at least once a day, even if they're not sure they're wrong. It's good practice to learn that you don't have to be perfect."

Burn the rule book. Many Type A's expect others to follow their rules, and they get very upset when those rules are broken. Being on time is a special bugbear. "It's important for Type A's to learn to be flexible and realize that some people don't value time as much as they do," says Jane Irvine, Ph.D., director of the Behavioral Cardiology Program at the Toronto Hospital.

Sweat away your anger. Moderate aerobic exercise such as bicycling, running or walking may reduce stress and relieve anger, but don't overdo it. "People with Type A personalities, particularly when they're angry, may actually exercise to a point that they hurt themselves," Dr. Babich says. She suggests exercising in the morning before the stresses of the day overwhelm you.

Slow down, you're going too fast. Make time for the three Ps—people, plants and pets, Dr. Friedman suggests. Have a long, thoughtful chat with your children, stroll through a botanical garden or play with a pet.

"Take time to observe them, learn from them, grow with them," he says.

Ulcers

If ever an ailment was designed to test our patience, it's this one. Ulcers are the ultimate hang-around, come-and-go, now-you-feel-it-now-you-don't kind of problem.

If you could peek inside your stomach, however, you'd see the problem at once. Ulcers are raw, craterlike spots in the stomach or just beyond the stomach in the part of the intestine called the duodenum.

They occur when, for one reason or another, the cells normally lining the stomach or intestine no longer provide protection against the caustic effects of stomach acid. The stomach literally digests itself.

Only a doctor can tell you for sure whether you have ulcers. And even the best of doctors can't tell you exactly when you're going to have a flare-up.

But here are some self-care steps to take when you feel your ulcers going into overdrive, along with some tips that could help your ulcers heal faster.

Multiply and divide your meals. Food neutralizes the stomach acid that causes ulcers, so you may be able to reduce ulcer pain by eating more frequently. Some people have less ulcer upset if they eat six small meals a day instead of three full-size meals, according to Thomas Brasitus, M.D., professor of medicine and director of gastroenterology at the University of Chicago Pritzker School of Medicine.

Banish the food culprits. Doctors used to supply a hit list of foods to strike from the diet, including a lot of yummy fare. No longer. Now it's up to you to decide.

"The foods that bother people seem to vary with each individual," says David Earnest, M.D., professor of medicine at the University of Arizona College of Medicine Health Sciences Center in Tucson and chairman of the Clinical Practice Section for the American Gastroenterological Association.

Those foods *might* be the classic arsonists such as pepperoni pizza and very hot chili. "Obviously, spicy foods may bother some people," says Dr. Earnest. But foods that sound soothing, such as milk, ice cream or chicken soup, could be part of the problem. So play watchdog with your diet, and drop the symptom aggravators from your menu.

Use over-the-counter antacids. These drugs can heal an ulcer, at least temporarily, according to Naurang Agrawal, M.D., staff gastroenterologist at the Ochsner Clinic in New Orleans. To help ease ulcer discomfort, try the following schedule: Take two tablespoons of antacid one hour after a meal, three hours after a meal, at bedtime and whenever you have pain.

Antacids are safe, although high doses may cause diarrhea or constipation, according to Dr. Agrawal.

Try stress relief. "Classic studies have presented strong evidence of a stress component in ulcer development," according to Steven Fahrion, Ph.D., clinical psychologist and director of the Center for Applied Psychophysiology at the Menninger Clinic in Topeka, Kansas.

When to See the Doctor

Don't count on pain to tip you off to the fact that you have ulcers. Doctors say you may have ulcers whether or not you have telltale discomfort in the stomach area.

It's true that the classic symptoms *can* be unmistakable. Often there's a burning, gnawing or aching pain just below the breastbone. You can begin to suspect ulcers (as opposed to heartburn) if the pain is relieved by eating food but recurs two to three hours after eating a meal. Sometimes that pain is so strong that it awakens you in the wee hours of the morning.

But doctors say that only about *half* of the people who develop ulcers have these symptoms. Ulcer pain is also described as soreness, an empty feeling or hunger, and some older people have no pain at all!

"For many ulcer sufferers, the first sign that something is wrong is stomach bleeding and perforation, a serious condition that requires prompt medical attention," says Howard Mertz, M.D., associate director of the University of California, Los Angeles, Center for Functional Bowel Disorders and Abdominal Pain.

For this reason, you should be aware of warning signs that blood is seeping into your digestive tract. If you spit up what looks like coffee grounds or have dark, tarry bowel movements, call the doctor immediately.

Not all researchers agree. But studies suggest that stress *increases* stomach acid production and *decreases* blood flow. And if there's anything an ulcer-prone stomach doesn't need, it's more acid.

Many stress relief techniques are recommended by doctors, including deep breathing, moderate physical exercise and mind relaxation techniques such as meditation, yoga, visualization or listening to relaxation tapes.

For ulcer sufferers, Dr. Fahrion recommends a stomach-warming technique. Spend some time every day in a quiet, relaxed state and try to visualize warmth, increased blood flow and decreased acid secretion in the stomach area. This technique can "relax" blood vessels, allowing greater blood flow to the stomach area.

Puff no more. Smokers are twice as likely to get ulcers as nonsmokers. And when they do get them, studies show, the ulcers take longer to heal and will be more than three times as likely to recur. What's the best way to quit smoking? "I offer my patients nicotine gum, but that's not enough," according to Howard Mertz, M.D., associate director of the University of California, Los Angeles, Center for Functional Bowel Disorders and Abdominal Pain. "Those who simply go cold turkey seem to be most successful."

Avoid aspirin and ibuprofen. Over-the-counter pain relievers that fall under the category of nonsteroidal anti-inflammatory drugs (NSAIDs) should be off-limits for anyone who has ulcers, according to Dr. Agrawal.

"Even when they're taken with food or taken in 'buffered' form, they can cause the stomach lining to deteriorate to the point where ulcers form," he says. If you need to use a pain reliever, try acetaminophen (Tylenol) instead: It's not an NSAID. *Note:* Some prescription drugs, including many of those used to treat arthritis, are also ulcer-aggravating NSAIDs. But check with your doctor before you stop taking any prescribed medication.

Underweight

Y ou say you'd like to *gain* a few pounds?
There's little doubt most people wish they could be underweight instead of overweight. But underweight can be just as tough on your looks—and your health.

"Gaining weight can involve as much effort as losing weight, especially if you are concerned about your health," says George Blackburn, M.D., Ph.D., chief of the Nutrition/Metabolism Laboratory at New England Deaconess Hospital in Boston. "After all, gaining ten pounds won't do much for your health or your looks if those pounds are added as fat. What you should aim for is gaining muscle mass. And for that, it takes the right kind of diet and exercise."

But before you decide to gain some pounds, make sure you really would benefit from more weight. Who says you're too skinny? Your husband? Your mother? A worrywart friend? The mirror? Not everyone who thinks he needs to gain really does.

When to See the Doctor

If you are normally thin and want to gain weight, that's one thing. But what if your weight drops suddenly?

"When people lose weight without trying, something is wrong," says Maryl Winningham, R.N., Ph.D., an exercise physiologist and a nurse specializing in the care of cancer patients at the University of Utah College of Nursing in Salt Lake City. It could indicate a wide range of problems, from cancer to depression—so don't delay seeing a doctor.

Also, don't automatically assume that people lose weight as they age. "People *don't* normally lose weight as they get older, although they do tend to lose muscle tissue," according to Dr. Winningham. So see a doctor if you've lost ten pounds or more without dieting.

Prescription drugs can deaden your appetite and cause weight loss, but of course you'll have to see a doctor before going off any prescribed drugs. See a doctor, too, if you are thin and get lots of colds, flu or infections or if you lack energy, says Dr. Winningham. Being underweight can compromise your immune system.

If you feel energetic all day long, then sleep well and wake up feeling great, if you have enough upper body strength to tote suitcases and children or grandchildren, then your light weight is probably not a problem, according to Dr. Blackburn. You're just naturally thin.

On the other hand, if you feel weak and lack energy, or if you'd like to try to build yourself up for strength, endurance and looks, weight gain might be for you. Here's what experts recommend.

Gain muscle, not fat. "Probably the best thing you can do to gain weight is start a weight-lifting program," says Adam Drewnowski, Ph.D., director of the Human Nutrition Program at the University of Michigan in Ann Arbor. "If you increase your exercise, particularly resistance training, your body requires more food, and you will eat more. But with weight training, you will gain weight in the form of *muscle* instead of fat."

Aim for 100 to 200 extra calories a day. That's all your body can use each day to build and sustain the muscle tissue you will develop in your exercise program, Dr. Blackburn says.

Be patient. Give your muscle-building program plenty of time. "You'll have to work at it consistently for 6 to 12 months to see a big difference, but you *will* see a difference in endurance and strength," says Larry Houk, M.D., a specialist in the treatment of rheumatic diseases and director of the Arthritis Fitness Center in Cincinnati.

Leave the milkshakes and hot fudge sundaes alone. You might feel this is the perfect opportunity to pig out on fattening foods. "But quality is as important as quantity in a weight-gain diet," Dr. Blackburn says. Excess fat in the diet causes excess fat on your body and, in the long run, can lead to serious health problems, such as heart disease. So your extra calories should come from healthy, low-fat foods: grain products such as bread, pasta and cereals; low-fat dairy products such as skim milk, yogurt and cottage cheese; and proteins such as chicken (without the skin), fish and lean meat.

(If your doctor has you on a recommended diet for medical reasons, be sure to check with him before changing.)

Don't go for concoctions. Look on the shelves of any health food store and you'll find many protein and amino acid concoctions that imply they'll make you look like the muscle-bound figures on the labels. But many doctors advise against these products. They are not proven to work, and the high amounts of protein in them can be hard on your kidneys, Dr. Blackburn says.

Urinary Incontinence

It's a problem many people are reluctant to mention, even to their doctors. And that's unfortunate, because *nearly everyone* who temporarily loses control of his bladder can be made better or cured, experts agree.

"Most people who have incontinence can be helped, and that includes the elderly," says Catherine DuBeau, M.D., an instructor in medicine at Harvard Medical School and a member of the Gerontology Division and the Continence Center at Brigham and Women's Hospital, both in Boston.

First of all, Dr. DuBeau points out, "it's important to have a medical evaluation to determine what kind of incontinence you have and what's causing it." During the evaluation, your doctor will suggest which treatments might work best for you. While drugs or surgery are sometimes called for, there are many other approaches that doctors recommend. Here are some of them.

Get on a schedule. Follow the clock as you schedule times to go to the toilet. Most people start by going every hour or so for a few days; then if they remain dry, they go on a two-hour schedule. If you feel an urge to go in between times, stop and relax, then walk slowly to the toilet. The goal is to go every three or four hours during waking hours, Dr. DuBeau says. "What you're doing, in a sense, is trying to retrain the brain to control the bladder, so the bladder doesn't contract unless you are on the toilet, ready to go." People on this daytime program are less likely to get the sudden urge to go at night, she observes, because the bladder is trained for a regular schedule.

Learn the Kegel squeeze. These exercises strengthen the pelvic floor muscles, which contract and relax to control the opening and closing of your bladder. When they are weak, urine may leak out when you sneeze, laugh, contract your abdomen, lift something heavy or simply get up out of a chair, explains Katherine F. Jeter, Ed.D., executive director of Help for Incontinent People (HIP) in Union, South Carolina, and assistant clinical professor of urology at the Medical University of South Carolina in Charleston.

This kind of wetting problem, called *stress* incontinence, often improves with Kegel exercises, Dr. Jeter says. "Doing these exercises regularly can build up pelvic muscle strength and, in some cases, help you regain bladder control."

First identify the muscles you'll be exercising: Without tensing the muscles of your legs, buttocks or abdomen, imagine you are trying to hold back a bowel movement by tightening the ring of muscles around the anus. Do this exercise only until you identify the back part of the pelvic muscles.

Next, when you're passing urine, try to stop the flow, then restart it. This will help you identify the front part of the pelvic floor.

Now you're ready for the complete exercise. Working from back to front, pull up and tighten the muscles while counting to four slowly, then release and relax while counting to four slowly. Do this for two minutes at least three times daily, for a total of approximately 40 to 50 repetitions.

If you're doing Kegel exercises right, expect improvement in a few weeks to months, Dr. Jeter says. If you're not certain you're doing them correctly, talk to your doctor or nurse.

For people who have stress incontinence, it helps to do a Kegel squeeze before you cough, laugh, get out of a chair or pick up something heavy. The muscle contractions help prevent wetting accidents.

Drop some weight. "Obesity does seem to make bladder control more difficult, and we've had letters from people who say they've lost weight and improved bladder control," says Cheryle B. Gartley, president of the Simon Foundation for Continence in Evanston, Illinois, and editor of the book *Managing Incontinence*.

Retire your pogo stick. Bouncy exercises don't *cause* stress incontinence, but in people who already have a problem, they can cause leakage, Gartley says. Learning Kegel exercises can help solve the problem for many. Don't avoid exercise, she advises, but try the kinds that are less jarring. Gartley often recommends swimming or biking.

Stay regular. If you're constipated, take steps to get your bowels moving. Constipation can impair bladder control, Dr. DuBeau says.

When you go, make sure you empty your bladder completely. Remain on the toilet until you feel your bladder is empty. If you feel there is still some urine in the bladder, stand up, sit back down, and lean foward slightly over your knees.

Check the drugs you're taking. "There are a host of medications that can contribute to urinary incontinence," says Dr. DuBeau. "We ask people to make a list of all the medications they take, including over-the-counter drugs. One of the first things we do is review that list. Antihistamines, antidepressants, even common pain relievers such as ibuprofen (Advil) can cause problems. It's extremely important to let your doctor know about any medication you are taking."

Keep a food diary. Coffee, milk, sugar, corn syrup, honey, alcoholic beverages, tea, soft drinks, chocolate, citrus juices and fruits, tomatoes or tomato-based products and highly spiced foods have all been associated with incontinence in some people, Dr. Jeter says. To find out whether incontinence follows consumption of certain foods, try going without one kind of food or drink for a week or so. If that helps, it's a sign that you should continue to keep that food off your diet.

Urinary Tract Infections

Your bladder and urinary tract usually do a great job of removing impurities from your bloodstream. But sometimes the bladder and its exit tubes get infected, making urination a slow, painful and bothersome experience.

Although men are by no means immune, women are much more likely to get urinary tract infections (UTIs). Half of all women get them sometime during their lives; one in five has several episodes. Usually the cause is bacteria that enter the vagina and move to the urethra, the tube that carries urine from the kidneys. Once there, they cause burning, stinging and general discomfort, especially during urination. Here's the sum of doctors' advice on how to get your urinary tract on the right track again.

Fill up on fluids. "Absolutely the best thing a woman can do is drink fluids to flush out the bacteria that are causing the inflammation," says Elliot L.

When to See the Doctor

Should you visit the doctor if you have a urinary tract infection? There are four major symptoms to watch out for.
- Blood in the urine
- Pain in the lower back or flank
- Fever
- Nausea or vomiting

Usually an antibiotic prescribed by the doctor can clear up the infection and put an end to the symptoms. But urologists warn that a very small number may develop more serious problems with the kidneys. So you should see a physician or urologist immediately if you have any of these symptoms.

The *Real* Juice on the Cranberry Cure

T he legend of cranberry juice for urinary tract infections (UTIs) is surpassed perhaps only by the old saying that Mom's chicken soup is the best thing for colds. So here's the latest (as we go to press) report from the cranberry juice front.

Researchers at Tufts University in Medford, Massachusetts, found that cranberry juice *does* help cure UTIs, but not because it's too acidic for bacteria to live in (as many believe). The real reason: It prevents bacteria from anchoring onto bladder walls. That means that drinking cranberry juice helps "sweep" the bacteria from your urethra.

Some experts believe that *any* juice has the same impact. But maybe cranberry has an edge because it contains quinolic acid *and* vitamin C, both of which have been shown to have an impact on the infection.

If you don't have an infection, cranberry juice may be a good preventive: "I recommend drinking 3 ounces of cranberry juice cocktail daily," says Varro E. Tyler, Ph.D., professor of pharmacognosy at Purdue University in West Lafayette, Indiana. "And if you develop a UTI? Drink 12 to 32 ounces a day."

Cohen, M.D., assistant professor of clinical urology at Mount Sinai Hospital in New York City. That's because the more nonalcoholic beverages you drink, the more often you'll urinate. And the more often you urinate, the faster you'll flush the bacteria from your system.

Up your vitamin C intake. "About 1,000 milligrams taken throughout the day will acidify the urine enough to interfere with bacterial growth," says Richard J. Macchia, M.D., professor and chairman of the Department of Urology at the State University of New York Health Science Center at Brooklyn. He recommends vitamin C especially if you have a recurrent problem with UTIs. But, he cautions, check with your doctor if you're taking antibiotics prescribed for bladder infections; some of them don't work well when urine is highly acidic.

Use pads instead of tampons. "I advise those of my patients experiencing chronic infection at the time of menstruation to quit using tampons and replace them with pads," says Joseph Corriere, M.D., director of the Division of Urology at the University of Texas Health Science Center at Houston. For the same reason, he cautions that some women may want to reconsider use of a diaphragm.

Wipe from front to back. Front-to-back wiping is a form of prevention that is often recommended to keep UTIs (as well as yeast infections and other problems) from getting out of hand, according to Jack W. McAninch, M.D., chief of urology at San Francisco General Hospital. "It's common advice for women with recurrent infections," says Dr. McAninch.

Give your libido a rest. "No one's absolutely certain why certain women seem more susceptible to reinfection, but vaginal manipulation of some sort—sex, using a diaphragm, putting a tampon in—always seems to precede it," says Dr. Corriere.

Vaginal Dryness

I t's hard to determine which aches more because of this condition—your vagina or your feelings. Sex becomes a lot less fun if you lack the natural lubrication to enjoy lovemaking. In fact, it may get downright painful. But there's also the self-doubt, depression and even anger that you and your partner might feel because of it.

Instead of blaming yourself (or him), you might want to point the finger at a lack of estrogen. During menopause, you can *expect* estrogen to be in short supply. But if that's not the only reason for the problem, other causes might include a low-grade vaginal infection, taking birth control pills or even the natural aging process. Besides getting estrogen replacement therapy from your doctor, here are some natural ways to make intercourse go more smoothly.

Toss out the cigs. "Smoking destroys estrogen in the body," says Ellen Yankauskas, M.D., director of the Women's Center for Family Health in Atascadero, California. Since the most common cause of vaginal dryness is lack of enough estrogen, smoking only makes the problem worse.

Choose the right lubricant. You can remedy vaginal dryness with a commercial lubricant, but avoid anything scented or oil-based. "You want a lubricant

When to See the Doctor

If vaginal dryness leads to bleeding or intense itching, these signs should be looked at by your gynecologist," says Yvonne Thornton, M.D., professor of clinical obstetrics/gynecology at Columbia University College of Physicians and Surgeons in New York City. They could be an indication of more serious problems.

that's water-soluble, unscented, colorless, odorless and tasteless," says John Willems, M.D., associate clinical professor of obstetrics/gynecology at the University of California, San Diego, and a researcher at the Scripps Clinic and Research Foundation in La Jolla. "After that, it's a matter of personal choice." He and other experts recommend Astroglide, SurgiLube, Lubrin vaginal inserts, Gyne Moisturin and the more familiar K-Y jelly. Another recommended product is Replens, a moisturizer that can be used on a regular basis.

The key is to stay away from oil-based products like petroleum jelly or cocoa butter—or homemade recipes. "Some people use whatever is on the night table—things like suntan oil," says Dr. Willems. "But they aren't good for the vagina and can cause problems."

Go for fatty acids. Eating foods that are rich in fatty acids can be a big help. Among the best sources are raw pumpkin, sesame and sunflower seeds. Also eat fish that contain lots of fatty acids: Salmon, tuna and mackerel are all good choices, because they help retain estrogen in the body, says Susan Lark, M.D., medical director of the PMS and Menopause Self-Help Center in Los Altos, California.

Don't douche. Most douche products have a drying effect, which contributes to vaginal dryness, adds Dr. Yankauskas. "In general, you shouldn't douche unless you feel it's absolutely necessarily—and it's usually not."

Savor the moment. "Give yourself more time for foreplay," says Dr. Willems. As women age, he points out, their response to sexual stimulus is slower. You don't lose sexual response—it just occurs at a different pace.

Vaginitis

s most women can attest, any itching or discomfort in the vaginal area is just one nuisance too many. Unfortunately, this area is a regular magnet for trouble. The dark, moist surroundings are the perfect breeding ground for a wide array of bacteria and other organisms that can cause a host of irritations, inflammations and infections.

"*Vaginitis* is basically a catch-all phrase for any kind of inflammation of the vaginal area," says Ellen Yankauskas, M.D., director of the Women's Center for Family Health in Atascadero, California. "Inflammations can result from an infection, a chemical irritation from douche products, spermicides or condoms or simply not having enough estrogen." Whatever the cause—and there are many—here are some cures. (And for tips on coping with the discomfort of yeast infections, see page 576.)

Obey the Zen Commandments. Women with recurring vaginitis might want to consider a usually unlikely suspect—stress. "For chronic cases, I ask the woman to breathe deeply and try to get completely relaxed, so she can ask herself what she needs to know," says Susan Doughty, R.N., who is a nurse practitioner at Women to Women, a clinic in Yarmouth, Maine.

When to See the Doctor

If you have deep pelvic pain or swollen glands in the groin area *and* you have a fever above 101°F, you need to visit your doctor, according to Ellen Yankauskas, M.D., director of the Women's Center for Family Health in Atascadero, California. A doctor should also look at any open sores in the vaginal area, whether or not they're painful.

And be sure to see the doctor if there is no improvement with home remedies after a few weeks.

A Solution for Some Monthly Problems

Some women experience vaginal itching just prior to their menstrual flow. Once their period ends, the itching seems to stop until the following month, observes Susan Doughty, R.N., a nurse practitioner at Women to Women, a clinic in Yarmouth, Maine. Your doctor may tell you that this condition, cytolytic vaginosis, is caused by an overgrowth of bacteria in the presence of estrogen. Since this is just an imbalance (not a true infection), you may be able to clear it up with a home-prepared remedy.

The remedy, according to Doughty: Mix two tablespoons of baking soda in one quart of warm water and douche twice daily. The first douching should be just before the time of the month when symptoms typically appear. After that, continue to douche twice daily as long as you have the symptoms.

After a few months, reassess whether you need to continue, suggests Doughty. You don't need to use the douche again unless the itching returns.

In Doughty's view, a regular, meditation-like evaluation of yourself can answer "internal" questions that could subconsciously be causing physical symptoms. Doughty also recommends looking at relationships: "We can keep treating the infections, but there's usually some issue in a woman's relationship with her sexual partner that needs to be addressed."

Double-rinse your underwear. Harsh laundry detergents can increase the amount of irritation that results from vaginitis, says John Willems, M.D., associate clinical professor of obstetrics/gynecology at the University of California, San Diego, and a researcher at the Scripps Clinic and Research Foundation in La Jolla. So make sure all detergents and soaps are thoroughly rinsed from underwear.

Go thigh-high in stockings. Panty hose may be a fashion godsend, but they're a contributing cause of vaginitis and yeast infections. "Panty hose do not allow the skin to breathe," says Dr. Yankauskas. When the crotch area is covered by panty hose, it becomes a better breeding ground for infections. "If you must wear stockings, I recommend the thigh-high types rather than the full cover-your-crotch styles," says Dr. Yankauskas.

Be Alert to Antibiotics

Many doctors recommend antibiotics to help clear up vaginitis—but antibiotics that are taken for other kinds of illnesses or infections can actually *trigger* vaginal infections.

You might be able to avoid or clear up some infections by using a nonprescription douche that contains Betadine, according to Susan Doughty, R.N., a nurse practitioner at Women to Women, a clinic in Yarmouth, Maine. Betadine, an iodine-like bactericide, is an ingredient in some douche preparations. It's also sold in separate packets, so you can make your own mixture. In both forms, it's available over the counter in drugstores.

Doughty recommends trying a douche containing Betadine either nightly or twice a day for one week.

But if you use the douche and there's no improvement after seven days, be sure to get a checkup with your doctor.

She and other experts also recommend wearing only cotton panties—and *not* blends—because cotton allows for better air circulation.

Practice brand loyalty in birth control. "Many women notice vaginitis when they switch brands of condoms or spermicides," says Dr. Yankauskas. "If you notice an irritation or infection after trying one brand, then obviously it's not the one for you." On the other hand, if you're not having any problems with a brand, stay with it.

Favor *bambino's* soap. "If you're prone to vaginitis, or when you have an irritation, use the same soaps to bathe with as you would use on a baby," says Dr. Yankauskas. "Avoid deodorant soaps or anything with heavy dyes and perfumes."

Don't treat it with yogurt! While the yogurt/yeast infection connection is known far and wide, realize that yeast infection is only *one* type of vaginitis—and yogurt may not be the cure.

"Some women try to treat vaginitis with a tampon dipped in yogurt," says Doughty, "but if the infection is bacterial, it'll grow like crazy when it comes in contact with yogurt."

Varicose Veins

Many people deal with varicose or "spider" veins the same way: They hide them. When those reddish or blue bulges appear on legs and thighs, there's a temptation to buy a wardrobe full of long skirts and pants and pretend this isn't happening.

But guess what? Many of the people you're hiding your legs from *also* have varicose veins. No fewer than 10 percent of men and 20 percent of women have varicose veins or the less prominent, weblike spider veins that show up on the thigh. That means more than 20 million Americans in all are involved in this cover-up.

Sometimes varicose and spider veins can be quite painful, but it's reassuring to know they usually are *not* serious and don't lead to other problems in the legs or circulatory system. You can't change the veins, but you *can* ease the pain. Here's what the experts recommend.

Take two aspirin every day. "One of the easiest ways to get relief is to take half an aspirin every morning and every night," says Luis Navarro, M.D., founder and director of the Vein Treatment Center and senior clinical instructor of surgery at Mount Sinai School of Medicine, both in New York City. "Not only does aspirin help relieve any pain you might have from varicose veins, it also increases blood mobility."

Tilt your bed. One simple remedy is to place bricks or blocks of wood under your bed's footboard, so your feet will be raised a few inches, suggests Andrew Lazar, M.D., assistant professor of clinical dermatology at Northwestern University Medical School in Chicago. But check with your doctor first if you have a history of heart trouble or difficulty breathing during the night.

Learn yoga. A simple yoga breathing practice can help relieve varicose vein pain, says John Clarke, M.D., a cardiologist with the Himalayan International Institute of Yoga Science and Philosophy in Honesdale, Pennsylvania. Simply

When to See the Doctor

If your varicose veins are *very* painful—and you can see red lumps in the veins that don't decrease in size, even when you put up your legs—this could be a sign of clotting. Even if you've had varicose veins for some time, doctors say you should seek medical attention if these new signs appear.

Also, you'll need medical attention immediately if you have varicose veins around the ankle area that rupture and begin to bleed. The danger is that you can lose blood very rapidly. If bleeding begins, doctors recommend putting finger pressure on the area. Press a gauze pad or clean washcloth on the open vein to stop the bleeding and get to your doctor right away.

lie flat on your back and prop your feet up on a chair. Breathe slowly by expanding your diaphragm—that is, the whole area just *under* your lungs. (With diaphragmatic breathing, your stomach should rise and fall.) While doing this, breathe through your nose. In this position, gravity pulls excess blood out of your raised legs, and your full, steady inhalations create negative pressure in your chest, Dr. Clarke says. This negative pressure helps pull air into the chest cavity, which also helps get the blood flowing from your legs into the trunk area of your body.

Put up your feet—a lot. Weakened veins lack the strength to return blood to the heart. Since veins in your legs are farthest from the heart, you're helping them out whenever you get gravity on your side.

For one exercise that brings relief, lie flat on your back, raise your legs straight up in the air, and rest them against a wall for two minutes. Or simply place your legs on an easy chair to raise them above hip level whenever they're aching. Using either of these leg-raising methods, the discomfort should start to go away, says Dudley Phillips, M.D., a family practitioner in Darlington, Maryland.

Get those legs moving. "Any exercise that helps strengthen the legs can help varicose veins," says Dr. Navarro. "That's because when muscles contract, their compression empties the superficial veins and sends the blood to the deep veins and toward the heart." Although some reports claim that bicycling and running *worsen* varicose veins, Dr. Navarro says that applies only to excessive amounts of exercise. "Unless you're a professional athlete, *any* exercise will help," he says.

Watch your salt intake. Salt in the diet contributes to swelling, according to Dr. Navarro. "So if you have a propensity toward swelling, you're better off restricting the amount of salt you consume." Avoid salting your meals, and look for low-salt or sodium-free packaged products. And watch out for fast food that's usually high in salt.

And watch your weight. Added body weight, especially excess abdominal fat, creates more pressure on your groin; this makes it harder for venous blood to return to the heart. Keep your weight down and chances are you'll have fewer problems with bulging veins, says Lenise Banse, M.D., a dermatologist and director of the Northeast Family Dermatology Center near Detroit.

Avoid constriction. Girdles and other constricting clothing can act like tourniquets and keep blood pooled in your legs. If you have varicose veins, it's advisable to wear loose-fitting clothing and give up knee highs.

Stock up on special stockings. Support stockings and compression stockings, available in pharmacies and department stores, resist the blood's tendency to pool in the small blood vessels closest to the skin, says Dr. Phillips. When you wear these stockings, the blood is pushed into the larger, deeper veins, where it is more easily pumped back up to the heart. Compression stockings exert twice as much pressure as support stockings. Dr. Navarro suggests you choose a pair with a rating of 20 to 25 millimeters of mercury compression. The higher the compression, the greater the support these stockings provide. But there is a trade-off: Stockings with higher compression are less comfortable to wear.

Join the nonsmokers. A report from the Framingham Heart Study says smokers have a higher incidence of varicose veins, and researchers suggest that smoking may be a risk factor.

Vomiting

Thank your stomach.

Every once in a while, it telegraphs a rejection notice that skips from the tips of your shaky fingers to the surface of your clammy forehead—"No! Don't want! Will not accept!" And when your stomach sends out that kind of blanket refusal, you know it's no use fighting nausea anymore.

The only *good* thing that can be said about vomiting is that you often feel a lot better after it's happened. In fact, vomiting is sometimes the *best* thing your body can do to get rid of whatever is ailing it. So if low-key queasiness turns to gotta-go nausea, try to relax—it is going to happen whether you want it to or not. And when you catch your breath, follow these tips to make the unpleasant a little better.

Don't do anything for one hour. When you feel that you are finished vomiting, let your stomach rest for at least one hour, suggests Mitchell C. Sollod, M.D., a pediatrician in San Francisco. It is doubtful that you will want to eat anything, but if hunger strikes, ignore it.

Keep a washcloth handy. "Dampen a washcloth and gently wipe the area around your mouth," says Dr. Sollod. "Scoop the unpleasant material from the inside of your mouth also." Wet washcloths are also handy when you want to cleanse your mouth by sucking on them.

Sip some soft drinks. You will lose excessive amounts of fluids when you vomit, so doctors agree that it is very important to replenish your water supply. How you do this is personal choice: Water and sports drinks are most often used to rehydrate, and flat soda is popular, as it also calms your stomach. Whatever you drink, be sure to wait one hour after vomiting before you start sipping.

Soothe your stomach with Pepto-Bismol. After your hour of rest, Dr. Sollod suggests a dose of the over-the-counter stomach medication Pepto-Bismol to

When to See the Doctor

Often it is hard to tell just why you are vomiting. It could be a viral infection, food poisoning or simply the result of overeating.

"But sometimes nausea and vomiting are signs of more serious problems, such as internal bleeding, obstruction or appendicitis," says Christa Farnon, M.D., associate director of Occupational Medical Services for SmithKline Beecham, a pharmaceuticals company in King of Prussia, Pennsylvania.

"Vomiting blood or coffee ground–like material may be a sign of internal bleeding. Unrelenting pain may be due to an obstruction, and pain in the right lower abdomen could be a sign of appendicitis," she says. If it's appendicitis, this pain might be accompanied by a fever.

Don't eat or drink anything if you suspect that you may have one of these more serious problems, advises Dr. Farnon. Instead, see your physician or go directly to an emergency room.

ease your stomach irritation. This well-known aid for indigestion won't *stop* you from vomiting, but it can have a soothing effect afterward.

Reintroduce bland foods. When you are ready to eat again, do it slowly. Begin with easily digestible foods such as crackers, bread, tea, cereal and broth. Avoid coffee, alcohol, dairy products and fried, smoked, salty and spicy foods, as well as raw vegetables and red meats, until your stomach feels normal again.

Warts

Sorry, folklore fanatics, but despite what you've heard, you *don't* get warts from the neighborhood toad. If you've got warts and are wondering why, cast your eyes toward your Prince or Princess Charming.

Warts are spread by various strains of the common papovaviruses, which don't affect amphibians. But when it comes to primates, warts are so common that at this moment, at least one in ten people has at least one wart; as much as 75 percent of our population will have warts sometime in their lives. In fact, after acne, warts are the most common dermatologic complaint—with Americans spending more than $125 million each year on wart treatments.

Save your money by paying attention to these tried-and-true remedies.

Keep it under wraps. Handymen and handywomen aren't the only ones who can attest to the wonders of duct tape. If you have warts around and/or under the fingernail, "wrap duct tape two times around the fingernail and leave the tape on for 6½ days. Then let the finger air out for a half-day," says Jerome Z. Litt, M.D., assistant clinical professor of dermatology at Case Western Reserve University School of Medicine in Cleveland. "If the wart isn't gone by then, wrap it again for another 6½ days." Dr. Litt says adhesive tape works just as well, "but you should wrap the finger four times instead of two."

Give it aspirin. "Crush aspirin and apply it to the wart, and then wrap it in cellophane tape or any other type of tape that won't allow air in," says Rodney Basler, M.D., a dermatologist and assistant professor of internal medicine at the University of Nebraska Medical Center in Omaha. "The important thing is to *not* use a Band-Aid or anything that allows air in. You want the skin to get pruny underneath, so that the aspirin is absorbed." *Warning:* This should not be attempted by those who are allergic or sensitive to aspirin.

Call in the A-team. A daily application of the liquid from a vitamin A capsule (25,000 international units) helps some people see improvement after several days, says Robert Garry, Ph.D., professor of microbiology and immunology at Tulane University School of Medicine in New Orleans. Just open the

---

Is It a Wart?

Warts are benign skin tumors that can occur singly or in "clusters" on just about any part of the body. They are generally pale, skin-colored growths with blackened surface capillaries, a rough surface and even borders. Normal skin lines *don't* cross a wart's surface, and contrary to popular belief, warts are very shallow growths—with *no* "roots" or "runners."

If you have warts, look but don't touch. Warts can easily spread to other parts of your body—even if you have just a small cut on your finger.

capsule and squeeze the contents directly onto the wart. *Note:* The vitamin should be applied only to the skin, since excess oral doses can be toxic.

Or try the C-team. A paste made from water and crushed vitamin C tablets applied to the wart and then wrapped in a bandage can also bring relief, adds Jeffrey Bland, Ph.D., a former researcher at the Linus Pauling Institute in Menlo Park, California. The theory is that the high acidity of vitamin C may kill the wart-producing virus.

Imagine them gone. Warts can be "visualized" away, according to studies by Nicholas Spanos, Ph.D., a professor of psychology at Carleton University in Ottawa, Ontario. "We tell patients to imagine that their warts are shrinking, that they can feel the tingling as their warts dissolve and their skin becomes clear," he says. "Initially we give them about two minutes of this type of imagery, then we have them practice on their own at home for five minutes a day." Results: Warts disappear in about one of three people this way.

Water Retention

When you feel as though you're too big for your skin, not to mention your britches, check for some other signs. Perhaps your face is puffy, especially when you first wake up. Your ring may feel tight, and your belly seems bloated. Do your shoes feel like they belong to Minnie Mouse? Does this awful, bloated, uncomfortable feeling seem to come out of the blue? What *is* going on?

It could be water retention, or *edema* (to use the medical name). It happens to all of us to some extent during a normal 24-hour period, says Norman C. Staub, M.D., a professor in the Department of Physiology at the University of California, San Francisco. "Our bodies are constantly adjusting fluid levels based on what we drink and eat."

Usually our bodies do an admirable job of quickly correcting fluid balance. But sometimes the balance gets temporarily thrown off. Too much salt or alcohol, long periods of inactivity and, for women, monthly hormone fluctuations or pregnancy can all tip the scale toward fluid retention. A sudden

569

weight gain of several pounds may be your first and only sign that you're retaining fluid. Swollen ankles are a common tip-off, too.

For mild fluid retention, here's what experts suggest.

Get into deep water. As any skin diver knows, water pressure forces fluid out of tissues and, ultimately, into the bladder. You can get similar results by exercising in a swimming pool, according to Vern L. Katz, M.D., associate professor of obstetrics and gynecology at the University of North Carolina Medical School at Chapel Hill. Try a half-hour, three times a week, of gentle water exercise in a pool that's 80° to 90°F, or about skin temperature. "Avoid water above 100° if you're pregnant," Dr. Katz warns.

Avoid using diuretics. While they're very effective at removing excess body fluid for patients who have heart, kidney or liver disease, diuretics set up the potential for something called rebound edema, says Robert Schrier, M.D., a professor and chairman of the Department of Medicine at the University of Colorado School of Medicine in Denver. If you're taking them steadily for minor fluid retention, the diuretics turn on a lot of salt- and water-retaining hormones, says Dr. Schrier. "When you stop taking them, the high levels of hormones cause a lot more sodium and water retention, and you get into a vicious cycle."

Shake the salt habit. Too much salt—from hot dogs, popcorn, olives, salted nuts, pickles or pepperoni pizza—makes your body retain fluid. That fluid stays with you until your kidneys have a chance to excrete the excess salt, which can take about 24 hours. So if you avoid salty foods, you are less likely to have noticeable fluid retention, Dr. Staub says.

When to See the Doctor

Occasionally fluid balance gets seriously thrown off. Heart and kidney problems, along with other serious diseases, can cause life-threatening fluid retention. Don't delay seeing your doctor if you have a sudden weight gain, swollen ankles or difficulty breathing.

If you find that an indentation remains when you press your skin, that's a sign of "pitting edema"—a type of fluid buildup that needs a doctor's attention.

While you're at it, shake a leg. Exercise can relieve the body of excess fluid and salt through sweating, increased respiration and, ultimately, increased urine flow, Dr. Staub says. Walking up and down the hallway, or climbing a flight of stairs every hour or so, will reduce the fluid retention you develop from sitting for long periods of time. If you must sit still, try this: Point your toes downward, then raise them up as high as you can. That pumps your calf and your foot muscles. Moving your arms around up over your head will help, too.

Drink plenty of water. Water moves through your kidneys and bladder, diluting the urine. And since urine has some fluid-retaining salt in it, the more it's diluted, the easier it is to remove salt and prevent or decrease edema.

"Plain water is definitely the best, because just about every other drink—juices, soda, milk—has salt in it," Dr. Staub says.

Sip an herbal tea. Several herbs have a mildly diuretic effect, according to William J. Keller, Ph.D., a professor and head of the Division of Medicinal Chemistry and Pharmaceutics at Northeast Louisiana University School of Pharmacy in Monroe. Parsley is the best known of these. Try two teaspoons of dried leaves per cup of boiling water. Steep for ten minutes. Drink up to three cups a day.

Lie down, put up your feet. Sometimes this is the simplest and best thing to do, Dr. Staub says. If you recline with your feet in a raised position, you allow fluid that has pooled in your legs to more easily make its way into the circulatory system and then to your kidneys, where it can be excreted.

Windburn

It seems so unfair. Right in the middle of winter, you find yourself suffering from something as painful as summer's sunburn. But how can you possibly have a burn when you can hardly see the sun at all and the temperature hovers well below 32°F?

The reason: windburn.

Despite its name, windburn is actually a skin irritation. But it looks like a burn, because your skin appears red and slightly swollen on some exposed areas of your body. "Wind causes the loss of the oil layer on your skin," explains Norman Levine, M.D., chief of dermatology at the University of Arizona College of Medicine Health Sciences Center in Tucson. "And when your skin dries out excessively, you get an irritation that looks and feels like a real burn. To reverse the effect of windburn, you need to add that oil layer back to your skin."

So here are some ways to make winter weather less damaging and to take the burn out of windburn.

Put out the flame with moisturizers. "Any type of injury to the skin causes an inflammatory reaction," says John P. Heggers, M.D., director of clinical micro-biology at the Shriners Burns Institute in Galveston, Texas. "A moisturizer such as Dermaid Aloe is a good anti-inflammatory." It restores oil to your skin but allows water to evaporate as usual.

Wash on the mild side. Go for mild soaps and cleansers that have moisturizers, suggests Dr. Levine. They leave necessary oils in the skin. Dr. Levine warns against strong soaps that don't contain moisturizers. "The more effective a soap is as a cleanser, the more drying it is," he says.

Gently rewarm the skin. If you treat damaged skin gently, it is more likely to heal quickly, according to Dr. Heggers. Avoid exposing your skin to extreme temperature changes, he warns, and when you come indoors, allow the heat of the room to defrost your body. Don't turn on the heat lamp or stand next to a roaring fire.

Add a little oil. If the burning sensation is too much to bear, rub an oily skin medication on the windburned area, advises Murray Hamlet, D.V.M., director of the Plans and Operations Division at the U.S. Army Research Institute of Environmental Medicine in Natick, Massachusetts. "Vaseline is good because it is heavy," he says. "Chap Stick will work, too."

Elevate it. Occasionally there is noticeable swelling in windburned areas. Dr. Heggers recommends elevating windburned hands and feet while they are being rewarmed to minimalize the swelling.

Wrap things up. Your nose, lips and ears are particularly susceptible to windburn, notes W. Steven Pray, Ph.D., R.Ph., professor at Southwestern

Oklahoma State University School of Pharmacy in Weatherford. So wear earmuffs or a woolly hat, with a scarf or face mask to cover your nose and lips.

Block the wind. "The best way to protect yourself from the wind is with a barrier," says Carol Frey, M.D., chief of the Foot and Ankle Service and associate clinical professor of orthopedic surgery at the University of Southern California School of Medicine in Los Angeles. She recommends wearing a shell made from Gore-Tex or other synthetics. Zipping it high over the chin and pulling the hood around your face will shield your skin from that parching arctic breeze.

Know the wind chill factor. The wind chill factor is sometimes more of an indication of the weather conditions than the temperature. As the wind chill sends the temperature plummeting, the chance of injury rises, says Dr. Frey. So check the weather report before you head outdoors for those bracing winter activities.

Wrinkles

Many things improve with age: wine, cheese and the value of real estate and baseball cards, to name a few. Unfortunately, skin isn't one of them. As skin ages, it naturally loses some of its elasticity and resiliency.

This gives us wrinkles—etched-in-skin reminders of how far we've come. But wrinkles can also show where we've been—in the sun too much, smoking cigarettes too long and scrubbing our faces too hard with harsh soaps. Here's how you can iron out at least some of those creases that make you look older.

Sleep on your back. "You can create wrinkles by sleeping on your side or belly, with your face on the pillow," says D'Anne Kleinsmith, M.D., a cosmetic dermatologist at William Beaumont Hospital near Detroit who is an expert on wrinkles. "You'll see this in people who have a diagonal crease on their forehead, running above their eyebrows. For some people, sleeping on their back eliminates this problem."

Take your vitamins. The best vitamins for your skin are B-complex vitamins, found in beef, chicken, eggs and whole wheat, and antioxidants—vitamins A, C and E—which are abundant in green leafy vegetables, carrots and fresh fruit. These vitamins help ensure healthy and young-looking skin, says Marianne O'Donoghue, M.D., associate professor of dermatology at Rush–St. Luke's–Presbyterian Medical Center in Chicago.

Stop the squint with shades. "One problem area for wrinkles is around the eyes—what we call crow's feet," says Dr. Kleinsmith. "These wrinkles often result from squinting, so one way to avoid them, or lessen their severity, is to wear sunglasses when you go outside."

Keep a stone face. "Excessive frowning or smiling, or any other much-repeated facial expression, emphasizes wrinkles," adds Dr. Kleinsmith. "I'm not saying you should not smile or frown, but try to be aware of how often you're doing it—especially frowning." She and other experts advise *against* facial exercises, because excessive facial contortions only "aggravate" wrinkles.

Don't open another pack. Smoking is a double whammy for wrinkles. "Smokers have more wrinkles than people who don't smoke, especially around their lips," says Dr. Kleinsmith. That's because smoking robs the complexion of oxygen, decreasing blood circulation to facial skin and resulting in premature lines and wrinkles. *Plus,* anyone puffing on a cigarette is essentially doing a lot of repetitive facial movements that add even more wrinkles.

Go light on the bottle. The sobering fact is, excessive drinking causes your face to "puff up" the morning after, which temporarily stretches the skin. Subsequent shrinking brings your face back to normal but also causes wrinkles, says Gerald Imber, M.D., a plastic surgeon at The New York Hospital–Cornell Medical Center in New York City.

Wash with the cool and mild. Excessive washing and scrubbing—particularly with hot water and harsh soaps—tends to dissolve oils that help nourish the skin, says Jerome Z. Litt, M.D., assistant clinical professor of dermatology at Case Western Reserve University School of Medicine in Cleveland. Dr. Litt says to wash with cool or lukewarm water, using a mild soap or cleanser such as Neutrogena soap or Moisturel sensitive skin cleanser.

Avoid the midday sun. It's no surprise that too much sun exposure is the leading cause of premature wrinkles. The trouble is, no one except Count

When You Should Wear Egg on Your Face

Big night out? Just because you want to paint the town doesn't mean you have to get ready by painting your face with expensive wrinkle-hiding creams. Here's a way to avoid the cosmetic shelf and still have smoother-looking skin.

"It will only last a couple of hours, but a couple of egg whites work as well as those $100-an-ounce wrinkle creams," says Jerome Z. Litt, M.D., assistant clinical professor of dermatology at Case Western Reserve University School of Medicine in Cleveland. "You beat the egg whites—*not* the yolks—into a meringue and put it all over your face just before your party. Leave it on for about 30 minutes and then wash it off with cool water. (*Don't* use hot water or you'll have scrambled egg all over your face!) Pat your face dry, and then go off to your party."

Dr. Litt says the protein in the egg whites helps tighten the skin. "There's nothing permanent about it, but it does help for an hour or two. It's also effective for shrinking pores," he says.

Dracula can avoid the sun all the time. But take note: About 95 percent of the sun's wrinkling rays occur when Old Man Sol is at his strongest—between 10:00 A.M. and 3:00 P.M.—says Stephen Kurtin, M.D., assistant professor of dermatology at Mount Sinai School of Medicine in New York City. As long as you avoid those maximum-intensity hours, you're doing your skin a favor.

Ban the tanning booth. Whether it's achieved indoors or out, today's tan leads to tomorrow's wrinkles. The synthetic sunshine found in tanning booths is just as bad as the real thing, wrinkle-wise, says Jeffrey H. Binstock, M.D., assistant clinical professor of dermatologic surgery at the University of California, San Francisco, School of Medicine.

Use a moisturizer. If you have dry skin, daily use of a moisturizing lotion can temporarily help hide smaller wrinkles that form on the skin surface, says Dr. Kurtin.

Yeast Infections

I t takes very little to get the normally docile *Candida albicans* fungus that lives in a woman's vagina to turn into a rampant troublemaker. Candida is encouraged by many things—getting pregnant, using spermicides or birth control pills or taking antibiotics. And if you nick the vaginal walls while inserting a tampon, that can also trigger this most common form of vaginitis.

Yeast infections are not dangerous, but they can be painful and embarrassing. The most common symptoms include a bothersome itch and burning that can become maddening. Often there's a white discharge that resembles cottage cheese, sometimes accompanied by a yeasty or fishy smell. Here's how to cease the yeast.

Watch your sweet tooth. Sugar can cause chronic yeast infections—which is one reason why women who binge on sweets are particularly prone. "Avoid candy, cakes and pies—anything with refined, white or powdered sugar," says Jack Galloway, M.D., clinical professor of obstetrics and gynecology at the University of Southern California School of Medicine in Los Angeles. If you must indulge your sweet tooth, use brown sugar or honey. Since these take longer to break down in your body, you'll lessen the amount of circulating blood sugars, which can trigger yeast infections.

And watch the rest of your diet. Take heed of the connection between yeast infections and yeasty foods. "Avoid things such as bread, mushrooms and alcoholic beverages," says Susan Doughty, R.N., a nurse practitioner at Women to Women, a clinic in Yarmouth, Maine. She says that patients with chronic yeast infections who avoid these foods for three to six months will often notice a significant improvement.

Take Yeast Infections to the Cleaners

Perhaps the best weapons for treating yeast infections are in your laundry room. But you have to use special tactics to conquer *Candida albicans,* which can survive regular wash-and-dry cycles. Here are the basics.

Go soak. Soak panties in water for 30 minutes or more before washing them.

Scrub-a-dub-dub. After soaking, scrub the crotch of your panties with unscented detergent before putting them into the washing machine, advises candida specialist Marjorie Crandall, Ph.D., of Yeast Consulting Services in Torrance, California.

Double-rinse. Make sure panties are rinsed thoroughly, since residues from soaps and detergents can intensify vaginitis, according to John Willems, M.D., associate clinical professor of obstetrics/gynecology at the University of California, San Diego, and a researcher at the Scripps Clinic and Research Foundation in La Jolla.

Get 'em hot. Studies have found that the heat-sensitive candida die when panties are touched up with a hot iron.

"C" an improvement. Eat plenty of foods that are high in vitamin C, such as potatoes, citrus fruits and broccoli, adds Dr. Galloway. Vitamin C helps boost your immune system, and "if your immunity is down, you're a prime candidate for a yeast infection."

Wear baggy clothing. Tight-fitting clothing doesn't allow for good air circulation in the vaginal area. So stay away from clingy polyester, Lycra spandex, leather and other fabrics that don't "breathe." "Yeast love it when it's moist, dark and warm," says John Willems, M.D., associate clinical professor of obstetrics/gynecology at the University of California, San Diego, and a researcher at the Scripps Clinic and Research Foundation in La Jolla.

If you must wear tight clothing or Lycra, do it for only a few hours—and then change into loose-fitting garb made from cotton and other natural fibers. Avoid panty hose when you can, because they're too restrictive in the vaginal area, suggests Dr. Willems.

Is It Another Yeast Infection?

You've consulted a doctor for a previous yeast infection, and now you seem to be getting the same symptoms again. You may be able to save the time and expense of a return visit to the doctor by going to the drugstore and buying a strip of pH paper—litmus paper.

Moisten the paper with a small amount of vaginal discharge. (The discharge *must* be wet to react to the paper.) "If you have a yeast infection, your pH will be between 4 and 4.5 or less," says Ellen Yankauskas, M.D., director of the Women's Center for Family Health in Atascadero, California. "With other types of vaginitis, the pH tends to be higher."

If the litmus test confirms your suspicions, you may simply want to resume treatment with an over-the-counter cream. But if it's not effective after three days, Dr. Yankauskas says, you should definitely see your doctor again.

Change wet clothing fast. Lounging around in a wet bathing suit? You're wearing a perfect environment for yeast growth, adds Dr. Galloway. So once you're out of the pool, change into a dry outfit.

Heal with yogurt. Most experts point to yogurt as *the* natural healer of yeast infections (though it shouldn't be used for other types of vaginitis). Yogurt's lactobacillus cultures fight the candida, says Eileen Hilton, M.D., an infectious disease specialist at Long Island Jewish Medical Center in New Hyde Park, New York, who has studied yogurt's effect on yeast infections. While some experts recommend inserting yogurt into the vaginal area, an easier way is to simply eat at least ½ cup of yogurt containing live cultures each day to prevent and treat infections. (Nearly all yogurt *does* contain live cultures).

"If you don't like the taste of yogurt, you can get a dose of the same helpful bacteria by drinking milk containing live lactobacillus," suggests Ellen Yankauskas, M.D., director of the Women's Center for Family Health in Atascadero, California. (This type of milk will be identified on the container as cultured milk, acidophilus milk or kefir milk.)

Sit in a sitz. Frequent douching should be avoided, since it can be too irritating to those with yeast infections. But there's an easy cleansing solution for your vaginal area. Fill the bathtub to hip height with warm water, then add ½ cup of salt (enough to make the water taste salty) and ½ cup of vinegar. Stay in this sitz for about 20 minutes.

Go for a nonprescription medication. "The best way to treat this infection is with an over-the-counter antiyeast vaginal cream," according to Dr. Yankauskas. The creams are available in most pharmacies. Just follow the directions on the package.

Give applicators a hot scrub. If you use an antiyeast cream, you're probably reusing the applicator. "Wash the reusable applicators in hot soapy water," says Dr. Galloway.

Try no-frills toiletries. Avoid bubble baths, scented tampons, colored toilet paper and other products with dyes, perfumes and other chemicals that can irritate vaginal tissue, says Dr. Willems. White toilet paper is your best bet.

Index

Underscored page references indicate text within boxes. Brand names of prescription medications are denoted by the symbol Rx.

M